Pocketpedia

Second Edition

MATTHEW M. SHATZER, DO
EDITOR

Physical Medicine & Rehabilitation Pocketpedia

Second Edition

MATTHEW M. SHATZER, DO
Residency Program Director
Physical Medicine and Rehabilitation
North Shore-Long Island Jewish Health System
New Hyde Park, New York

Chief of Physical Medicine and Rehabilitation
North Shore University Hospital
Manhasset, New York

Assistant Professor
Hofstra North Shore-Long
Island Jewish School of Medicine
Hempstead, New York

Wolters Kluwer | Lippincott Williams & Wilkins
Health
Philadelphia • Baltimore • New York • London
Buenos Aires • Hong Kong • Sydney • Tokyo

Acquisitions Editor: Robert Hurley
Product Manager: Elise M. Paxson
Production Manager: Bridget Dougherty
Senior Manufacturing Manager: Benjamin Rivera
Marketing Manager: Lisa Lawrence
Design Coordinator: Doug Smock
Production Service: Integra Software Services

Two Commerce Square
2001 Market Street
Philadelphia, PA 19103 USA
LWW.com

Printed in China

Library of Congress Cataloging-in-Publication Data

Physical medicine & rehabilitation pocketpedia. – 2nd ed./[edited by] Matthew M. Shatzer.
p. ; cm.
Physical medicine and rehabilitation pocketpedia
Includes bibliographical references and index.
ISBN 978-1-60913-240-8 – ISBN 1-60913-240-8
I. Shatzer, Matthew M. II. Title: Physical medicine and rehabilitation pocketpedia.
[DNLM: 1. Physical Medicine–methods–Handbooks. 2. Rehabilitation–methods–Handbooks. WB 39]
615.8'2–dc23

2012002828

To purchase additional copies of this book, call our customer service department at (800) 638-3030 or fax orders to (301) 223-2320. International customers should call (301) 223-2300.

Visit Lippincott Williams & Wilkins on the Internet: at LWW.com. Lippincott Williams & Wilkins customer service representatives are available from 8:30 am to 6 pm, EST.

RRS1204

10 9 8 7 6 5 4 3 2 1

PREFACE

The second edition of the *Physical Medicine & Rehabilitation Pocketpedia* expands many of the chapters of the original edition. There is more evidence-based discussion in most chapters and further detail in the chapter on pain medicine. This edition also includes new chapters, including pediatric rehabilitation and burn rehabilitation.

In order to keep this text as accessible as possible, abbreviations are used for most terms familiar to the field. An index of abbreviations is included in the back of the book for easy reference.

It is hoped that this new edition will further enhance the readers' understanding of all relevant topics necessary to learn about physical medicine and rehabilitation.

Matthew M. Shatzer, DO

ACKNOWLEDGMENTS

I would like to express my sincere and deep gratitude to all readers for their interest in this handbook. The feedback received from the first edition of the *Physical Medicine & Rehabilitation Pocketpedia* was extremely helpful in allowing me to write a second edition. Additionally, I would like to thank all of the contributors to the second edition. Your hard work in helping me put this together is greatly appreciated. I would also like to thank several other people:

My beautiful wife Hania and adorable boys Zachary, Jeremy, and Skyler, for their continued support and love.

My parents, Aaron and Arlene Shatzer, who always taught me to do the right thing and the value of hard work.

Dr. Howard Choi, whose tireless efforts in making the first edition of this book laid the groundwork for this second edition.

Drs. Adam Stein and Steve Kirshblum, who have been wonderful mentors to me.

Additional thanks to the following people who have been instrumental in the completion of this book: Elise Paxson, and Robert Hurley.

Matthew M. Shatzer, DO

CONTENTS

Contributors

Malathy Appasamy, MD
Chief Resident
Department of Physical Medicine and Rehabilitation
Hofstra North Shore-Long Island Jewish Health System
Hempstead, New York

Rawa Araim, DO
Resident Physician
Department of Physical Medicine and Rehabilitation
Nassau University Medical Center
East Meadow, New York

Edward Barawid, DO
Resident Physician
Department of Physical Medicine and Rehabilitation
Nassau University Medical Center
East Meadow, New York

Maria Louise Barilla-LaBarca MD
Attending Rheumatologist
North Shore University Hospital
Manhasset, New York

Hilary Berlin, MD
Pediatric Physiatrist
North Shore-Long Island Jewish Health System
Hempstead, New York

Rodrigo Cayme, MD
Resident Physician
Department of Physical Medicine and Rehabilitation
Hofstra North Shore-Long Island Jewish Health System
Hempstead, New York

Ricardo Cruz, MD
Director, Brain Injury Program
Nassau University Medical Center
East Meadow, New York

Jessica Daigle, MA, OTR/L
North Shore-Long Island Jewish Health System
Hempstead, New York

Renee Enriquez, MD
Resident Physician
Department of Physical Medicine and Rehabilitation
Hofstra North Shore-Long Island Jewish Health System
Hempstead, New York

Negin Gohari, DO
Resident Physician
Department of Physical Medicine and Rehabilitation
Hofstra North Shore-Long Island Jewish School of Medicine
Hempstead, New York

Navdeep Jassal, MD
Resident Physician
Department of Physical Medicine and Rehabilitation
Hofstra North Shore-Long Island Jewish School of Medicine
Hempstead, New York

Sylvia John, MD
Assistant Professor
Department of Physical Medicine and Rehabilitation
Hofstra North Shore-Long Island Jewish School of Medicine
Hempstead, New York

Sharmatie Lal, MD
Resident Physician
Department of Physical Medicine and Rehabilitation
Hofstra North Shore-Long Island Jewish School of Medicine
Hempstead, New York

Dayna McCarthy, DO
Resident Physician
Department of Physical Medicine and Rehabilitation
Hofstra North Shore-Long Island Jewish School of Medicine
Hempstead, New York

John Michalisin, MD
Resident Physician
Department of Physical Medicine and Rehabilitation
Hofstra North Shore-Long Island Jewish School of Medicine
Hempstead, New York

Anthony Oreste, MD
Division Chief
Department of Physical Medicine and Rehabilitation
Long Island Jewish Hospital
New Hyde Park, New York
Assistant Professor
Department of Physical Medicine and Rehabilitation
Hofstra North Shore-Long Island Jewish School of Medicine
Hempstead, New York

Arti Panjwani, DO
Resident Physician
Department of Physical Medicine and Rehabilitation
Hofstra North Shore-Long Island Jewish School of Medicine
Hempstead, New York

Nisha Patel, MD
Resident Physician
Department of Physical Medicine and Rehabilitation
Hofstra North Shore-Long Island Jewish School of Medicine
Hempstead, New York

Shaheda Quraishi, MD
Assistant Professor
Department of Physical Medicine and Rehabilitation and Neurosurgery
Hofstra North Shore-Long Island Jewish School of Medicine
Hempstead, New York

Paulinder Rai, DO, MPH
Assistant Professor
Hofstra North Shore-Long Island Jewish School of Medicine
Hempstead, New York
Attending Physiatrist
Southside Hospital
Bay Shore, New York

Craig Rosenberg, MD
Assistant Professor
Department of Physical Medicine and Rehabilitation and Neurosurgery
Hofstra North Shore-Long Island Jewish School of Medicine
Hempstead, New York

Amy Schneider-Lyall, DO
Former Resident
Department of Physical Medicine and Rehabilitation
Hofstra North Shore-Long Island Jewish School of Medicine
Hempstead, New York

Jennifer Schoenfeld, DO
Resident Physician
Department of Physical Medicine and Rehabilitation
Hofstra North Shore-Long Island Jewish School of Medicine
Hempstead, New York

Sameer Sharma, MD
Resident Physician
Department of Physical Medicine and Rehabilitation
Hofstra North Shore-Long Island Jewish School of Medicine
Hempstead, New York

Gurtej Singh, MD
Attending Physiatrist
Greater Baltimore Medical Center
Baltimore, Maryland

Adam Stein, MD
Chairman
Department of Physical Medicine and Rehabilitation
Hofstra North Shore-Long Island Jewish School of Medicine
Hempstead, New York

Renat Sukov, MD
Clinical Associate Professor
Department of Rehabilitation Medicine
New York University
New York, New York

Thuy Vu, MD
Resident Physician
Department of Physical Medicine and Rehabilitation
Hofstra North Shore-Long Island Jewish School of Medicine
Hempstead, New York

Jay Weiss, MD
Associate Professor of Clinical Physical Medicine and Rehabilitation
Medical Director
Long Island Physical Medicine and Rehabilitation
New York, New York

Lyn Weiss, MD
Professor of Clinical Physical Medicine and Rehabilitation
Chair and Director of Residency Training
Department of Physical Medicine and Rehabilitation
Nassau University Medical Center
East Meadow, New York

James Wyss, MD
Assistant Attending Physiatrist
Hospital for Special Surgery
New York, New York

Contributors to Chapter 17

Rafael Abramov, DO
Maryam Rafael Aghalar, DO
Rawa Araim, DO
Edward Barawid, DO
Deborah Friedman, MD
Luke Garcia, DO
Derek Higgins, DO
Sasha Iversen, DO
Harry Lenaburg, MD
Celine Mathew, DO
Jose Mathew, DO
Yulia Maystrovskaya, DO
Anuradha Mutyala, MD
Adaku Nwachuku, DO
Weibin Shi, MD
Farah Siddiqui, MD
Teena Varghese, MD

Chapter 1

NEUROLOGIC EXAMINATION

1. Mental status

Orientation	Time, person, and place
Attention/concentration	Serial 7s Spelling "world" backward
Memory	Remote and recent memory New learning ability with three objects
Mood	"How are you feeling?"
Insight/judgment	"Why are you in the hospital?"
Speech/language	Rate, articulation, fluency, naming, word comprehension, repetition, writing, and reading
Higher cognitive functions	Calculations, abstract thinking, and drawing a clock

2. Cranial nerves

No.	Cranial nerve	Function
I	Olfactory	Sense of smell
II	Optic	Vision
III	Oculomotor	Pupillary constriction, opening the eye, and most extraocular movements
IV	Trochlear	Downward, inward movement of the eye
V	Trigeminal	Motor – temporal and masseter muscles (jaw clenching); also lateral movement of the jaw Sensory – facial. The nerve has three divisions: (1) ophthalmic, (2) maxillary, and (3) mandibular
VI	Abducens	Lateral deviation of the eye
VII	Facial	Motor – facial movements, including those of facial expression, closing the eye, and closing the mouth Sensory – taste for salty, sweet, sour, and bitter substances on the anterior two-thirds of the tongue
VIII	Acoustic	Hearing (cochlear division) and balance (vestibular division)

(Continued)

(Continued)

No.	Cranial nerve	Function
IX	Glossopharyngeal	Motor – pharynx Sensory – posterior portions of the eardrum and ear canal, the pharynx, and the posterior tongue, including taste (salty, sweet, sour, and bitter)
X	Vagus	Motor – palate, pharynx, and larynx Sensory – pharynx and larynx
XI	Spinal accessory	Motor – the sternocleidomastoid and upper portion of the trapezius
XII	Hypoglossal	Motor – tongue

3. Muscle tone (resistance to passive stretch)

Flaccidity	No resistance to muscle stretch Clinical indication of lower motor neuron involvement Observed in Guillain-Barré syndrome, acute phase of stroke, and spinal cord injury
Spasticity	Increased resistance to muscle stretch that is velocity dependent Clinical indication of upper motor neuron involvement Observed in multiple sclerosis, chronic phase of stroke, and spinal cord injury Measured using the modified Ashworth Scale
Rigidity	Increased resistance to muscle stretch that is independent of velocity Clinical indication of basal ganglia involvement Observed in parkinsonism
Clonus	Alternate involuntary muscular contraction and relaxation in rapid succession

4. Muscle strength testing (a tool used to grade a specific, symmetric group of muscles)

Grade	Description
0	No muscular contraction
1	Trace contraction that is visible or palpable
2	Full active range of motion with gravity eliminated
3	Full active range of motion against gravity
4	Full active range of motion against gravity with minimal to moderate resistance
5	Full active range of motion against gravity with maximal resistance

5. Muscle stretch reflexes are tested by tapping the tendon with a hammer to elicit muscle contraction (To optimize the response ask, distract the patient by asking him or her to interlock their flexed fingers [Jendrassik maneuver].)

Grade	Description
0	No response
1+	Diminished response – hypoactive
2+	Normal response
3+	Brisk response – hyperactive without clonus
4+	Hyperactive with clonus

- Upper extremity: biceps reflex (C5, C6); brachioradialis reflex (C5, C6); triceps reflex (C6, C7)
- Lower extremity: patella or knee-jerk reflex (L2, L3, and L4); Achilles or ankle-jerk reflex (S1); plantar reflex (L5, S1)

6. Sensation should examine superficial and deep sensation by comparing symmetric dermatome distributions with the patient's eyes closed
   - Light touch: use a cotton tip applicator
   - Pain: use a safety pin
   - Temperature: use two different test tubes of hot and cold liquids
   - Joint position or proprioception: move the patient's finger or toe by the side and test the ability to distinguish between the upward and downward movements
   - Vibration: use a 128-Hz or 256-Hz tuning fork over a bony prominence and ask the patient when the stimulus ends
   - Point localization: lightly touch the patient and ask for identification of the area
   - Two-point discrimination: ask the patient to distinguish between one point and two points of stimulus on the fingertips or palm
   - Stereognosis: place a common object in the patient's hand for identification
   - Graphesthesia: draw a number or letter on the patient's palm for identification
7. Coordination, stance, and gait assessment can reveal cerebellum involvement with clumsy movements, ataxia, and balance instability
   - Finger-to-nose test and heel-to-shin test
   - Rapid alternating movements
   - Pronator drift: ask the patient to keep arm held up with eyes closed; if there is a downward drift, it indicates a positive sign
   - Romberg test: ask the patient to stand with feet together and close their eyes; if there is any swaying, it indicates a positive sign and lack of position sense

- Observe the individual walk down hallway, do a tandem walk, walk on the heels/toes, hop on each foot, and perform shallow knee bend

RECOMMENDED READING

Bickley L. *Bates' Guide to Physical Examination and History Taking.* 8th ed. Philadelphia, PA: Lippincott Williams & Wilkins; 2003.

Chapter 2

GAIT AND GAIT AIDS

Gait Cycle

The normal gait cycle has two primary components: *stance phase*, which represents the duration of foot contact with the ground, and *swing phase*, which represents the period in which the foot is in the air. The typical gait pattern consists of approximately 60% stance phase and 40% swing phase. Figure 2-1 shows the components of gait.

A *Step* is defined as the time measured from an event in one foot to the subsequent occurrence of the same event in the ***other*** foot.

A *Stride* is defined as the time measured from an event in one foot to the subsequent occurrence of the same event in the ***same*** foot.

The Six Determinants of Gait

Saunders et al.[1] began by assuming that gait is most efficient when vertical and lateral excursions of the body's COG are minimized. They identified six naturally occurring "determinants" in normal gait that reduced these excursions and suggested that pathologic gait could be identified when these determinants were compromised.

1. **Pelvic rotation in the horizontal plane** – The pelvis rotates 4° to each side, which occurs maximally during double support, elevating the nadir of the COG pathway curve by about 3/8".
2. **Pelvic tilt in the frontal plane** – The pelvis drops 5° on the side of the swinging leg controlled by the hip abductors, shaving 3/16" from the apex of the COG pathway curve.
3. **Knee flexion** – KF at midstance (10° to 15°) lowers the apex of the COG by 7/16".

4, 5. **Knee and ankle motion** – The rotation over the calcaneus in early stance with rotation over the metatarsal heads in late stance combined with KF in late stance produces a smooth sinusoidal pathway for the COG.

6. **Lateral pelvic displacement** – Normal anatomic valgus at the knee and varus at the hip decreases lateral sway, reducing total horizontal excursion from about 6" to <2".

Muscle Activity during Nondisabled Gait

Ankle Dorsiflexors – These muscles (primarily the tibialis anterior, but also the extensor digitorum longus and the extensor hallucis longus) eccentrically contract to smoothly lower the foot from heel strike to foot flat. They also concentrically contract during the swing phase to dorsiflex the ankle and effectively shorten the swinging limb in order to clear the ground.

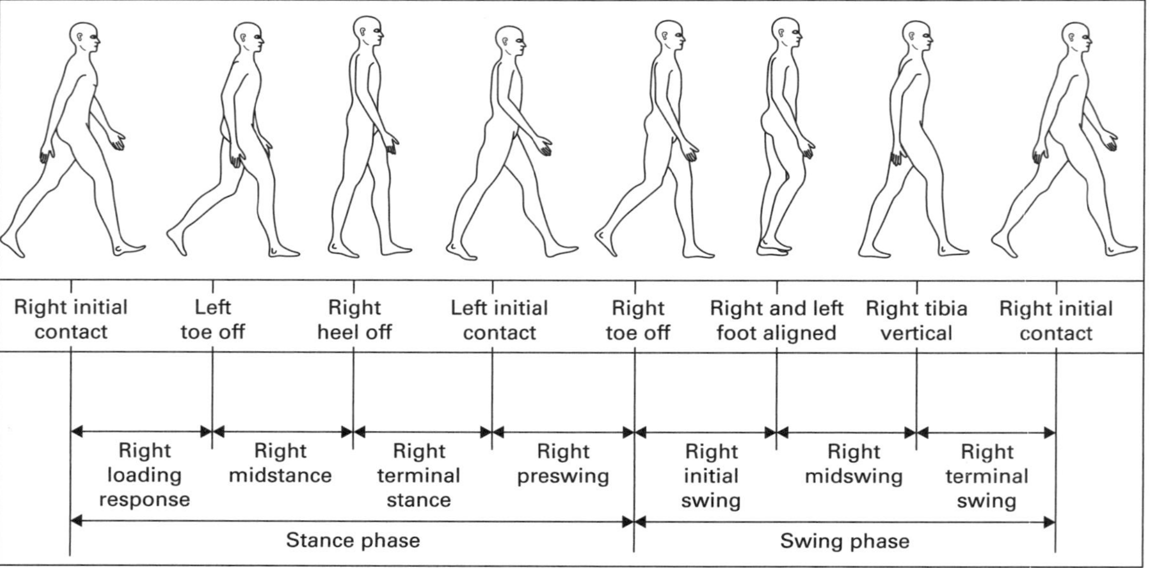

Figure 2-1 Components of the gait cycle.

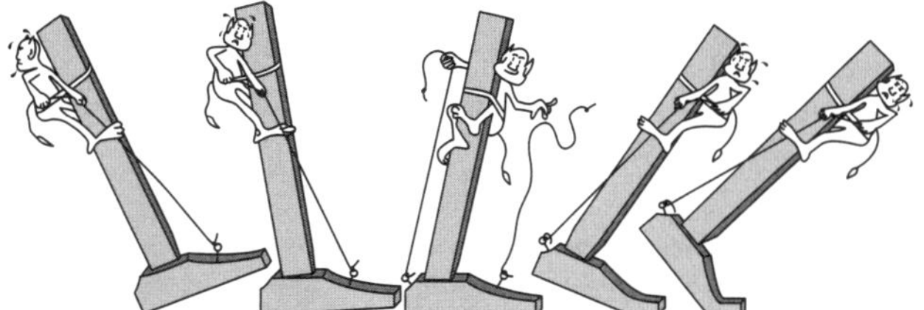

Figure 2-2 The actions of the ankle dorsiflexors/plantar flexors in normal gait.

Adapted from Inman V. *Human Walking*. Philadelphia, PA: Williams & Wilkins; 1981.

Ankle Plantar Flexors – The triceps surae act eccentrically during midstance to control ankle dorsiflexion caused by the body's forward momentum. At push-off, they act concentrically to lift the heel and toes off the ground (see Fig. 2-2).

Hip Abductors – The gluteus medius and minimus contract eccentrically during stance phase to limit pelvic tilt of the swing phase leg.

Hip Flexors – The hip flexors (primarily the iliopsoas) contract eccentrically after midstance phase to slow truncal extension caused by the GRF passing behind the hip. The tensor fasciae latae, pectineus, sartorius, and iliopsoas contract concentrically to flex the hip and shorten the limb for effective ground clearance during swing phase.

Hip Extensors – The gluteus maximus and hamstrings start to eccentrically contract just before heel strike to maintain hip stability and slow down the forward momentum of the trunk, since the GRF is anterior to the hip at this stage. They become essentially inactive after foot flat, once the GRF passes posterior to the hip. The hamstrings may weakly contract during the swing phase to flex the knee for ground clearance.

Hamstrings have a double peak of activity just prior to and after heel strike. The first peak occurs during swing phase when there is an open kinetic chain (foot not in contact with ground). This peak decelerates the forward swing of the leg by eccentrically contracting during hip extension and flexing at the knee. At the moment of heel strike, the open kinetic chain is converted to a closed kinetic chain (foot in contact with ground), while the hamstrings act predominantly as a hip extensor preventing both hip and knee buckling.

There is a less consistent peak of activity during late stance phase when hip extension by the gluteus maximus helps propel the COG forward.

Knee Extensors – The quadriceps act primarily to absorb shock during heel strike and keep the knee stable by eccentric contraction. They are also active just before toe-off to help initiate the forward swing of the limb.

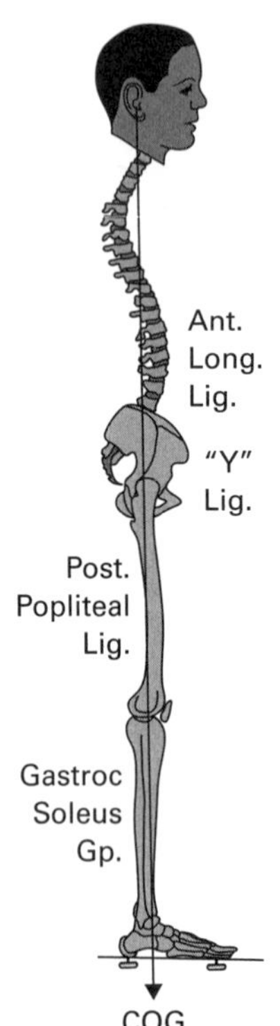

Figure 2-3 The gastroc–soleus complex.
Adapted from Cailliet R. *Low Back Pain Syndromes.* 5th ed. Philadelphia, PA: FA Davis; 1995.

The gastroc–soleus complex (primarily the soleus) is the only muscle normally active during quiet standing. Ligaments and bony articulations maintain the stability of the other joints. The COG is located ~2" anterior to S2 (Fig. 2-3).

Gait Deviations and Prescriptions

Muscle Deficit Gait

Antalgic Gait – To reduce pain, there is avoidance of WB on the affected limb. The examiner may note a decrease in the stance phase, a reduced step length on the unaffected side, and a prolonged period of double support.

Gastrocnemius Gait – Weak plantar flexors during terminal stance and toe-off prevent adequate heel lift. To limit the drop in the COG that occurs without heel lift during terminal stance, the step length of the contralateral leg is shortened. *Treatment*: a solid or semisolid AFO with a full-length footplate simulates plantar flexion during terminal stance.

Gluteus Medius–Minimus (Trendelenburg) Gait – In an uncompensated Trendelenburg gait (Fig. 2-4A), there is contralateral pelvic drop secondary to the inability of the hip abductors to stabilize the pelvis during stance. In a compensated Trendelenburg gait (Fig. 2-4B), the patient compensates for weak abductors by having a lateral lurch over the affected side as a compensatory maneuver to reduce the stress on the weak muscles. *Treatment*: a cane used in the contralateral hand widens the base of support and decreases the hip abductor strength needed to keep the pelvis level. In b/l abductor weakness, b/l canes with a four-point gait may be used.

Gluteus Maximus (Extensor Lurch) Gait – This may be seen following injury to the inferior gluteal nerve or a subtrochanteric hip fracture. Weakened hip extensors are unable to decelerate the forward momentum of the body (hip flexion moment) at heel strike. To compensate, the subject adopts a prominent posterior lean and locks the

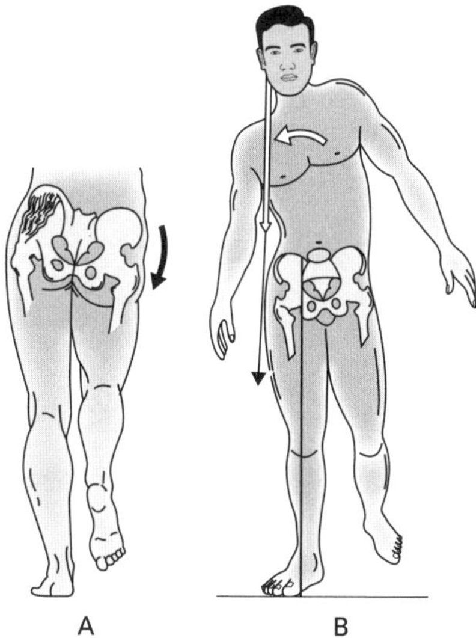

Figure 2-4 Uncompensated (**A**) and compensated (**B**) Trendelenburg gait.

hip joint in extension against the iliofemoral ligament, which keeps the body's COG behind the hip. *Treatment*: two crutches or canes are used for a three-point gait (Fig. 2-5).

Quadriceps (Back Knee) Gait – With weakness or inhibition of the quadriceps (e.g., distal femoral fracture), the patient will adopt measures to prevent buckling of the knee. One compensation is the use of the hands to force the knee into extension. Also, patients may lurch their trunks forward at initial contact and strongly contract their ankle plantar flexors to bring the COG in front of the knee and force it into extension. Another compensatory technique might be to externally rotate the leg at initial contact and early stance to bring

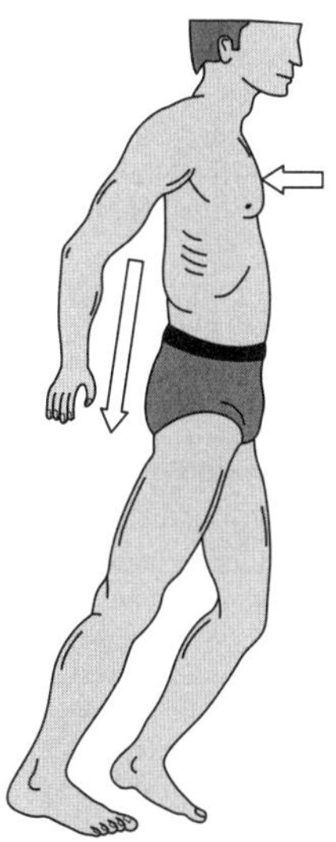

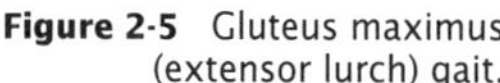

Figure 2-5 Gluteus maximus (extensor lurch) gait.

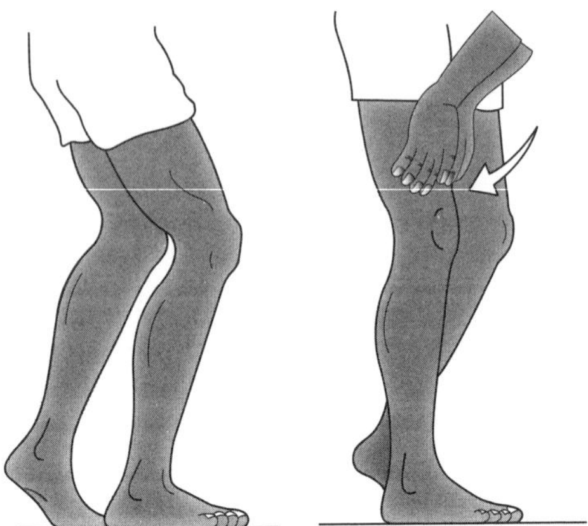

Figure 2-6 Quadriceps (back knee) gait.

the medial collateral ligament anteriorly and prevent knee buckling. *Treatment*: a knee brace may be used to provide knee stability at heel strike (Fig. 2-6).

Tibialis Anterior Gait – Pretibial muscle weakness that is at least antigravity (≥3/5 grade) may cause *foot slap* after heel strike. If the muscles are <3/5 grade, foot slap is generally *not* heard because a steppage gait is more likely. The hip and knee are hyperflexed in a steppage gait to clear the foot during swing phase, which may otherwise drag. The affected limb may alternatively be circumducted during swing phase. *Treatment*: a standard PLSO, which allows plantarflexion and assists in dorsiflexion. An AFO is often used both to prevent foot slap and to allow clearance of the foot during swing phase. Note that ankle plantarflexion stabilizes the knee. Thus, a standard hinged AFO (with plantarflexion posterior stop) may destabilize the knee. An alternative is a PLSO, which allows plantarflexion and assists in dorsiflexion (Fig. 2-7).

Central Nervous System Gait Deviations

Hemiplegic Gait – Patients with extensor synergies will typically ambulate independently. The typical extensor synergy pattern is toward knee extension, ankle plantarflexion, and inversion. Therefore, extensor tone effectively makes the plegic limb longer than the nonplegic side. Patients compensate with a circumduction gait via excessive hip abduction to allow for toe clearance and ending with toe strike. Despite the circumduction, there is a decreased step length and swing phase on the plegic side. Gait speed will be reduced in order to maintain an acceptable rate of energy expenditure. *Treatment*: a solid AFO or a hinged AFO with a

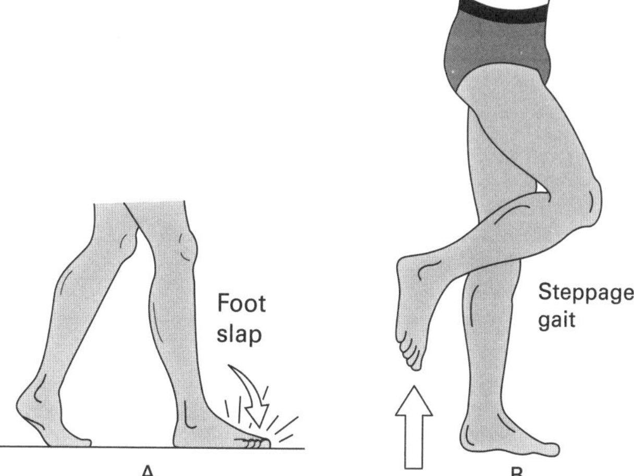

Figure 2-7 Tibialis anterior gait. **A.** Foot slap. **B.** Steppage gait.

posterior stop to decrease effective limb length may be helpful. A small degree of plantarflexion, however, should be maintained to promote knee stability for patients with quadriceps weakness. If patients demonstrate genu recurvatum, a small degree of dorsiflexion or addition of a heel lift will be indicated (Fig. 2-8).

Parkinsonian Gait – The classic triad of Parkinson's disease is tremor, bradykinesia, and instability, with at least the last two affecting gait. While standing, the knees, trunk, and neck are typically flexed and the body appears stiff. When there is ambulation, there is a characteristic shuffling gait with short quickening steps, as if the patient were racing after the COG (festination). Turns are made "en bloc." Decreased arm swing further compromises balance. *Treatment*: heel lifts and assistive devices may help reduce the tendency to fall backward. Walkers with added weight may provide additional stability. Physical therapy to address postural issues can be helpful (Fig. 2-9).

Spastic Paraplegia or Diplegia/Crouched Gait – Often seen in CP patients. While standing, the hip

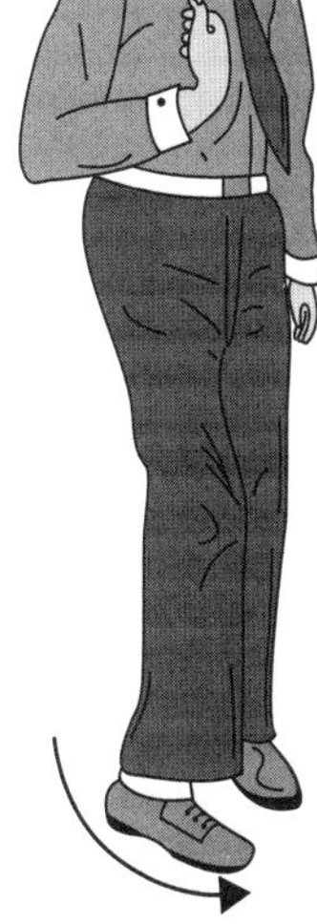

Figure 2-8 Hemiplegic gait.

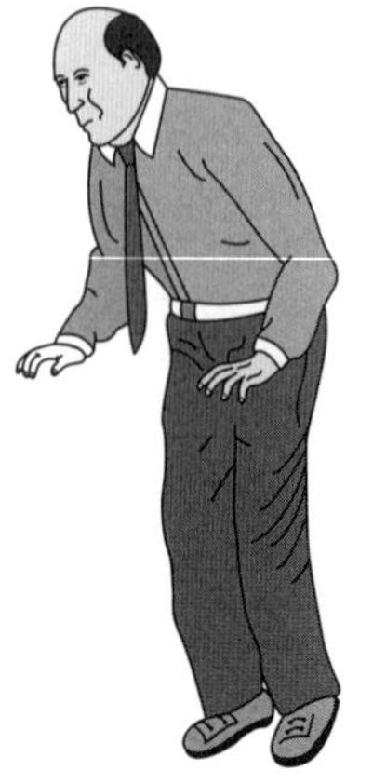

Figure 2-9 Parkinsonian gait.

and knees are flexed and internally rotated and the foot is held in equinovarus. When there is ambulation, the increased adductor tone at the thighs causes the knees to scissor in front of each other with each step. Hip adduction causes short step lengths, making the feet to seem like they are sticking to the floor. Balance may be impaired as a result of a narrowing base of support, and to compensate for this, the patient tends to lean forward and toward the supporting side. The upper extremities tend to be semiflexed with elbows held out to the sides. Diagnostic nerve blocks may help establish whether or not a contracture is present. *Treatment*: AFOs can be used to address equinovarus. Botox may be helpful for adductor scissoring and equinovarus. Use of an assistive device (e.g., walker) may provide additional stability.

Gait Aids

Cane Basics

In general, a cane should be held in the hand opposite to the lower limb with neuromuscular weakness or joint pathology and is advanced with the affected limb together in a *three-point gait* pattern. Stairs are usually ascended with the stronger lower limb first, then the cane and affected limb. The affected lower limb and cane proceed down first during stair descent. ("Up with the good, down with the bad.") In practice, however, there are no hard and fast rules.

Cane length should be from the bottom of the shoe's heel to the upper border of the *greater trochanter* with the patient standing. The shoulders should be level and the arm holding the cane should be *flexed ~20° to 30° at the elbow*, to provide proper push-off. A cane can unload up to 20% of body weight off the affected lower limb, depending on cane design and the patient's level of training.

The basis for holding a cane on the opposite side of hip joint pathology is elegantly described elsewhere.[2]

In essence, the cane provides a rotatory moment (**C** [see Fig. 2-10]) that counteracts the weight of the body (**W**) and reduces the force of the gluteus medius (**F**) necessary to maintain equilibrium at the hip fulcrum (**H**) when the affected lower limb is in single support stance phase.

Crutch Basics

Crutches have two points of contact with the body and are thus more stable than canes. Shoulder depressors (latissimus dorsi and pectoralis major) are important muscles in ambulation with crutches. Other important muscles that need to be strengthened in preparation for crutch use include the

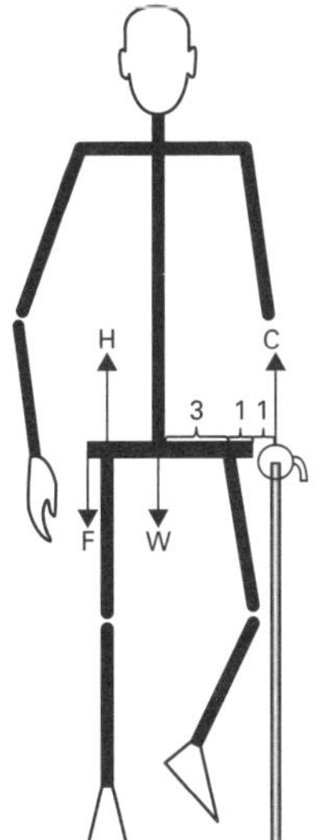

Figure 2-10 The basis for holding a cane on the opposite side of the affected hip.

triceps brachii, biceps brachii, quadriceps, hip extensors, and hip abductors.

Axillary crutch: Length is 1" to 2" plus the distance from the anterior axillary fold to a point on the ground 6" lateral to the bottom of the heel while standing. The handpiece is placed with the *elbow flexed 30°*, the wrist in extension, and the fingers forming a fist. The patient should be able to raise the body 1" to 2" by complete elbow extension. Use of heavy padding on the axillary area of the crutch, although a popular practice, should be discouraged. This encourages the habit of resting the body on the crutches, which increases the risk of *compressive radial neuropathies*. When used properly, b/l crutches can provide total WB relief to a lower limb (Fig. 2-11A).

Forearm crutches (Lofstrand): These are indicated if pressure in the axilla is contraindicated, e.g., open wound and compression neuropathy. They provide less trunk support than axillary crutches. A single forearm crutch can relieve up to 40% to 50% of body weight off a lower limb. B/l forearm crutches can provide total WB relief to a lower limb (Fig. 2-11B).

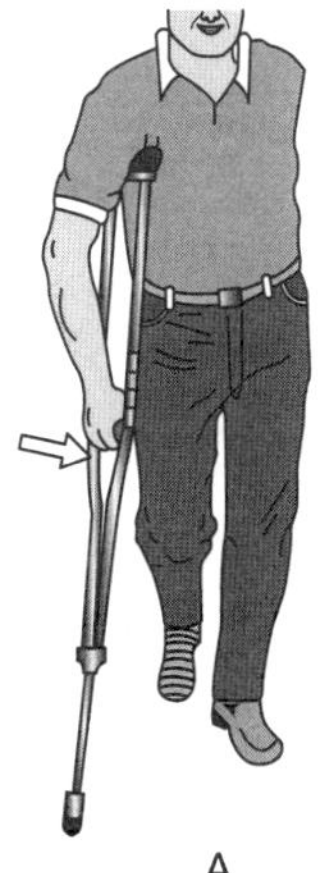

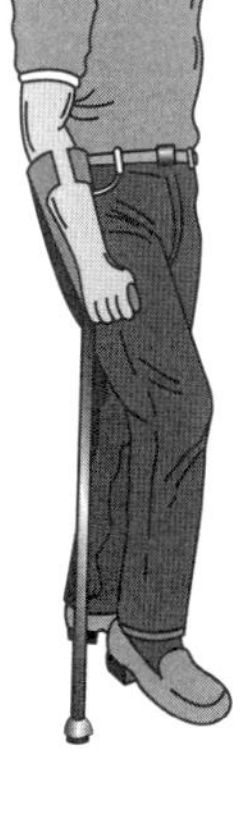

Figure 2-11 Crutches. **A.** Axillary crutch. **B.** Forearm crutch.

Crutch gaits: The crutches and involved limb serve as point 1, while the uninvolved limb is point 2 in the *2-point* (or *"hop-to"*) *gait.* In the *3-point gait* (i.e., the involved limb is PWB), the crutches (1 point) and each limb (points 2 and 3) are advanced separately, with any two of the three points maintaining contact with the ground at all times. In the *4-point gait,* point 3 is the involved leg. Each point is advanced separately. Efficiency is forsaken for increased stability or balance (Fig. 2-12A). When negotiating

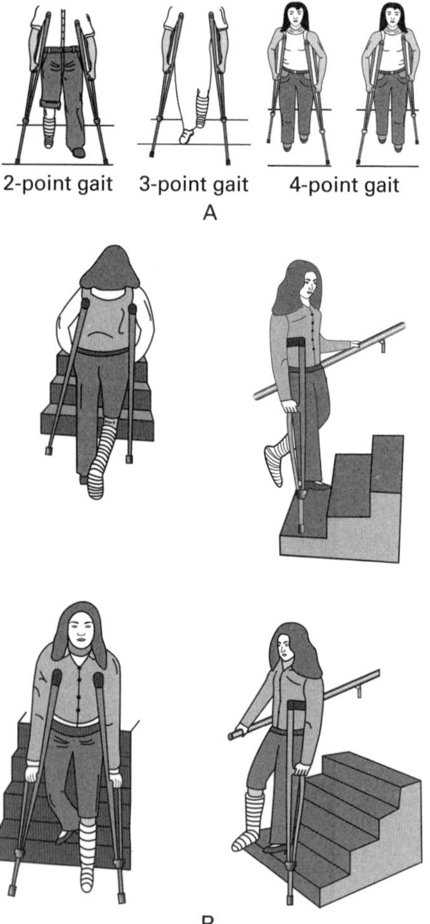

Figure 2-12 Crutch gaits. **A.** Two-, three-, and four-point gaits. **B.** Negotiating stairs using a banister for support.

stairs w/o a banister, one method might be stronger limb → weaker limb → crutch → crutch for ascent and crutch → crutch → weaker limb → stronger limb for descent. A rail or banister, if present, replaces one of the crutches in the above method (Fig. 2-12B).

Walker Basics

Walkers provide a wider base of support and safer gait than canes or crutches (Fig. 2-13A). They allow up to 100% WB relief from an affected lower limb depending on how they are used. A walker is fitted by placing it about 10" to 12" in front of the patient. The proper height is set with the patient standing straight, shoulders relaxed, and the elbows flexed about 20°. The main disadvantages are that they cause a slow and awkward gait and in the long term can promote bad posture.

Rolling walkers are indicated for patients who lack the coordination or strength in the upper limbs to lift and advance a standard walker and are preferred in the rehab of total joint replacement because of the smoother gait.

A *hemiwalker* is used by a hemiplegic. It is wide based, provides more lateral support than a quad-cane, and is advanced by the nonplegic side.

Platform walkers (Fig. 2-13B) are used in a variety of situations including distal upper extremity joint deformities, grip weakness, and flexion contractures of the elbow. They allow WB at the elbow, bypassing the hand, wrist, and part of the forearm, and are useful for patients with multiple fractures that may preclude use of a nonplatform device.

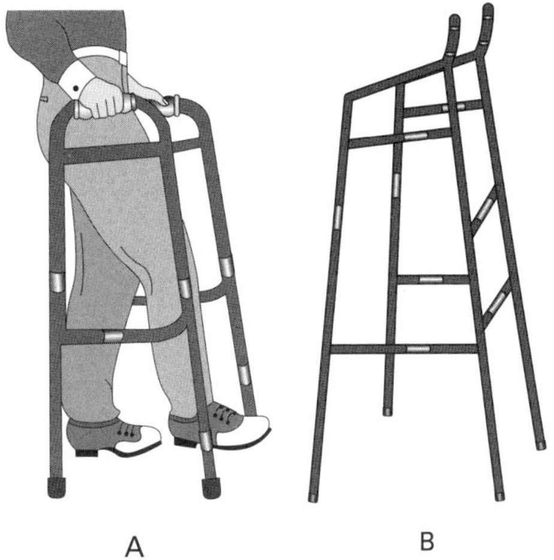

Figure 2-13 Walkers. **A.** Basic walker. **B.** Platform walker.

REFERENCE

1. Saunders JB, Inman VT, Eberhart HD. The major determinants in normal and pathological gait. *J Bone Joint Surg Am.* 1953;35:543-548.
2. Kottke F, ed. *Krusen's Handbook of Physical Medicine and Rehabilitation.* 4th ed. Philadelphia, PA: WB Saunders; 1990.

RECOMMENDED READING

Blount WP. Don't throw away the cane. *J Bone Joint Surg Am.* 1956;38:695-698.

Deathe AB. The biomechanics of canes, crutches, and walkers. *Crit Rev Phys Med Rehab.* 1993;5:15-29.

Kottke F, ed. *Krusen's Handbook of Physical Medicine and Rehabilitation.* 4th ed. Philadelphia, PA: WB Saunders; 1990.

Chapter 3

WHEELCHAIR

Manual Wheelchairs

Typical Measurements

Back height	Self-propeller, good trunk control	2" below inferior angle of scapula
	Self-propeller, poor trunk control	2" below scapular spine
	Poor UEx strength, poor trunk control	Standard (typically 16.5")
Seat width	Widest point, usually hip, plus 1"	18"
Seat depth	Buttock to popliteal fossa, minus 2"	16"
Seat height	Popliteal fossa to floor, plus 2"	19"
WC width	18" seat width usually corresponds to 27" WC width. (Doorways need to have a clearance that is ≥32" wide to be ADA compliant)	
WC weight[a]	Standard (no set definition)	~43–50 lbs
	Lightweight	<35 lbs
	Ultralightweight (i.e., sports chairs)	<28 lbs
	Heavy duty (for users >250 lbs)	45–60 lbs
Wheel size	Standard	24"
	"Hemichair"	20"

[a]Decreasing the weight of a manual WC does not necessarily increase propulsion efficiency on level surfaces, but a difference is appreciable on uphill grades.

Courtesy of Redford J, ed. *Orthotics Etcetera.* 3rd ed. Philadelphia, PA: Williams & Wilkins; 1986.

A mat evaluation is also done to determine joint angles (hip, knee, or ankle), to assess postural deformities (e.g., joint contractures, pelvic obliquities, spinal kyphosis, or scoliosis), and to assess the effects of gravity on sitting balance.

The following components are needed as part of a comprehensive WC and seating evaluation (Fig. 3-1):

- Medical history
- Home environment
- Method of transportation

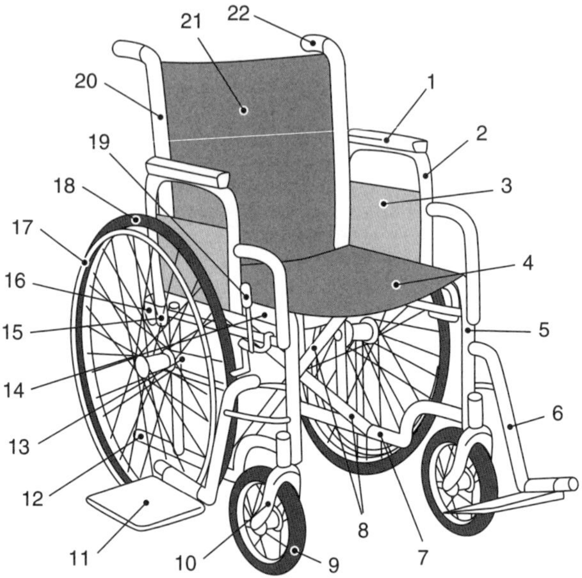

Figure 3-1 Components of a typical outdoor sling-seat WC. *1.* Arm pad; *2.* Desk-style removable arm rest; *3.* Clothes guard; *4.* Sling seat; *5.* Down tube; *6.* Footrest; *7.* Bottom rail; *8.* Cross brace, X bar, or X frame; *9.* Caster; *10.* Caster fork; *11.* Footplate; *12.* Tipping lever; *13.* Axle; *14.* Seat rail; *15.* Arm rest bracket or hole for non-wraparound arm rest; *16.* Arm rest bracket or hole for wraparound arm rest; *17.* Handrim; *18.* Wheel; *19.* Wheel lock; *20.* Back post; *21.* Sling back; *22.* Push handle.

- Employment/school requirements for mobility
- Functional/sensory processing skills
- Communication
- Sensation/skin issues
- Current seating/mobility
- WC skills
- Patient measurements
  - Hip/trunk/shoulder width
  - Knee-to-seat depth
  - Knee to heel
  - Shoulder height
  - Axilla height
  - Top of head
  - Range of motion

Prescription Considerations

Frame – Folding frames are easier to transport but may be heavier, be less durable, and require more energy to propel. Rigid frame chairs are more durable and energy efficient during propulsion, but may be more difficult to transport. Rigid frame WCs are not particularly useful for ambulatory patients because they do not typically come with swing-away footrests, making it difficult for them to perform sit-to-stand transfers.

Axle – Posterior placement is advantageous for users with poor trunk control, amputees, and reclining/posterior tilt WCs, but increases turning radius, rolling resistance, and the difficulty in doing wheelies. Anterior placement decreases rolling resistance and improves maneuverability (decreased turning radius and easier wheelies), but also increases the risk of tipping over backward.

Molded Plastic (Mag) versus Wire-Spoked Wheels – Mag wheels are slightly heavier but more durable than spoked wheels. Spoked wheels are preferred in most sports chairs, but require more maintenance and are less safe for some individuals whose fingers may get caught in the spokes.

Pneumatic versus Rubber Tires – Pneumatic (air-filled inner tube) tires offer a comfortable ride on uneven terrain but are susceptible to going flat and have a higher resistance to propulsion. Solid rubber tires may be preferred if the WC is mostly to be used indoors (e.g., office work, hospitals, and nursing homes) due to the easier propulsion and low maintenance.

Camber – (typically range from 3° to 5°) Increasing camber decreases turning radius, improves side-to-side and forward stability, decreases rolling resistance at high speeds (no effect at normal speeds), and protects user hands during sports. Disadvantages include difficulty in tight spaces due to increased overall WC width, increased tire/wheel-bearing wear, and decreased rear stability.

Handrims – Small-diameter handrims (sports WCs) increase the distance covered with each stroke, but require greater force. Pegged handrims ("quad knobs") improve ease of use for tetraplegics and users with hand deformities but increase risk of trauma during attempts to stop and may limit accessibility.

Casters – Small (≤5" diameter), narrow casters are appropriate for smooth, level surfaces and are less likely to shimmy. Smaller casters are more likely to get caught in sidewalk cracks and elevator thresholds.

Large (≤6" diameter), wide casters are advantageous in rougher, outdoor terrain, but have increased rolling resistance on smooth surfaces and are more likely to shimmy.

Cushions – *Foam cushions* are lightweight and inexpensive, but are not washable and dissipate heat poorly. These cushions do not offer adequate pressure relief. They are appropriate for ambulatory patients with intact sensation.

Gel/foam combo cushions (i.e., Jay and Jay-3) consist of a firm gel emulsion enclosed in a nonbreathable plastic that provides good postural stability. They are durable, are easy to maintain and clean, and offer a high capacity to dissipate skin heat buildup, but are expensive and heavy, and the contouring can interfere with transfers. The new Jay-3 has "memory," which maintains optimal configuration. This is good for patients with poor pelvic/trunk control and insensate skin.

Air-filled villous cushions, such as the Roho, consist of multiple balloonlike air cells that assure maximum skin contact and provide the best pressure relief. The design is favorable for pressure ulcer prevention or healing. These cushions are lightweight, good at heat dissipation, and easy to clean and transport, but expensive and poor at providing postural stability. The cells also need constant maintenance to maintain the air pressure and repair punctures.

Recline/Tilt-in-Space – Reclining and tilt-in-space chairs are helpful for patients who lack the ability to do adequate pressure relief otherwise and for patients with orthostatic instability. These chairs are frequently prescribed as backups for patients using power WCs. The addition of these features, however, can significantly increase the size and weight of the WC. Users of reclining WCs may be susceptible to increased spasms and shear forces during the reclining motion. Tilt-in-space WCs offer pressure relief w/o shear and also reduce the likelihood of triggering a spasm during the tilt. Backflow of urine in the tilted position, however, may be an issue in patients with indwelling catheters. The patient that uses the reclining or tilt-in-space WC is usually dependent. Manual recline/tilt-in-space positioning and WC propulsion must be done by a caregiver.

Special WCs

"Hemichair" – This may be an option for some patients following stroke. The seat height is lowered ≈2" and a footrest is removed to allow the neurologically intact foot to propel and steer.

Lower Limb Amputee – The rear axle is moved posteriorly ≈2" to compensate for the rearward displacement of the patient's center of gravity. Turning radius is increased.

One-Arm Drive – This is for unilateral arm amputees or hemiplegics. Both hand rims are on one side. Turning both rims propels the WC; one rim turns the WC. WC width and weight are increased. Good strength and coordination are required.

Standing WC – These chairs have frames that allow the user to passively assume a standing position. The standup position provides pressure relief and weight bearing (which may reduce osteoporosis[1]) and can promote improved bowel/bladder function.

Electrically Powered Mobility Systems

Powered WC

Indications – This is for patients with physical limitations not compatible with manual WC propulsion (e.g., C1-4, many C5-6 tetraplegics, or severe weakness) and for those with endurance deficits (e.g., severe COPD and cardiac failure) who must conserve their energy for other functions.

User Requirements – Patients must have at least one reproducible movement to access the control system, adequate cognitive and visuoperceptual function, proper judgment, and motivation. Ideally, a trial is given to power WC candidates to see if they can eventually learn how to control the WC.

Contraindications – Failing to meet the user requirements; involuntary motions or inattention that might result in inadvertent activation of the controls.

Electric Carts (Scooters)

Indications – For patients who can ambulate and transfer but have poor endurance or poor tolerance for prolonged manual WC use secondary to arthropathy or other diseases.

User Requirements – Good sitting balance, intact cognitive and visuoperceptual skills, good hand–eye coordination, and adequate function of at least one upper limb to operate the controls are needed.

Caution – Some models tip over fairly easily, especially at high speeds.

Scooters are not recommended for patients with progressive diseases such as multiple sclerosis. If a patient receives a scooter and has a functional decline that prevents them from using the scooter, it is very difficult to get another mobility device paid for by their insurance company before they are eligible. (Medicare guidelines state that an individual will be considered "eligible" for a new mobility device every 5 years.) It is extremely important to consider the progressive nature of an individual's illness when prescribing a mobility device.

REFERENCE

1. Goemaere S. Bone mineral status in paraplegic patients who do or do not perform standing. *Osteoporosis Int.* 1994;4:138-143.

Chapter 4

AMPUTATION/PROSTHETICS

Epidemiology, Etiology, and Levels of Amputation

In the United States, an estimated 185,000 people undergo an amputation of an upper or lower limb each year. It is estimated that 1.2 million people are living with the loss of a limb.[1] Amputation due to dysvascular disease accounts for 54% of cases, and of these, two-thirds have a diagnosis of DM. Trauma accounts for 45% of cases and cancer for the remaining less than 2%.

Over the next 45 years, the number of persons living with loss of a limb is predicted to more than double. Figures 4-1, 4-2, and 4-3 illustrate some of these data.

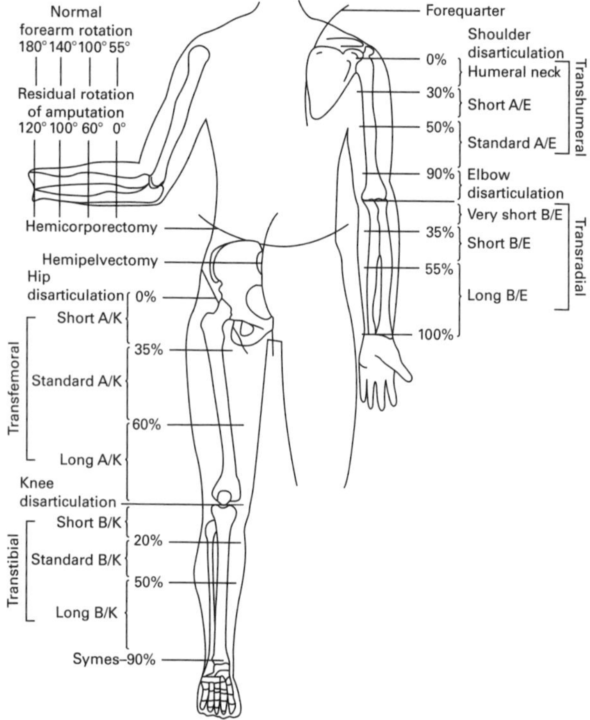

Figure 4-1 Amputation terminology.

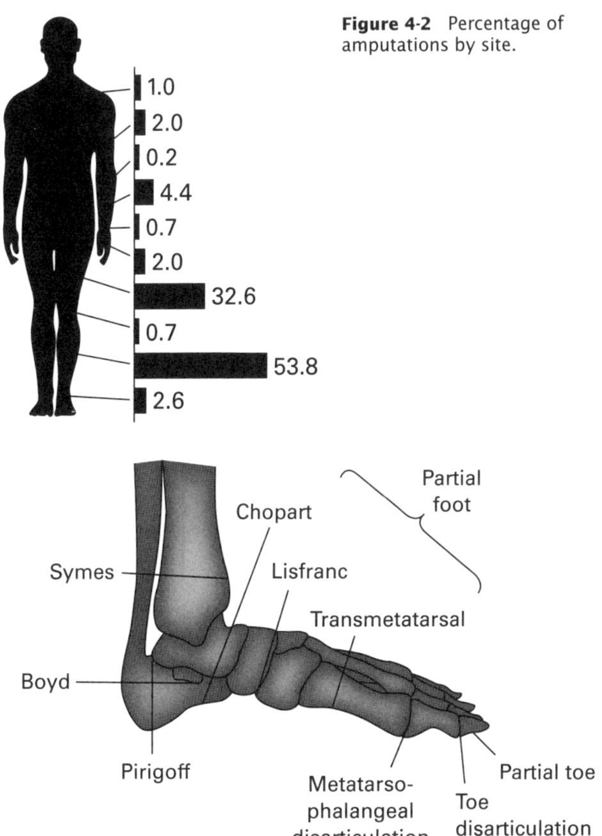

Figure 4-2 Percentage of amputations by site.

Figure 4-3 Foot amputation levels. Mnemonic: The *Cho*part is *shorter*; the *Lis*franc is longer.

Preferred Mature Residual Limb Length and Shape

Transhumeral – Cylindrical appendage with retention of the deltoid tuberosity. Generally, the longer the better (up to 90% of normal length).

Transradial – Ideal shape follows the contours of the natural limb. Longer appendages provide better lever arms and more pronation/supination and are optimal for body-powered prostheses and heavy labor. Retention of the brachioradialis improves elbow flexion. Medium length limbs are optimal for externally powered prostheses.

Transfemoral – Ideal shape is conical. Longer residual limbs improve seating balance and tolerance. For shorter limbs, maintaining the greater trochanter and its attachment to the hip abductors is key.

Transtibial – Ideal shape and length is a cylindrical appendage about one-third the original tibial length, with retention of the patellar tendon attachment to the tibial tuberosity. The fibula should be shorter than the tibia. In vascular disease, longer limbs may not have adequate circulatory supply and fitting of the below-knee socket may be problematic. The ideal length recommended from medial tibial plateau to bony end is 5" to 7".

Basic LEx Postamputation Preprosthetic Care

Wound Care – Keep limb clean and protected and debride any nonviable tissue.[2]

Edema Control

- Elastic wraps: Most commonly Ace bandages. Must use *figure-of-8 elastic wrapping*, which should begin immediately after surgery and should ideally be rewrapped qid. May be time consuming.
- Elastic socks: Alternative to wraps. Not expensive and easy to apply.
- Rigid dressings: Protective. Allow for weight bearing to desensitize the limb. Examples include the *immediate postoperative-fitting prosthesis*, which is not removable and therefore inhibits ability to check and desensitize the skin. The *removable rigid dressing* is custom made and allows for wound inspection and desensitization.

Scar mobilization massage should be instituted as soon as tolerated to help prevent adherence of the scar to the underlying soft tissues and bone. Once the sutures are removed, the massage can be performed more aggressively.

Anticontracture Management – Due to muscle imbalance. AKA commonly develop HF, hip abduction, and hip external rotation contractures. In addition, BKA develop KF contractures. Prevent with a firm mattress, prone lying 15 minute tid, and promoting knee extension while resting. A posterior splint to maintain knee extension can be considered for patients at higher risk.

Preprosthetic and Prosthetic Training – Hip AROM and strengthening exercises are key. A good test to determine cardiovascular tolerance for prosthesis use is ambulation with a walker (without a prosthesis). Prosthetic gait training should begin with parallel bars and progress to walkers or canes. Crutches should be avoided since they promote poor gait patterns. The *definitive prosthesis* is usually created at 3 to 6 months.

Transtibial Prosthetics

Socket Designs

The socket connects the residual limb to the rest of the prosthesis and plays an important role in the transfer of body weight to the ground (Fig. 4-4).

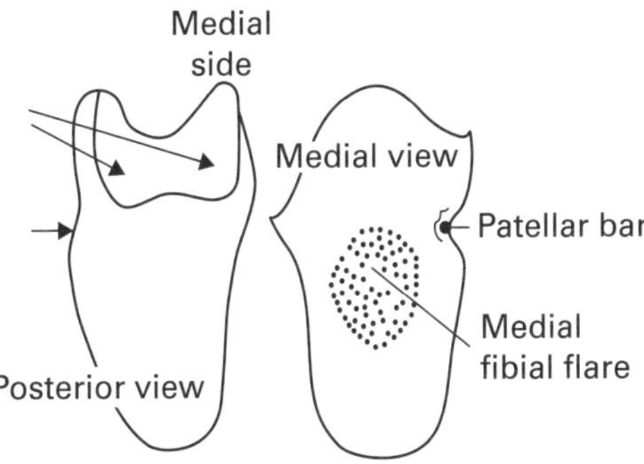

Figure 4-4 Total contact socket.

The PTB socket is an old term for the *total contact socket.* The patellar tendon actually only bears a moderate load. Weight is distributed over many areas (see "pressure-tolerant areas" in Fig. 4-5), but not over the bony prominences.

For any socket, soft inserts made of polyethylene foam or silicone gel provide extra protection, e.g., for cases of PVD or extensive scarring. The inserts, however, reduce the intimacy of contact between the limb and prosthesis, which is important for proprioception. A soft foam distal end discourages verrucous hyperplasia formation.

Selected Suspension Options

Differential Pressure (Silicone Suction with Shuttle Lock) – A flexible, molded silicone liner is rolled directly onto the residual limb and secured to the socket with a pin. This provides optimal suspension and proprioception, but requires stable limb volumes and good hand dexterity for donning/doffing.

Anatomic – A *brim suspension* is an extension of the socket over the femoral epicondyles. This design is easy to don/doff, provides mediolateral knee stability, and is useful for short limb lengths.

The *supracondylar cuff* clips on above the epicondyles and is a common suspension option. This design is not indicated in patients with very short residual limbs or with mediolateral knee instability. A supracondylar cuff with fork strap and waist belt suspension provides additional stability for very active patients, e.g., manual laborers.

Sleeve – An elastic sleeve can serve as a primary or secondary suspension via longitudinal tension and negative pressure during swing phase. It can provide additional security for short residual limbs, when mediolateral knee stability is questionable, or when hyperextension control is required (Fig. 4-6).

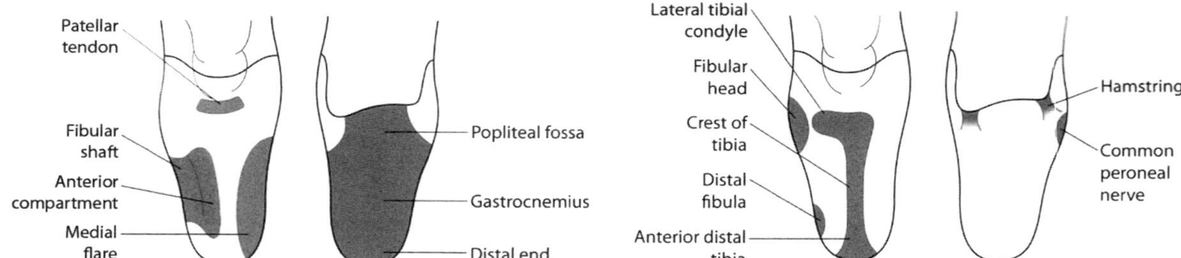

Figure 4-5 Pressure-tolerant/sensitive areas in the transtibial total contact socket.
From Braddom RL. *Physical Medicine & Rehabilitation.* 4th ed. Philadelphia, PA: Elsevier; 2011, with permission.

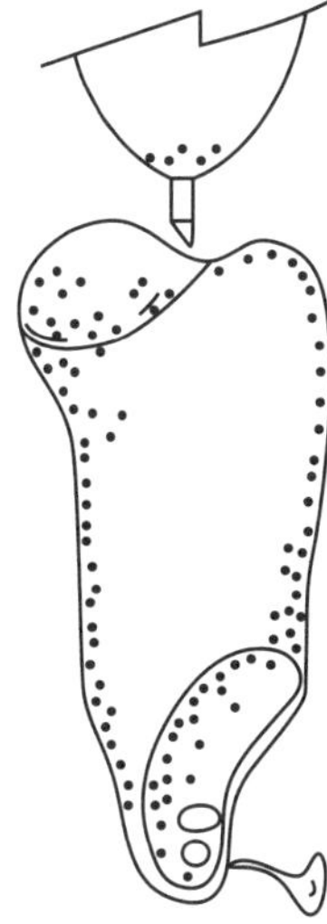

Figure 4-6 Sleeve

Selected Foot-Ankle Assembly Options

Solid Ankle Cushioned Heel Foot – SACH feet are light, durable, inexpensive, and stable. The soft heel simulates PF during heel strike (Fig. 4-7A).

Single-Axis Foot – These feet are heavier but less durable than the SACH feet. They are most commonly used for TF amputees, i.e., when knee stability is desired (a quick foot flat improves knee stability). Only sagittal axis movement is allowed.

Multiaxis Foot (Greissinger, Endolite Multiflex, SAFE II, TruStep) – The multiaxis foot allows PF/DF, inversion/eversion, and rotation, which improve balance and coordination. It provides good shock absorption and is good for uneven ground, but is heavy, costly, and needs relatively frequent adjustments or repairs.

DER Foot (Seattle Light, Carbon Copy II, Quantum Foot, Flex-Foot, SpringLite) – These feet were formerly called "energy-storing feet," but they have *not* demonstrated a reduction in the energy cost or rate of energy expenditure during level walking, compared with the SACH foot.[3] They may, however, be more efficient than other feet at higher speeds. Geriatric amputees benefit from the light weight of these feet (Fig. 4-7B).

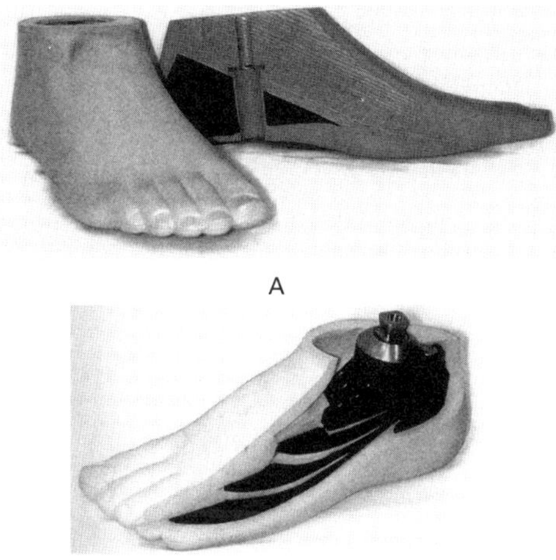

A

B

Figure 4-7 Foot-ankle assembly options. **A.** SACH foot. **B.** DER foot.

From Braddom RL. *Physical Medicine & Rehabilitation.* 4th ed. Philadelphia, PA: Elsevier; 2011, with permission.

TF Prosthetics

Traditional Socket Designs

TF sockets are often fitted in slight (5°) flexion and adduction to stretch the hip extensors and abductors and give them a mechanical advantage.

QUADRILATERAL DESIGN

This ischial–gluteal weight–bearing, *narrow anteroposterior* design was originally designed by Inman and Eberhart at UC Berkeley in the 1950s. It has four sides and four corners. It is easy to make and fit but less stable for shorter residual limbs and less comfortable when sitting than the ischial containment design (Fig. 4-8A).

ISCHIAL CONTAINMENT DESIGN

A "bony lock" incorporates the ischial tuberosity, pubic ramus, and greater trochanter. The posterior rim provides ischial–gluteal weight bearing and is contoured for the ischial tuberosity and gluteal muscles. These features improve stability, particularly for shorter residual limbs. The *narrow mediolateral* design also provides a more efficient energy cost of ambulation than the narrow anteroposterior design at high speeds (Fig. 4-8B).

Selected Suspension Options

Suction – Subatmospheric socket pressure maintains prosthetic attachment during swing phase. The sock bandage is pulled through a one-way valve hole. Its use is indicated in active amputees with well-shaped, nonfluctuating residual limbs.

Silesian Belt or Bandage – A belt that attaches from the socket at the greater trochanter and wraps around the opposite iliac crest (Fig. 4-9A).

Total Elastic Suspension (Belt) – Wraps around the proximal prosthesis and waist, enhancing rotational control. It retains body heat and has limited durability (Fig. 4-9B).

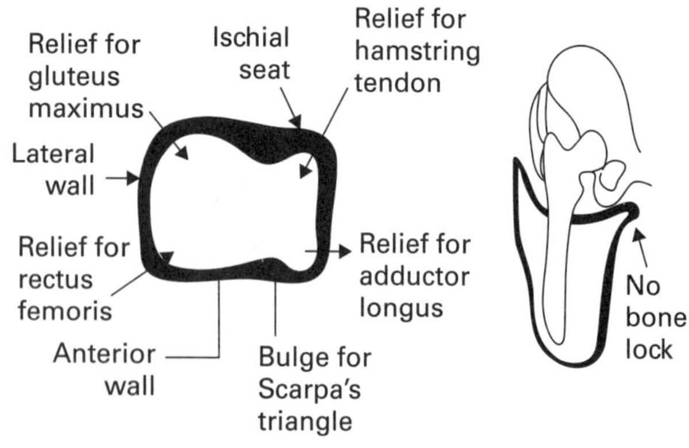

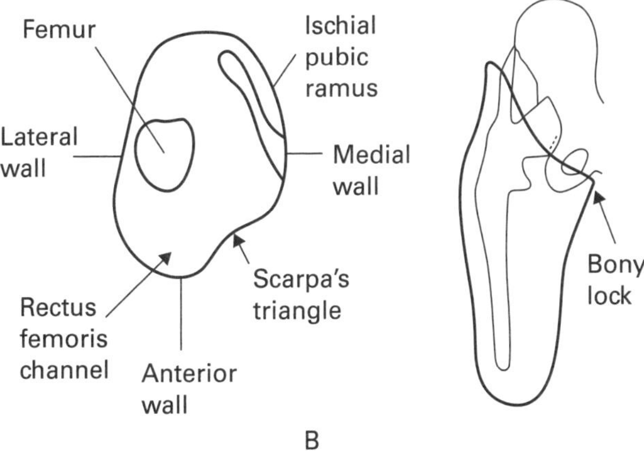

Figure 4-8 TF prosthetics. **A.** Quadrilateral design. **B.** Ischial containment design.

Pelvic Band and Belt Suspension – A rigid belt is connected to a metal hip joint on the lateral side of the socket. It is indicated for improving rotational and mediolateral pelvic stability in obese patients with significant redundant tissue or weak abductors with short or poorly shaped amputations. It is heavy and bulky and tends to interfere with sitting (Fig. 4-9C).

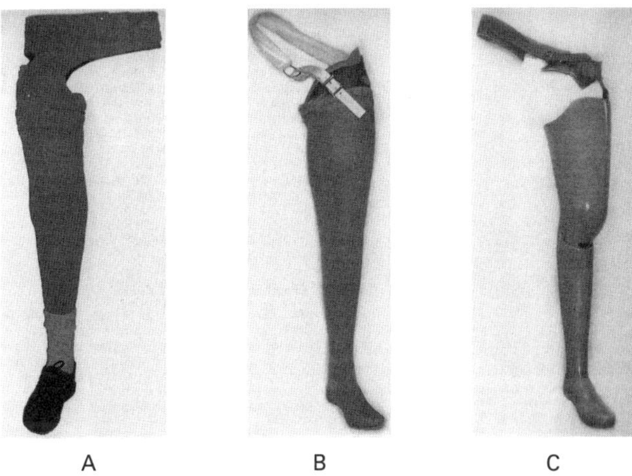

Figure 4-9 Three TF belts. **A.** Total elastic suspension belt. **B.** Silesian belt. **C.** Hip joint with pelvic band.

From Braddom RL. *Physical Medicine & Rehabilitation.* 4th ed. Philadelphia, PA: Elsevier; 2011, with permission.

Selected Knee Components: Key Features

Single-Axis or Constant friction – This knee is durable and inexpensive, but the cadence is fixed, or else the swing phase will be asymmetric. Stability is poor. It is indicated for level surfaces (Fig. 4-10).

Stance Phase Control or Safety Knee Joint – The stance phase control knee can control KF during weight bearing, which provides stability during stance phase. It is a common initial prosthesis used in geriatrics, general debility, and poor hip control. It allows ambulation on uneven surfaces. A delayed swing phase is noted, as full unloading is needed to flex the knee.

Polycentric – This typically has a 4-bar linkage design and a shifting instantaneous center of rotation that remains behind the GRF, providing increased stability during stance phase. The center of rotation moves proximally and posteriorly to the anatomic knees. Cosmesis is excellent, especially during sitting, but polycentrics are heavy, costly, and require high maintenance. It is indicated for knee disarticulations and short TF amputees (Fig. 4-10B).

Fluid Controlled (Pneumatic or Oil) – The design uses a piston in a fluid-filled cylinder, which provides automatic swing phase control at variable cadences. It provides a smooth and natural gait, but is heavy, costly, and requires high maintenance.

Manual Locking or Fixed Lock – The knee of last resort, this design provides the ultimate in stability. The gait, however, is awkward and energy consuming.

Microprocessor-Controlled Hydraulic Knee Joint – The C-Leg is composed of a complex system of sensors that records stresses every 0.02 seconds,

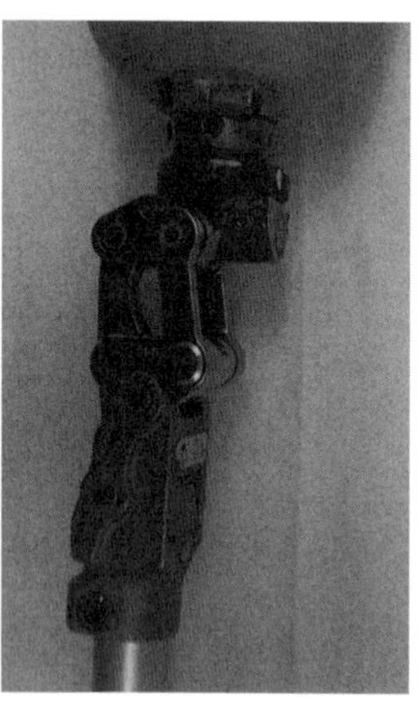

A

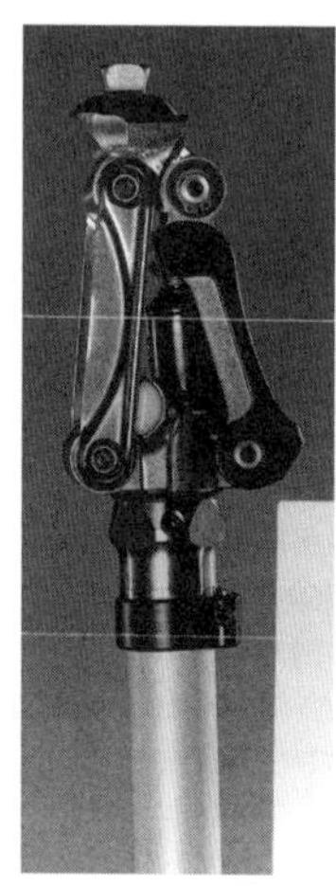

B

Figure 4-10 Selected knee components. **A.** Manual locking knee. **B.** Polycentric knee.

From Braddom RL. *Physical Medicine & Rehabilitation.* 4th ed. Philadelphia, PA: Elsevier; 2011, with permission.

measuring both the ankle movement and the angle and angular velocity of the knee joint. With this information, the joint continuously recognizes which walking phase the wearer is currently in and adjusts automatically. There is a high level of resistance in stance phase, allowing for the ability to bear weight on the prosthesis during flexion, yielding low-energy expenditure and improved gait symmetry on stairs, inclines, and uneven terrain. Disadvantages include having to recharge the battery every night, increased cost, and high maintenance.

Selected Postamputation Complications

Pain – Multiple causes

Prosthetic use: Skin irritation, prosthetic fit.

Phantom Pain – Phantom limb sensation, phantom limb pain, and generalized limb pain are maintained by afferent, central, and efferent dysfunction.[4]

Phantom limb pain can be described as sharp, burning, stabbing, tingling, shooting, electric, or cramping.[5] Treatment options include desensitization (e.g., massaging and tapping), neuropathic pain agents, topical anesthetics, modalities (e.g., TENS units), and injections into neuromas.

Choke Syndrome – Distal limb edema and painful *verrucous hyperplasia* may develop due to proximal limb pressure and a lack of total contact with the prosthesis. An underlying vascular disorder is usually present. Treatment involves adding a distal pad to the socket, correcting the suspension, removing proximal pressure, and/or refitting the socket.

Prosthetic Gait Analysis

Relationship between amputation level(s) and energy cost and speed is shown in Fig. 4-11.

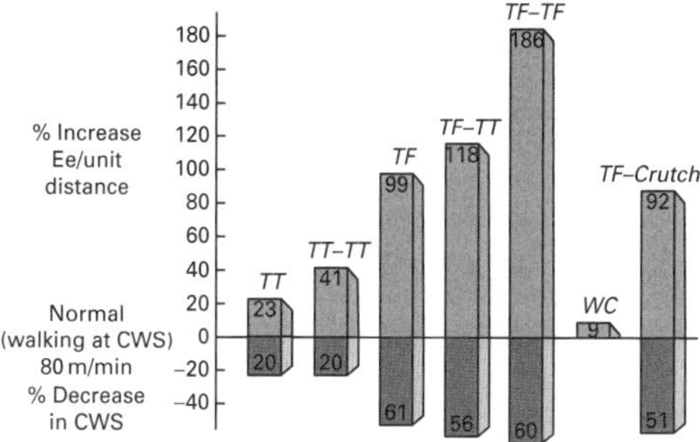

Figure 4-11 Graph showing relationship of amputation level(s) with energy cost and speed. CWS corresponds to the minimum energy cost per unit distance. Ee (Energy Expenditure)/unit distance and CWS for amputees using prostheses are compared with able-bodied subjects at a CWS of 80 m/min (≈3 mi/h). The energy cost of ambulation at CWS for able-bodied subjects is 4.3 kcal/min.

Adapted from Gonzalez EG, ed. *Downey and Darling's The Physiological Basis of Rehabilitation Medicine.* 3rd ed. Boston, MA: Butterworth Heinemann; 2001.

Causes of Stance Phase Problems

Excessive Trunk Extension/Lumbar Lordosis During Stance Phase – A poorly shaped posterior wall may cause patients to forwardly rotate their pelvis for pressure relief, with compensatory trunk extension. Other causes include insufficient initial flexion built into socket, HF contracture, and weak hip extensors.

Foot Slap – Foot slap may be noted with a TF locked-knee prosthesis if the foot is posteriorly placed or if socket flexion is excessive.

Knee Buckling/Instability – Causes include knee axis too anterior, insufficient PF, failure to limit DF, weak hip extensors, hard heel, large HF contracture, and posteriorly placed foot. Stability is achieved with a plantarflexed foot, a soft heel (i.e., SACH), or a more anteriorly placed foot.

Lateral Bending – Causes include a prosthesis that is too short, insufficient lateral wall, abducted socket, abduction contracture, and poor amputee balance.

Vaulting – Vaulting of the nonprosthetic limb may be due to a prosthesis that is too long, too much knee friction, or poor suspension.

Whip – A whip is an abrupt rotation of the heel occurring at the end of stance phase as the knee of a TF prosthesis is flexed to begin swing. If the heel moves medially, it is a medial whip; if laterally, a lateral whip. Causes include improper rotatory alignment of the knee axis, a knee axis not parallel to the floor, or flabby muscles about the femur with the prosthesis rotating freely within the underlying soft tissue.

Causes of Swing Phase Problems

Abducted Gait – Causes include a prosthesis that is too long, an abduction contracture, or a medial socket wall encroaching the groin.

Circumducted Gait – Causes include a prosthesis that is too long, too much knee friction making it difficult to bend the knee during swing-through, or an abduction contracture.

Excessive Heel Rise – Causes include insufficient knee friction or excessive KF moment (i.e., posterior foot or insufficient PF at heel strike).

Foot Drag – Causes include inadequate suspension, a prosthesis that is too long, insufficient HF or KF, or weak PF of the nonprosthetic limb.

Terminal Swing Impact – Insufficient knee friction may cause the amputee to deliberately and forcibly extend the knee.

Upper Limb Prosthetics

Unilateral amputees typically learn to perform most ADLs with their intact hand. B/l amputees often use their feet for many ADLs. Functional UEx prostheses should be prescribed for highly motivated patients with realistic expectations. Residual limb shaping with bandages may be required for 1 to 2 months before prosthetic fitting. If fitting is not performed within a 3- to 6-month window after unilateral amputation, long-term prosthesis use is infrequently seen.

TR Prosthetics

Body-powered prostheses with hooks or hands are typically prescribed for manual laborers (the typical patient who is going to suffer a traumatic UEx

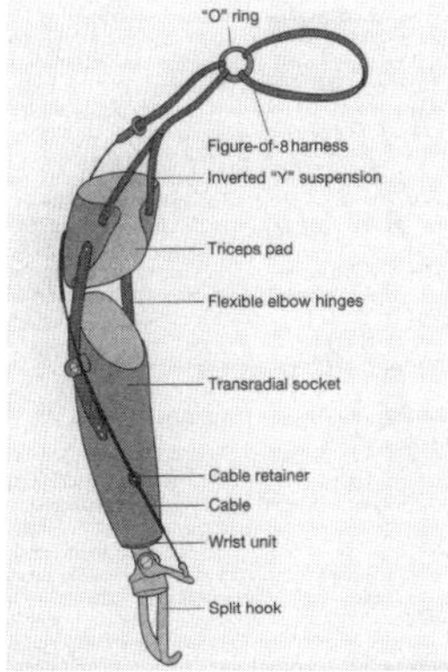

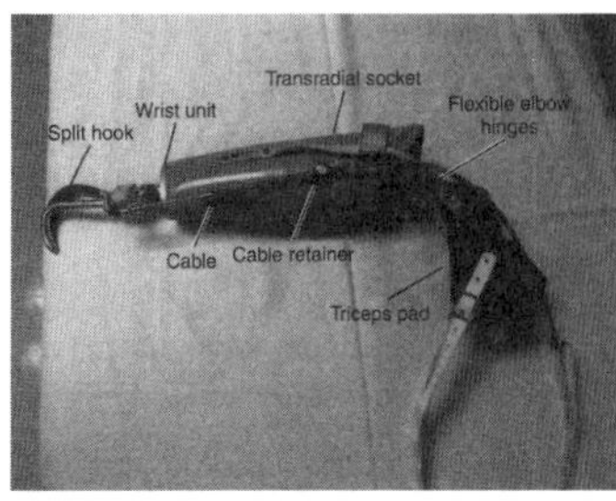

Figure 4-12 Commonly seen components in a TR prosthesis.

From Braddom RL. *Physical Medicine & Rehabilitation.* 4th ed. Philadelphia, PA: Elsevier; 2011, with permission.

amputation in the first place). Lifting up to 20 to 30 lbs can be expected. Longer residual limbs provide more lever arm and more pronation/supination and are better suited for heavy labor. Myoelectric prostheses are often appropriate for relatively sedentary amputees (Fig. 4-12).

TH Prosthetics

Longer residual limbs (up to 90% of original/expected length) are preferred. Function is usually much poorer than with a TR. A key difference for TH prostheses users is the need for an elbow unit. Harnessing and control systems are also different. Lifting between 10 and 15 lbs can be expected (more with a shoulder saddle). Length estimates for b/l TH amputees are 19% of patient height for the upper arm and 21% for the forearm component.

Functional TDs

TDs are the most important functional part of the UEx prosthesis. They are classified as active or passive.

Active TDs are broken into hooks and artificial hands. Hooks may have prehensors with thumb- and fingerlike components. The proximal limb/prosthesis essentially functions to position the TD in space. *Body-powered VO split-hooks* are the most common and practical TDs. In these devices, the TD is closed at rest. Prehensile force is predetermined by the number of rubber bands in place (each rubber band requires 5 lbs of force to provide 1 lb of pinch force). Up to 10 bands can be used (typical nonamputee male pinch force is 15 to 20 lbs) (Fig. 4-13A).

VC TDs provide a better control of closing pressure, but active effort is required to maintain closure of the TD or items may be dropped (Fig. 4-13B).

Myoelectric hands offer spherical/palmar grasp with grip forces higher than body-powered TDs. They can have a lifelike appearance but are relatively fragile. Two-site two-function controllers use different muscles to open and close the TD, while one-site two-function controllers use weak versus strong contractions of the same muscle to operate the TD.

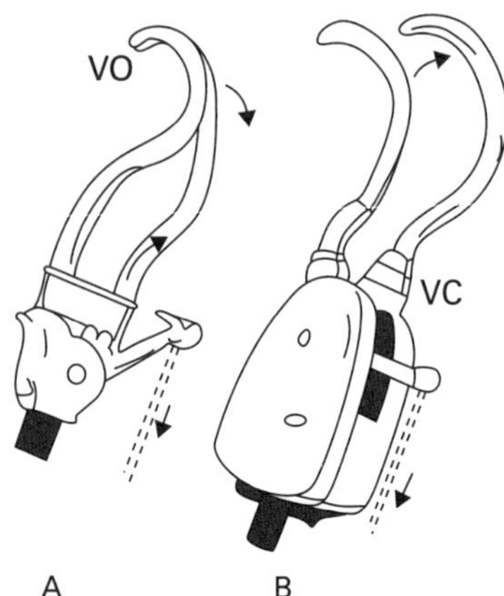

Figure 4-13 Functional terminal devices. **A.** Voluntary opening. **B.** Voluntary closing.

Upper Limb/UEx Prosthetic Systems

These have a number of basic needs (Table 4-1).

TABLE 4-1 UEx Essential Components

	Control		Shape	
	Body powered/myoelectric		Hook/hand	
Function				
Fine tip prehension	—	—	√	—
Cylindrical grip (large diameter)	—	—	—	√
Cylindrical grip (small diameter)	—	—	√	—
High grip force	—	√	—	—
Delicate grip force	—	√	—	—
Hook and pull	—	—	√	—
Pushing/holding down	—	—	—	√
Ruggedness	√	—	√	—
Comfort				
Low weight	√	—	√	—
Harness comfort	—	√	—	—
Low effort	—	√	—	—

(Continued)

	Control		Shape	
	Body powered/myoelectric		Hook/hand	
Reliability/convenience	√	—	√	—
Cosmesis	—	—	—	√
Low cost	√	—	—	—

Adapted from Dillingham T (specialist ed.). *Rehabilitation of the Injured Combatant Part IV.* Office of the Surgeon General, Department of the Army; 1998.

Other Components

The most common prosthetic **wrist** is the *friction wrist,* which allows passive pronation/supination but rotates when holding heavy objects. B/l amputees require at least one mechanical spring-assisted *flexion wrist* for access to the body midline. Most TH prosthetic **elbows** have an *alternator lock,* which alternately locks and unlocks with the same movement. With the elbow unlocked, body movements will flex or extend the elbow using a cable; when locked, the same cable operates the TD.

The traditional suspension employs straps and cables, with a double-walled **socket** for optimal fit. The outer wall is rigid and connects to other components; the inner wall must fit with the residual limb precisely or else the prosthesis may fail. The *suction socket* can provide self-suspension w/o straps and is ideally preferred for the TH amputee. The *Munster supracondylar socket* provides self-suspension for a very short TR or elbow disarticulation by encasing the humeral condyles and can be used for externally powered prostheses. Proper fit of the Munster socket, however, precludes full elbow extension.

The **body harness** uses cables to allow body motion and effort to operate prosthetic components. The *figure-of-8,* generally for a short TR or more proximal amputation, also holds the socket firmly in place, usually with an elbow hinge and half-arm cuff or triceps pad. The *figure-of-9,* generally for a long TR or wrist disarticulation, requires a self-suspending socket but is more comfortable than the *figure-of-8.* The *shoulder saddle with chest strap* frees the opposite shoulder and relieves the pressure caused by the axillary loop of the *figure-of-8.* Heavy loads are better tolerated, but donning is difficult and cosmesis is inferior.

Body-Powered Prosthesis Control

Glenohumeral (GH) Forward Flexion (TR, TH) – This natural movement provides excellent power and reach and can activate the TD or flex an elbow joint (Fig. 4-14A).

Biscapular Abduction (forequarter, shoulder disarticulation, TH, TR) – This movement can activate a TD, but the TD must stay relatively stationary. The forces generated are relatively weak (Fig. 4-14B).

GH Depression, Extension, Abduction (TH) – This movement locks or unlocks an elbow, but may be unnatural for some users and difficult to master (Fig. 4-14C).

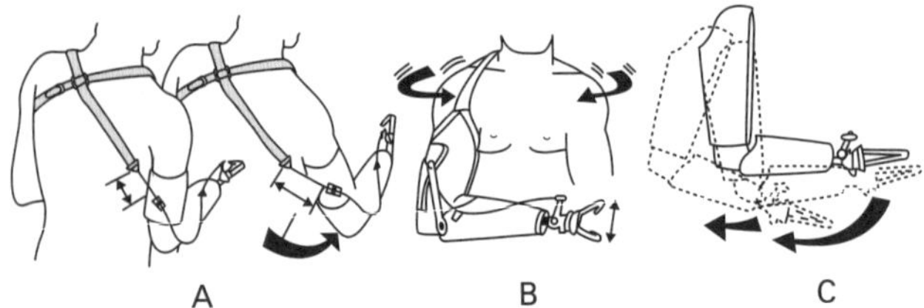

Figure 4-14 Body-powered prosthesis control. **A.** GH. **B.** Biscapular abduction. **C.** GH depression, extension, abduction.

Scapular Elevation (not pictured) – This locks or unlocks the elbow and is easy to master. It requires a waist belt.

Chest Expansion/Scapular Adduction (not pictured) – This locks or unlocks the elbow. It is an awkward motion, but does not interfere with TD operations.

REFERENCES

1. Eftekhari N. Amputation rehabilitation. In: O'Young BJ, ed. *Physical Medicine & Rehabilitation Secrets.* 2nd ed. Philadelphia, PA: Hanley & Belfus; 2002:553.
2. Garrison SJ. *Handbook of Physical Medicine and Rehabilitation Basics.* Philadelphia, PA: JB Lippincott; 1995.
3. Torburn L, Perry J. Energy expenditure during ambulation in dysvascular and traumatic BKAs: a comparison of 5 prosthetic feet. *J Rehabil Res Dev.* 1995;32:111-119.
4. Ehde DM. Chronic phantom sensations, phantom pain, residual limb pain, and other regional pain after lower limb amputation. *Arch Phys Med Rehabil.* 2000;81:1039-1044.
5. Jensen TS. Immediate and long-term phantom limb pain in amputees: incidence, clinical characteristics, and relationship to preamputation limb pain. *Pain.* 1985;21:267-278.

PEDIATRICS: CEREBRAL PALSY

Definition – A group of disorders of the development of movement and posture, causing activity limitations that are attributed to a nonprogressive disturbance that has occurred in the developing fetal or infant brain.[1]

Epidemiology

- Affects 3.6 per 1,000 school-aged children
- 2/1,000 live births for term infants
- 5/1,000 live births for 33 to 36 weeks gestation
- 30/1,000 live births <28 weeks

Risk factors include prenatal, perinatal, and postnatal infection, stroke, toxins, neonatal encephalopathy, complications of prematurity (SGA, BW < 800 g, IVH), maternal chorioamnionitis, fever during labor, coagulopathy or bleeding, placental infarction, thyroid disease, hyperbilirubinemia, and trauma.

The greatest risk factor is prematurity; neonatal encephalopathy is the best predictor of CP in term infants.

Classification

Movement Type

- Spastic (70% to 85%)
- Dyskinetic
- Hypotonic
- Ataxic
- Mixed

Anatomic Distribution

- Hemiparesis (UEx > LEx, one side of body)
- Diparesis (LEx > UEx)
- Quadriparesis (entire body)

GROSS MOTOR FUNCTION CLASSIFICATION SYSTEM

Level 1. Walks indoors and outdoors and climbs stairs without limitations

Level 2. Walks indoors and outdoors, climbs stairs with a rail, and has limitations walking on uneven surfaces and inclines

Level 3. Walks indoors and outdoors on a level surface with an assistive device; may climb stairs with a rail and use a manual wheelchair

Level 4. May walk short distances with assistive device but may rely on power mobility

Level 5. Self-mobility severely limited

>80% have abnormal neuroimaging, most often PVL following IVH in premature infants, focal cortical infarcts secondary to MCA stroke

in hemiparesis, basal ganglia and thalamic lesions in dystonic CP, brain malformations, and generalized encephalomalacia in spastic quadriparesis.

MRI more likely to show an abnormality compared with CT[2]

Persistence of primitive reflexes after 6 months, asymmetry or obligatory response

Early handedness/failure to use the involved hand

Early rolling (from tone)

Associated Disorders

- Sensory impairments, especially in hemiparesis
- Hearing, visual, cognitive, psychological, oralmotor, nutritional, genitourinary, respiratory, bone mineral density, and dental impairments
- Seizures in 15% to 55%[3]
- Hip dysplasia and dislocation
- Spine – kyphosis, lordosis, and scoliosis
- Spasticity and contractures
- Gait impairment: scissoring due to adductor tone, anteversion – intoeing, and psoas and hamstring tightness – crouch gait. Stiff knee ankle PF tone toe gait

Treatment

- Therapy: no clear evidence for any particular approach
- Stretching, strengthening, tone management, and functional training
- Spasticity management
  - Oral medications
  - Chemical neurolysis
  - Intrathecal baclofen
  - Selective posterior rhizotomy
    - Sectioning of a portion of abnormal L2-S1 sensory nerve rootlets to reduce excitatory input
    - Favorable in patients aged 3 to 8 years who have selective motor control and functional strength and lack significant contractures
    - Negative effects: hypotonia usually transient, weakness, bladder dysfunction (usually transient), spine deformity including spondylolysis/listhesis, and hip dislocation
  - Botulinum toxin: different dosing guidelines for children
    - Reported distant side effects in children with CP
- Orthopedic surgery: lengthening, transfers, and osteotomy

Outcomes

Good prognosis for ambulation[4–7]

Molnar: independent sitting by age 2 years

Badell: reciprocal crawl at 1½ to 2½ years

Fedrizzi transition: supine to prone by 18 months

Poor prognosis for ambulation

Bleck: presence of three or more primitive reflexes at 18 to 24 months

Life expectancy: reduced with immobility and inability to self-feed[8]

Congenital Brachial Plexus Palsy

Epidemiology

- 1 to 2/1,000 live births (United States)

Risk Factors

- Increase in birth weight
- Shoulder dystocia
- Traumatic delivery
- Breech
- Multiparous

Clinical Presentation

- "Waiter's tip" (shoulder irritation and adduction, elbow extension and pronation, wrist flexion) – Erb palsy – C5, 6, 7 – 80%
- Klumpke C7, 8, T1, rare to occur exclusively
- Spontaneous recovery in 50% to 90%

Associated Injuries

- Facial palsy
- Cephalohematoma
- Clavicle or humerus fracture
- Torticollis
- Cervical spine injury
- Diaphragmatic paralysis
- Horner syndrome (with lower plexus injury)

Examination and Testing

- Sensory
- Reflexes
- ROM
- EDX studies in the first few days, then after several months for reinnervation[9]; SNAP present in insensate areas; preganglionic lesion/root avulsion
- MRI

Treatment

- Goals are to normalize limb function, optimize nerve regeneration, and allow elbow flexion and shoulder stabilization
- Early pinning to avoid shoulder stretch and gentle ROM to consider pain due to traumatic neuritis
- Position to increase awareness, ROM, splinting, and developmental training
- Surgery indicated if antigravity strength not present at the elbow at 6 months[10]

- Other literature cites early surgical intervention between age 3 and 9 months
- Neurosurgery – neurolysis of scar and fibrotic tissue, end-to-end anastomosis, nerve transfer sural or great auricular, and end-to-side neurorrhaphy
- Orthopedic: tendon releases and transfers

Complications

- Muscle atrophy
- Contracture
- Developmental concerns
- Glenoid dysplasia with posterior subluxation (reduced ER)
- Cosmetic
- Pain may be indicated by biting the limb (possibly more in children who had surgery)

Prognosis

- Recovery by 3 months is a good indicator for normal function[11–12]
- Poor-grade elbow flexion at 6 months may be predictive

Developmental Milestones

2 months
- Raises head when prone
- Turns to voice, coos, and responsive smile

4 months
- Lifts head and chest in prone and rolls over prone to supine
- Reaches for objects and brings hand to midline and mouth
- Laughs

6 months
- Sits without support
- Grasps objects and transfers
- Babbles

9 months
- Sits alone and tries to crawl and stand
- Emerging pincer grasp with index finger and thumb
- Understands no and bye and babbles repeated sounds (da-da)

10 months
- Pulls to stand and cruises
- Finger feeds

12 months
- Walks alone
- Points at objects and neat pincer
- Single words

15 months
- Comes to stand unsupported
- Builds tower of two cubes
- Says four to six words

24 months
- Walks on stairs with rail
- Follows two-step commands

30 months
- Jumps

3 years
- Pedals tricycle and ascends stairs with alternating feet
- Copies a circle
- Knows name and gender

4 years
- Descends stairs with alternating feet
- Tripod pencil grip

SCI Specific to Pediatrics

Epidemiology and Risk Factors

- 3% to 5% of all SCIs occur in children under age 15 years[13]
- 20% of SCIs under age 20 years
- In children under age 9 years, boys are four times more likely to be affected compared with girls
- Racial difference in those over 15 years: overall increased risk for African Americans and Hispanic Americans

Causes:

1. Motor vehicle accident
2. Falls, under 10 years
3. Sports, 15 to 16 years

50% < age 10 years had occiput C1 injury, 50% were neurologically intact SCI without radiographic abnormality

5% to 67% incidence in pediatric SCI, higher in age < 9 years[14]
C5-C8 level most common
Developing spine is more mobile, favoring stretch injury to ligaments without bony fracture
Head size relatively large, resulting in higher cervical injuries

Management – area of difference from adult

Deep vein thrombosis prophylaxis not clear in children[15,16]

Younger children with high lumbar or thoracic levels may be ambulatory with bracing but become more wheelchair dependent at adolescence (more energy efficient).

Spina Bifida

Epidemiology

- Risk of having a child with NTD – 0.1% to 0.2%
- Recurrence if one child has NTD – 2% to 5%
- Recurrence if two children have NTD – 10% to 15%

Risk Factors

- Environmental – hyperthermia in first 28 days from maternal fever, hot tubs, or sauna
- Occupation – solvent exposure, health care workers, and agriculture
- Nutritional – folate deficiency
  - American Academy of Pediatrics guidelines for folate supplementation[17]:
    - folate 0.4 mg/day for women of child-bearing years
    - 4 mg/day prior to conception and through first trimester if previous child with spina bifida or high risk (has maternal diabetes or on valproate)
- Maternal – obesity and diabetes
- Maternal medications: valproic acid, antiretroviral drugs, isotretinoin, and methotrexate

Etiology

- Failure of neural tube closure
- Neural tube closure starts mid-cervical and proceeds caudal and rostral by day 27

Diagnosis

Prenatal screening
- α-fetoprotein elevated
- high-resolution US splaying of pedicles and lemon and banana sign
- amniocentesis

Spina bifida occulta
- bony defect without herniation of neural elements
- incidental in 5% to 36% of adults
- may have hair patch, dimple, sinus, or nevus
- may be associated with tethered cord and bowel/bladder

Meningocele
- bony defect with herniation of meninges but not neural tissue
- <10% of cases
- examination normal

Meningomyelocele
- herniation of meninges and neural elements
- associated with Chiari type 2 malformation in 90%
- hydrocephalus in 80% to 90%
- 75% lumbosacral

Caudal regression
- absence of sacrum and parts of lumbar spine
- risk factor – maternal diabetes
- syrinx, anorectal stenosis, renal, cardiac, and external genitalia

Management

Closure in the first 24 to 48 hours of life

In utero repair reported

Rehabilitation management for developmental training, mobility, and deformity prevention

Use of bracing depending on level of deficit, wheelchair, seating, and standers

Deficits

Motor and sensory deficits can be asymmetric

Thoracic – UEx spared except T1
- kyphoscoliosis from weak trunk occurs in 80% to 100%
- LEx contractures from position and wheelchair mobility

L1-3
- hip flex and abd present; leads to early hip dislocation and scoliosis
- may ambulate with bracing (HKAFO and RGO) and AD if young but stop due to high energy cost[18]

L4-5
- late hip dislocation and scoliosis in 5% to 10%
- L5 calcaneus foot, L4 calcaneovarus

Bladder Peds
- bladder capacity
  - first year of life: weight in kg × 7 to 10 mL
  - age 1 to 12 years: (age + 2) × 30 mL
  - teens/adult: 400 mL
- bladder studies
  - newborn – baseline US, urodynamics, and VCUG
  - repeat sono every 3 months in first year, 2×/year in second year, and then yearly
  - urodynamics and VCUG at 3 months, then at 1 year, 2 to 3 years, and then every 2 years or for change in status

Neurogenic bladder treatment – CIC (self-catheterization by age 5 years if adequate hand use and cognition), oral medications, Botulinum toxin, vesicostomy, bladder augmentation.

Other Concerns

Neurogenic bowel, fecal incontinence, and constipation

Obesity

Latex allergy, cross-reactivity with kiwi, banana, avocado, and chestnut

Cognitive function, learning problems – higher level > T12 with hydrocephalus having more severe structural brain anomalies[19]

Shunt malfunction – headaches, vomiting, personality changes, concentration difficulty, or other neurological findings

Tethered cord – spasticity, decreased strength, scoliosis, deterioration in neurological status, bowel/bladder changes, contractures, gait deviations, and back pain in only 20% but is the symptom that can improve after surgery[20]

Diastematomyelia – sagittal cleavage of the spinal cord

Syringomyelia – in up to 40%, most often cervical
- Scoliosis or decreased function above lesion level

REFERENCES

1. Bax M, Goldstein M, Rosenbaum P, et al. Proposed definition and classification of cerebral palsy. *Dev Med Child Neurol.* 2005;47(8):571-576.
2. Ashwal S, Russman BS, Blasco PA, et al. Practice parameters: diagnostic assessment of the child with cerebral palsy: report of the Quality Standards Subcommittee of the American Academy of Neurology and the Practice Committee of the Child Neurology Society. *Neurology.* 2004;62(6):851-863.
3. Wallace SJ. Epilepsy in cerebral palsy. *Dev Med Child Neurol.* 2001;43(10):713-717.
4. Molnar GE, Gordon SU. Cerebral palsy: predictive value of selected clinical sign of early prognostication of motor function. *Arch Phys Med Rehabil.* 1976;57:153.
5. Badell A. Cerebral palsy: postural locomotor prognosis in spastic diplegia. *Arch Phys Med Rehabil.* 1985;66:614-619.
6. Fedrizzi E, Facchin P, Marzaroli M, et al. Predictors of independent walking in children with spastic diplegia. *J Child Neurol.* 2000;15:228-234.
7. Bleck EE. Locomotor prognosis in cerebral palsy. *Dev Med Child Neurol.* 1975;17:18.
8. Strauss D, Brooks J, Rosenbloom R, Shavelle R. Life expectancy in cerebral palsy: an update. *Dev Med Child Neurol.* 2008;50(7):487-493.
9. Pitt M, Vredeveld JW. The role of electromyography in the management of the brachial palsy of the newborn. *Clin Neurophysiol.* 2005;116:1756-1761.
10. O'Brien DF, Park TS, Noetzel MJ, et al. Management of birth brachial plexus palsy. *Childs Nerv Syst.* 2006;22:103-112.
11. Noetzel MJ, Park TS, Robinson S, et al. Prospective study of recovery following neonatal brachial plexus injury. *J Child Neurol.* 2001;16:488-492.
12. National Spinal Cord Injury Statistical Center. *Spinal Cord Injury: Facts and Figures at a Glance.* Birmingham, AL: University of Alabama; 2008.
13. Massagli TL. Medical and rehabilitation issues in the care of children with spinal cord injury. *Phys Med Rehabil Clin N Am.* 2000;11(1):169-182.
14. Levy ML, Granville RC, Hart D, Meltzer H. Deep venous thrombosis in children and adolescents. *J Neurosurg: Pediatr.* 2004;101(2):32-37.
15. Truitt AK, Sorrells DL, Halvorson E, et al. Pulmonary embolism: which pediatric trauma patients are at risk? *J Pediatr Surg.* 2005;40:124-127.
16. Krach LE, Gormley, ME, Jr., Ward M. Traumatic brain injury. In: Alexander M, Matthews D, eds. *Pediatric Rehabilitation: Principles and Practice.* 4th ed. New York, NY: Demos Medical Publishing; 2010:231-260.
17. Diamond M, Armento M. Children with disabilities. In: DeLisa JA, Gans BM, Walsh NE, et al., eds. *Physical Medicine and Rehabilitation: Principles and Practice.* 4th ed. Philadelphia, PA: Lippincott Williams & Wilkins; 2005.
18. Williams EN, Broughton NS, Menelaus MB. Age related walking in children with spina bifida. *Dev Med Child Neurol.* 1999;41(7):446-449.
19. Fletcher JM, Copeland K, Frederick JA, et al. Spinal lesion level in spina bifida; a source of neural and cognitive heterogeneity. *J Neurosurg.* 2005;102(3):268-279.
20. Schoenmakers MA, Goosekens RH, Gulmans VA, et al. Long-term outcome of neurosurgical untethering on neurosegmental motor and ambulation levels. *Dev Med Child Neurol.* 2003;45(8):551-555.

RECOMMENDED READING

Alexander M, Matthews D. *Pediatric Rehabilitation; Principles and Practice.* 4th ed. New York, NY: Demos Medical Publishing; 2010.

Children with disabilities. In: DeLisa JA, Gans BM, Walsh NE, et al., eds. *Physical Medicine and Rehabilitation; Principles and Practice.* 4th ed. Philadelphia, PA: Lippincott Williams & Wilkins; 2005.

Kliegman RM. *Nelson Textbook of Pediatrics.* 18th ed. Philadelphia, PA: WB Saunders; 2007.

Kliegman RM. *Nelson Textbook of Pediatrics*. 18th ed. Philadelphia, PA: WB Saunders; 2007.

Molnar G, Alexander M. *Pediatric Rehabilitation*. 3rd ed. Philadelphia, PA: Hanley & Belfus; 1999: chap 2.

Simson V, Hornyak JE. Spinal cord injuries. In: Alexander M, Matthews D, eds. *Pediatric Rehabilitation: Principles and Practice*. 4th ed. New York, NY: Demos Medical Publishing; 2010:261-276.

Chapter 5.2

PEDIATRICS: NEUROMUSCULAR DISORDERS

Caused by an abnormality of any component of the lower motor neuron
- anterior horn cell
- peripheral nerve
- neuromuscular junction
- muscle

Frequently associated with systemic effects, as some of the pathologic changes may affect skeletal, smooth, and cardiac muscles, the brain, and mitochondria in multiple organs.

May be progressive, acquired, or hereditary.

The most common etiology is genetic. It is crucial to obtain a detailed family history and if possible to obtain diagnostic evaluation of the affected relatives.

Diagnostic evaluation of a child with suspected neuromuscular disorder:
- meticulous physical examination
- detailed family history
- comprehensive past medical history and surgical history
- request for additional laboratory and genetic data that may be costly and not readily available must be considered following ascertainment of developmentally appropriate assessment and history

THE MOST COMMON NEUROMUSCULAR DISORDERS IN INFANTS AND CHILDREN

The most common cause of referral for possible neuromuscular disorder is when the infant appears floppy. See Table 5.2-1 on Duchenne muscular dystrophy.

TABLE 5.2-1 Comparison of Duchenne Muscular Dystrophy vs. Becker Muscular Dystrophy

	Duchenne muscular dystrophy	**Becker muscular dystrophy**
US prevalence (est.)	15,000	2,200
Incidence rate	1/3,500 male births	Unknown
Inheritance	X-linked	X-linked
Gene location	Xp21 (reading frame shifted)	Xp21 (reading frame maintained)
Protein	Dystrophin	Dystrophin

	Duchenne muscular dystrophy	**Becker muscular dystrophy**
Onset	2–6 years	4–12 years (severe BMD) Late teenage to adulthood (mild BMD)
Severity and course	Relentlessly progressive Reduced motor function by 2–3 years Steady decline in strength Life span <35 years	Slowly progressive Severity and onset correlate with muscle dystrophin levels
Ambulation status	Loss of ambulation: 7–13 years (no corticosteroids) Loss of ambulation: 9–15 years (corticosteroids)	Loss of ambulation > 16 years
Weakness	Proximal > distal Symmetric Legs and arms	Proximal > distal Symmetric Legs and arms
Cardiac	Dilated cardiomyopathy first to second decade Onset of signs second decade	Cardiomyopathy (may occur before weakness); third to fourth decade frequent
Respiratory	Profoundly reduced vital capacity in second decade Ventilatory dependency in second decade	Respiratory involvement in subset of patients Ventilatory dependency in severe patients
Muscle size	Calf hypertrophy	Calf hypertrophy
Musculoskeletal	Contractures: ankles, hips, and knees Scoliosis: onset after loss of ambulation	Contractures: ankles and others in adulthood
CNS	Reduced cognitive ability (reduced verbal ability)	Some patients have reduced cognitive ability
Muscle pathology	Endomysial fibrosis and fatty infiltration Variable fiber size and myopathic grouping Fiber degeneration/ regeneration Dystrophin: absent Sarcoglycans: secondary reduction	Variable fiber size Endomysial connective tissue and fatty infiltration Fiber degeneration Fiber regeneration Dystrophin: reduced (usually 10%–60% of normal)
Blood chemistry and hematology	CK: Very high (10,000–50,000) High AST and ALT (normal GGT) High aldolase	CK: 5,000–20,000 Lower levels with increasing age

Anterior Horn Disorders in Children

Spinal Muscular Atrophy

The SMAs comprise a group of autosomal recessive disorders characterized by progressive weakness of the lower motor neurons.

SMA type I (acute infantile or Werdnig-Hoffmann): Onset is from birth to 6 months.
SMA type II (chronic infantile): Onset is between 6 and 18 months.
SMA type III (chronic juvenile): Onset is after 18 months.
SMA type IV (adult onset): Onset is in adulthood (mean onset, mid-thirties).

SMA TYPE I – ACUTE INFANTILE OR WERDNIG-HOFFMANN DISEASE

- Presents before 6 months of age – 95% of patients have signs and symptoms by 3 months. Severe, progressive muscle weakness and flaccid or reduced muscle tone.
- Reports of impaired fetal movements are frequently observed.
- Prolonged cyanosis may be noted at delivery.

Clinical signs:

- severe limb and axial weakness
- frog posture
- weak cry
- marked hypotonia
- diaphragmatic breathing
- bell-shaped chest
- internal rotation of arms
- no evidence of cerebral involvement
- severe nonprogressive weakness
- prone to respiratory infections

Diagnostic workup:

- CK is normal.
- EMG/NCV – decreased amplitude and possibly decreased velocity in motor conduction studies, a normal sensory conduction study, and a mild increase in amplitude and duration of motor unit potential and fibrillation potential.
- Muscle biopsy – early stages may be inconclusive. Large group atrophy and clusters of large fibers (type I) are noted at later (6 to 8 weeks) stages.

Prognosis:

- Poor. Vast majority die within the first 3 years of life.

Treatment:

- Supportive
- Suctioning

SMA TYPE II – CHRONIC INFANTILE FORM

Clinical signs:

- The most common manifestation – developmental motor delay between 6 and 18 months
- Unusual feature of the disease – postural tremor affecting the fingers, attributed to fasciculations in the skeletal muscles

- May see tongue fasciculations
- Normal–advanced intellect
- Joint laxity

Diagnostic workup:

- CK is normal–elevated.
- EMG/NCV – decreased amplitude and possibly decreased velocity in motor conduction studies, a normal sensory conduction study, and a mild increase in amplitude and duration of motor unit potential and fibrillation potential.
- Muscle biopsy – large group atrophy as well as clusters of large fibers (type I).

Prognosis:

- The life span of patients with SMA type II varies from 2 years to the third decade of life.

SMA TYPE III – CHRONIC JUVENILE OR KUGELBERG-WELANDER SYNDROME

Clinical signs:

- Mild form of autosomal recessive SMA.
- Appears after age 18 months.
- Characterized by slowly progressive proximal weakness.
- Patients can stand and walk but have trouble with motor skills, such as going up and down stairs. This is due to weakness of hip extensors.

Diagnostic workup:

- CK – normal–elevated.
- EMG/NCV – decreased amplitude and possibly decreased velocity in motor conduction studies, a normal sensory conduction study, and a mild increase in amplitude and duration of motor unit potential and fibrillation potential.
- Muscle biopsy – large group atrophy as well as clusters of large fibers. Also, focal small group atrophy may be seen.

SMA TYPE IV – ADULT-ONSET FORM

Clinical signs:

- Onset after age of 20 years
- Slowly progressive proximal weakness
- Normal life expectancy

There are other forms of anterior horn disorders that have been described in the medical literature. These disorders are rare and beyond the scope of this manual.

Bulbar hereditary motor neuronopathy (HMN) types I and II: bulbar HMN I (Vialetto-van Laere syndrome) and bulbar HMN II (Fazio-Londe disease), distal SMA (spinal Charcot-Marie-Tooth [CMT] or HMN type II), X-lined recessive bulbo-SMA (Kennedy disease), scapuloperoneal SMA type I autosomal recessive and type II autosomal dominant, X-linked form scapuloperoneal SMA, Davidenkow syndrome, facioscapulohumeral (FSH) SMA, scapulohumeral SMA, oculopharyngeal SMA, Ryukyuan SMA.

PERIPHERAL NERVE DISORDERS

Acute Inflammatory Demyelinating Polyradiculoneuropathy

- Also known as GBS
- A primarily demyelinating neuropathy
- The most common cause of acute motor paralysis in children
- An autoimmune-mediated disease with environmental triggers
- Heterogeneous condition with a number of different variants

Clinical Presentation

- Characterized by an acute monophasic, nonfebrile, postinfectious illness manifesting as ascending weakness and areflexia
- Pain and dysesthesias
- Triggers of GBS:
  - Epstein-Barr virus
  - Cytomegalovirus
  - Enteroviruses
  - Hepatitis A and B
  - Varicella
  - Mycoplasma pneumonia
  - *Campylobacter jejuni*

A variant of GBS, Miller Fisher syndrome, which is characterized by the triad of ophthalmoplegia, ataxia, and areflexia, is also linked to preceding infection with *C. jejuni*. Most of these patients have antibodies against the GQ1b ganglioside.

Outcome

- More favorable in children than in adults
- Recurrence is relatively uncommon in children (5% to 12%)

Differential Diagnosis of GBS in Children

1. **Botulism** – In infants, botulism should be considered. Botulism is characterized not only by (descending) weakness but also by involvement of the extraocular muscles (ophthalmoplegia), miosis of the pupil, and constipation.
2. **Myasthenia Gravis** – Can be present with primarily proximal weakness in childhood. A good history, testing for acetylcholine receptor antibodies, and electrophysiologic studies with nerve conduction studies (NCSs) and EMG, including repetitive stimulation, can help to distinguish myasthenia gravis from GBS.
3. **Infectious Processes** – GBS-like syndromes can occur in certain infections, such as Lyme disease or HIV.
4. **Peripheral Neuropathies** – Vincristine, glue sniffing, heavy metals, organophosphate pesticides, HIV, diphtheria, Lyme disease, inborn errors of metabolism, Leigh disease, Tangier disease, porphyria, and critical illness polyneuropathy.
5. **Neuromuscular Junction Disorders** – Tick paralysis, myasthenia gravis, botulism, and hypercalcemia.

Pediatric Aspects of Treatment and Management of GBS

a. The most effective form of therapy is generally considered to be intravenous immunoglobulin (IVIG).
b. Plasmapheresis may decrease the severity and shorten the duration of GBS.

Results of plasmapheresis and IVIG are similar, with possibly fewer side effects seen with IVIG.

In patients, care should be taken to monitor respiratory and cardiac function, especially in the acute, progressive stage of the disease.

Respiratory compromise is the most concerning and life-threatening aspect of GBS in childhood.

Hereditary Motor Sensory Neuropathy

- Inherited disorders of peripheral nerves, both motor and sensory
- Progressive neuromuscular impairments
- Onset usually in the first or second decade of life

Seven Types

- Hereditary motor sensory neuropathy (HMSN) types 1A and 1B (dominantly inherited hypertrophic demyelinating neuropathies) CMT type 1
- HMSN type 2 (dominantly inherited neuronal neuropathies) CMT type 2
- HMSN type 3 (hypertrophic neuropathy of infancy [Déjerine-Sottas])
- HMSN type 4 (hypertrophic neuropathy [Refsum] associated with phytanic acid excess)
- HMSN type 5 (associated with spastic paraplegia)
- HMSN type 6 (with optic atrophy)
- HMSN type 7 (with retinitis pigmentosa)

The most common form of CMT1, known as CMT1A, was associated with a duplication within chromosome 17p11.2.

The second most common form of CMT1 (CMT1B) and some cases of Déjerine-Sottas syndrome were found to be associated with mutations in the myelin protein zero (*MPZ*) gene in chromosome 1.

Mutations of each of these genes have been associated with multiple, overlapping phenotypes. For example, myelin protein zero mutations are associated with CMT1B, Déjerine-Sottas syndrome, and the axonal CMT2 phenotype.

Inheritance of HMSN Disorders

- CMT1 is a dominantly inherited, hypertrophic, predominantly demyelinating form.
- CMT2 is a dominantly inherited predominantly axonal form.
- Déjerine-Sottas is a severe form with onset in infancy.
- CMTX is inherited in an X-linked manner.
- CMT4 includes the various demyelinating autosomal recessive forms of CMT disease.

CMT is nearly always slowly progressive.

Clinical Features

- Motor signs tend to develop before sensory signs.
- Weakness and atrophy are first seen in intrinsic foot muscles, followed by ankle and toe dorsiflexors.
- Mismatch between strength in the affected peroneal-innervated muscles and the less affected tibial-innervated muscles results in development of typical high-arched feet, hammer toes, and difficulty with heel walking seen early in physical examination.
- Sensory impairment tends to follow motor impairment and remains less severe.
- Patients are more susceptible to compression neuropathies and radiculopathies.
- Sprains and fractures are disabling and avoidable.

Treatment

The common foot deformities of CMT can lead to discomfort, impaired ambulation, and disability. Ankle weakness and instability can be treated with orthoses or shoe modifications. Moderate activity is recommended. Overexertion should be avoided.

Neuromuscular Junction Disorders

Transient Neonatal Myasthenia

- It occurs in 10% to 30% of neonates born to myasthenic mothers.
- It may occur any time during the first 7 to 10 days of life, and infants should be monitored closely for any signs of respiratory distress.
- If treated and monitored, it is a self-limiting condition in vast majority of the cases.

The major cause is transplancental transfer of circulating acetylcholine antibodies from mother to fetus.

Congenital or Infantile Myasthenia

Occurs in infants of nonmyasthenic mothers and may have an autosomal recessive inheritance. Antibodies to ACh receptor are usually absent.

Juvenile Myasthenia

Juvenile myasthenia gravis has a similar pathophysiologic origin as adult myasthenia gravis, but there are important differences, mostly relating to epidemiology, presentation, and therapeutic decision making.

Several considerations should be emphasized, such as postponement of corticosteroid therapy from an early age, which is associated with growth retardation, and avoidance of thymectomy due to the risks of induced immunodeficiency.

It particularly affects adolescent girls and is severe and labile in presentation. Clinically presents with weakness of other muscles including facial and mastication. It can affect swallowing, speech, respiration as well as neck, trunk, and limb muscles.

Myopathies

Facioscapulohumeral Muscular Dystrophy (FSHD)

- Slowly progressive dystrophic myopathy
- Predominant involvement of facial and shoulder girdle musculature
- Autosomal dominant inheritance; 10% to 30% is caused by sporadic mutation
- Presents before age 20 years
- Serum CK levels are normal or slightly elevated in the majority of patients

Diagnosis – confirmed in more than 90% by molecular genetic testing.

Clinical Presentation

- Facial weakness
- Difficulties with eye closure
- Expressionless appearance
- Scapular stabilizers, shoulder abductors, and shoulder external rotators are affected
- Deltoids are spared if tested with scapulae stabilized
- Contractures of joints are uncommon
- Scoliosis is mild and nonprogressive
- Evidence for mild restrictive lung disease in 50% of patients

Coates syndrome – early onset of FSHD characterized by sensorineural hearing deficit and progressive exudative telangiectasia of the retina.

Rapid in progression.

Emery-Dreifuss Muscular Dystrophy (EMD)

Characterized by

- Weakness
- Contractures
- Cardiac conduction abnormalities

EMD-1

- X-linked recessive progressive dystrophic myopathy.
- Typically presents in the second decade of life but age of presentation may vary.
- Evolving contractures are more limiting than weakness.
- Elbow flexion contractures are a hallmark of disease.
- Functional limitations with ambulation and stair negotiation. However, due to slow progression, loss of ambulation is rare.
- Progressive cardiac disease is almost invariably present with onset in the early second decade to the fourth decade.
- Arrhythmia may lead to emboli or sudden death, cardiomyopathy leads to progressive left ventricular myocardial dysfunction.

EMD-2

- Abnormality due to lamin A/C protein linked to chromosome 1q21.2
- Inheritance may be dominant or recessive or missense
- Missense mutation leads to childhood onset
- Clinical feature is scapuloperoneal and facial distribution of weakness
- Contractures are rare

Congenital Myopathies

A group of heterogeneous disorders usually presenting with infantile hypotonia due to genetic defects, causing primary myopathies with the absence of any structural abnormality of the central nervous system or peripheral nerves.

Chapter 5.3

PEDIATRICS: JUVENILE IDIOPATHIC ARTHRITIS

- JIA is the most common rheumatic disease of childhood
- Diagnosis should fulfill the following criteria:
  - occur before age 16 years
  - persist for at least 6 weeks
  - diagnosis of exclusion

JIA affects bone and joints. It can lead to overgrowth, undergrowth, or aberrant growth. Possible anomalies related to JIA include micrognathia, leg length discrepancy, and hip dysplasia.

Indicators of poor outcome include

- Greater severity and extension at the onset of disease
- Symmetrical disease
- Early wrist and hip involvement
- Serologic evidence of RF
- Persistent active disease
- Early radiographic changes

There are seven subtypes of JIA:

1. Systemic arthritis
2. Oligoarthritis
3. RF-negative polyarthritis
4. RF-positive arthritis
5. Psoriatic arthritis
6. Enthesitis-related arthritis
7. Undifferentiated arthritis

Key Points

Systemic Arthritis

Diagnosis requires both

- Presence of arthritis
- Arthritis preceded by fever (periodic spike to 102° F) or at least 2 weeks of fever

One or more of the following signs:

- Evanescent salmon-colored rash
- Lymphadenopathy
- Hepatomegaly
- Splenomegaly
- Serositis

A small subset of children can develop macrophage activation syndrome, a life-threatening complication.

Half of the patients with systemic JIA follow a relapsing–remitting course with good long-term prognosis.

Another half have unremitting course with poor clinical and functional prognosis leading to joint destruction.

Oligoarthritis

Two subtypes

- Persistent (four joints affected)
- Extended (more than four joints after first 6 months)

Early onset before 6 years of age, asymmetric predominately in females, and good outcome. Presence of ANA is a risk factor for the development of iridocyclitis.

Silent uveitis can develop within 4 years of the onset of the disorder.

Polyarthritis

Affects five or more joints

- RF positive: affects adolescent girls, symmetric joint involvement
- RF negative: variable outcome in the subset of ANA-positive patients; development of chronic uveitis is possible

Psoriatic Arthritis

Diagnostic criteria:

- Presence of arthritis and psoriatic rash
- If rash is absent, a positive history of psoriasis in a first-degree relative, dactylitis, and nail pitting

Enthesitis-Related Arthritis

- Affects HLA-B27-positive males after 6 years of age

Enthesitis locations:

- Calcaneal insertion of the Achilles tendon
- Plantar fascia
- Tarsal area
- Hip involvement (common)

The disease may progress to ankylosing spondylitis.

JUVENILE ANKYLOSING SPONDYLITIS

- Not part of JIA subclassification
- Associated with HLA-B27
- Affects adolescent boys
- Oligoarthritis and episodic asymmetric
- Sacroiliac joint involvement
- "Bamboo" spine

Principles of Rehabilitation of Children with JIA

- Prevent joint damage
- Achieve normal growth and development
- Maintain and improve function

Treatment includes resting the joint, splinting in functional position, ROM, modalities, and adaptive equipment.

Ultrasound is *contraindicated* in children with open growth plates.

Special Considerations

Joints

- Cervical spine is more often involved than in adults
- TMJ is commonly affected and can lead to mandibular and facial growth disturbance (polyarticular form)
- Wrist involvement is common and requires splinting, ROM, and modalities
- Shoulder joint involved in polyarticular and psoriatic arthritis
- Hip flexion contractures with internal rotation and adduction unlike adults
- Knee is the most commonly involved joint; quadriceps weakness due to early contracture may not resolve (active quad strengthening is recommended)
- Leg length discrepancy due to bony overgrowth can lead to pelvic asymmetry and scoliosis

Treatment

FIRST LINE

- NSAIDs in initial phase
- Steroid intra-articular joint injections
- Up to 75% of children may achieve remission with NSAIDs and methotrexate

SECOND LINE

- TNF inhibitors (etanercept and adalimumab)
- T-cell blockers (abatacept) for TNF inhibitor nonresponders

RECOMMENDED READING

Alexander MA, Matthews DJ, eds. *Pediatric Rehabilitation: Principles and Practice.* 4th ed. New York, NY: Demos Medical Publishing, LLC;2010.

Davis PJC, Mc Donagh JE. Principles of management of musculoskeletal conditions in children and young people. *Best Pract Res Clin Rheumatol.* 2006;20(2):263-278.

Hofer M. Spondyloarthropathies in children – are they different from those in adults? *Best Pract Res Clin Rheumatol.* 2006;20(2):315-328.

Chapter 6

PAIN MEDICINE

Key Definitions

Pain

An unpleasant sensory and emotional experience associated with actual or potential tissue damage or described in terms of such damage. Pain is always subjective. Many people report pain in the absence of tissue damage or any likely pathophysiologic cause; usually, this happens for psychologic reasons. There is usually no way to distinguish their experience from that due to tissue damage if we take the subjective report (see Table 6-1).

TABLE 6-1 The Implications of Some of the Pain Medicine Definitions[a]

Term	Implication(s)
Allodynia[b]	Lowered threshold: stimulus and response mode differ
Hyperalgesia	Increased response: stimulus and response mode are the same
Hyperpathia	Raised threshold: stimulus and response mode may be increased
	Response: same or different
Hypoalgesia	Raised threshold: stimulus and response mode are the same Lowered response

[a]The essentials of the definitions do not have to be symmetrical and are not symmetrical at present.

[b]Lowered threshold may occur with allodynia but is not required. Also, there is no category for lowered threshold and lowered response (if it ever occurs).

Nociceptor

A receptor preferentially sensitive to a noxious stimulus or to a stimulus that would become noxious if prolonged.

Allodynia

Pain due to a stimulus that does not normally provoke pain.

Dysesthesia

An unpleasant abnormal sensation, whether spontaneous or evoked.

Hyperalgesia

An increased response to a stimulus that is normally painful. For pain evoked by stimuli that usually are not painful, the term *allodynia* is preferred, whereas the term *hyperalgesia* is more appropriately used for cases with an increased response at a normal threshold or at an increased threshold, e.g., in patients with neuropathy.

Hyperesthesia

Increased sensitivity to stimulation.

Hyperpathia

A painful syndrome characterized by an abnormally painful reaction to a stimulus, especially a repetitive stimulus, as well as an increased threshold.

Hypoalgesia

Diminished pain in response to a normally painful stimulus.

Hypoesthesia

Decreased sensitivity to stimulation, excluding the special senses.

Neuralgia

Pain in the distribution of a nerve or nerves.

Neuropathic Pain

Pain initiated or caused by a primary lesion or dysfunction in the nervous system.

Neuropathy

A disturbance of function or pathologic change in a nerve: in one nerve, mononeuropathy; in several nerves, mononeuropathy multiplex; if diffuse and bilateral, polyneuropathy.

Paresthesia

An abnormal sensation, whether spontaneous or evoked.

Complex Regional Pain Syndrome I versus II

CRPS I

- A relatively common disabling disorder
- Unknown pathophysiology
- Underlying mechanisms: changes in the peripheral and central somatosensory, autonomic, and motor processing systems and a pathologic interaction of sympathetic and afferent systems

Clinical Picture of CRPS

- Disproportionate extremity pain
- Swelling
- Autonomic (sympathetic) and motor symptoms

The condition can affect the upper or lower extremities, but it is slightly more common in the upper extremities.

CRPS I (also known as RSD) is the definition given in the setting of known trauma to an area without specific nerve injury. CRPS II (also known as causalgia) is defined by a known injury to a nerve.

Causes may include trauma, underlying neurologic pathology, musculoskeletal disorders, and malignancy.

The characteristics of CRPS I/II according to the IASP are as follows:

- Pain
  - Pain is reported in more than 90% of patients.
  - Most patients describe worsening of pain or other symptoms after exercising the affected limb.
- Edema
  - Vascular abnormalities (often abnormal vasodilation and skin warming in the early phase and vasoconstriction in the later stages) are characteristic symptoms of RSD/CRPS I.
  - Typically, patients with CRPS I exhibit a warm and vasodilated affected extremity in the early stages and cold and pale skin in the later stages.
- Alteration in motor function
  - Although the IASP did not include motor dysfunction within their formal criteria for diagnosing RSD (because it is not universal), they acknowledged that such dysfunction is common. The abnormal motor symptoms that are reported most classically in RSD include the following:
    - Inability to initiate movement
    - Weakness
    - Tremor
    - Muscle spasms
    - Dystonia of the affected limb
  - In one study, weakness was reported in 95% of patients, tremor of the affected limb in 49% of patients, and muscular incoordination in 54% of patients. In chronic RSD, severe spasms were present in 25% of patients.
- Alteration in sensory function – Although the IASP also decided not to include sensory dysfunction within their formal criteria for diagnosing RSD (due to variability), such symptoms, including hypoesthesia, hyperesthesia, and allodynia, may occur.

CRPS is subdivided into the following three phases:

- Acute stage: Usually warm phase of 2 to 3 months
- Dystrophic phase: Vasomotor instability for several months
- Atrophic phase: Usually cold extremity with atrophic changes

Diagnosis/Workup

- No single special investigation has been proven sensitive and specific enough to diagnose CRPS
- Radiographic findings
  - X-ray imaging may show osteoporosis
  - The *triple phase bone scan* has also been useful in diagnosis. According to Kozin et al.,[1] scintigraphic abnormalities were reported in up to 60% of RSD patients and may be useful in arriving at the diagnosis of RSD. The most suggestive and sensitive findings on bone scan include diffuse increased activity in the *delayed (third) phase,* including juxta-articular accentuation
  - Skin thermography: can reveal temperature disparities between limbs

- QSART[2]
- Electrodiagnostic studies: NCV/EMG is usually normal
- Laser Doppler imaging

Treatment/Medications

The mainstay of treatment for CRPS involves early restoration of function. Initiation of PT/OT program with focus on the affected limb. Oral steroids early in course can help quell symptoms.

Sympathetic Blocks – good for diagnostic and therapeutic purposes:
- Stellate ganglion block: good for UEx CRPS;
- Lumbar sympathetic block: good for LEx CRPS.

Sympathectomy – can be performed interventionally (radiofrequency and cryoablation) or surgically.

Dorsal Column Stimulation – can be a tremendous help with UEx/LEx CRPS. Appropriate diagnosis (good response to sympathetic block) and patient screening help to improve outcomes of neuromodulation.

Examination

A comprehensive history and physical examination is fundamental to the diagnosis and treatment of patients with pain. Pain assessments and diagrams help the physician in stratifying a patient's pain, especially the recognition of red flags that warrant emergent treatment (e.g., progressive numbness, weakness, bowel/bladder incontinence, and saddle anesthesia).

Anatomy

As neck and low back pain are often encountered by physiatrists in myriad settings, it is important to understand spinal anatomy when evaluating a patient and forming a differential diagnosis. Cervical and lumbar vertebral bodies are complex structures, with multiple possible pain generators present (Fig. 6-1).

The spinal cord gives off spinal nerves in pairs: 8 cervical, 12 thoracic, 5 lumbar, 5 sacral, and 1 coccygeal. The spinal cord and nerves are surrounded by a sac called the *dura mater*, which contains the CSF.

Knowing and understanding the dermatomal distributions of each nerve root is also important and this aids in obtaining history and during examination and treatment. As will be discussed, different types of spine pathology and radicular irritation/dysfunction can be treated differently. As a rule of thumb, in the cervical spine, a nerve root comes out *above* its corresponding vertebral body, meaning that at C6/7, the C7 nerve root exits. *At C7/T1, the C8 nerve root exits.* The presence of C8 translates to *the thoracic and lumbar nerve roots exiting below their corresponding vertebral body* (Fig. 6-2).

Similarly, the direction of the disc herniation can impact which nerve root is impacted. Posterolateral disk herniations typically spare the root that exits at that level and affect the root exiting at the next level below. The majority of disk herniations are posterolateral, given the additional support provided by the posterior longitudinal ligament (Fig. 6-3). Far lateral disk herniations can affect the nerve root at that level as it exits via the lateral recesses (Fig. 6-4).

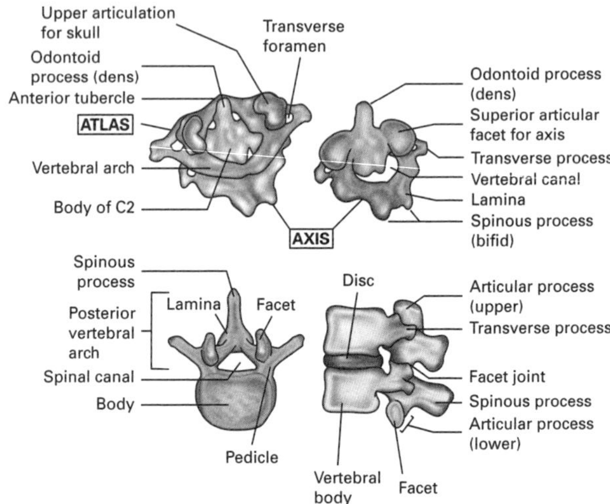

Figure 6-1 Cervical and lumbar vertebral anatomy.

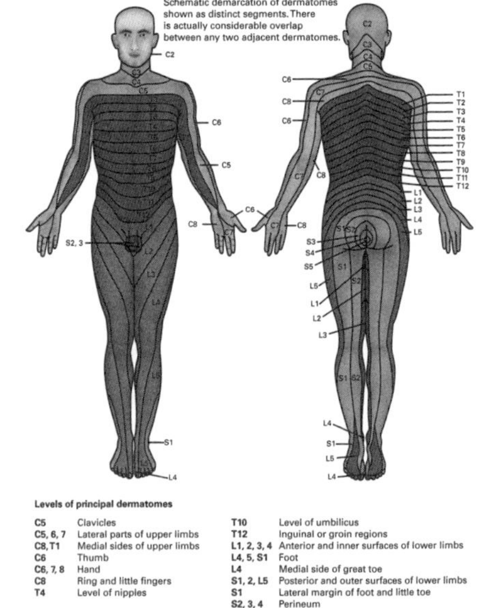

Figure 6-2 Dermatomal distribution of spinal nerve roots.

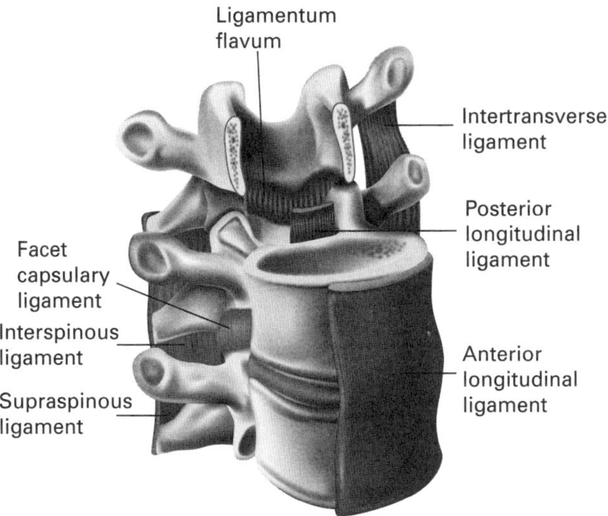

Figure 6-3 Support structures of the lumbar spine.

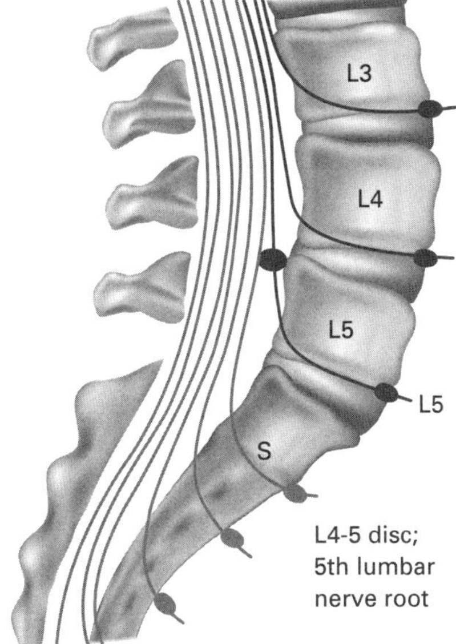

Figure 6-4 Disk herniation in relation to level affected.

Imaging

Imaging of the spine plays a large role in the workup/evaluation of low back pain. X-rays are often the first-line imaging obtained. It is important to know how the normal anatomy appears in x-ray/CT/MRI to better appreciate spinal pathology when present (Fig. 6-5).

X-rays can demonstrate multiple pathologics including

- Spondylytic changes
- Instability (best seen with flexion/extension films)
- Compression fractures
- Intervertebral disk degeneration
- Lytic/blastic lesions
- Pathologic finding in spine diseases (e.g., ankylosing spondylosis)

CT and MRI are usually the next modalities ordered if further radiographic evaluation is warranted (Figs 6-6 and 6-7). Unless contraindicated, MRI is often ordered to evaluate for soft tissue pathology (i.e., disk disease) and to better evaluate bony pathology (e.g., assessing acuity of fracture).

The main MRI types are T1, T2, sagittal STIR, and T1 with fat suppression. Different tissues appear differently on different types, however.

Water and pathology: white on T2, dark on T1
Fat: white on T1 and T2
Bone cortex, stones, and ligaments: dark on every type. Contusions are white

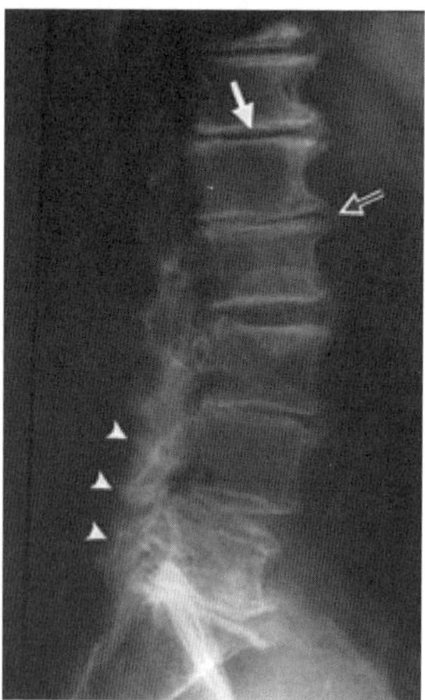

Figure 6-5 X-Ray demonstrating spondylosis and intervertebral disk degeneration.

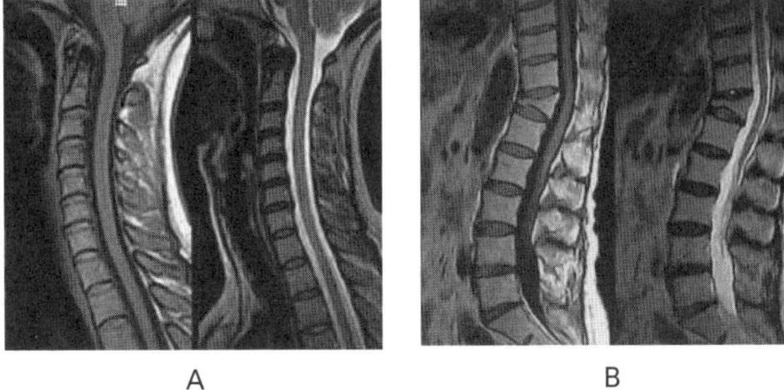

Figure 6-6 T1 (**Left**) versus T2 (**Right**) MRI of cervical spine (**A**) and lumbar spine (**B**).

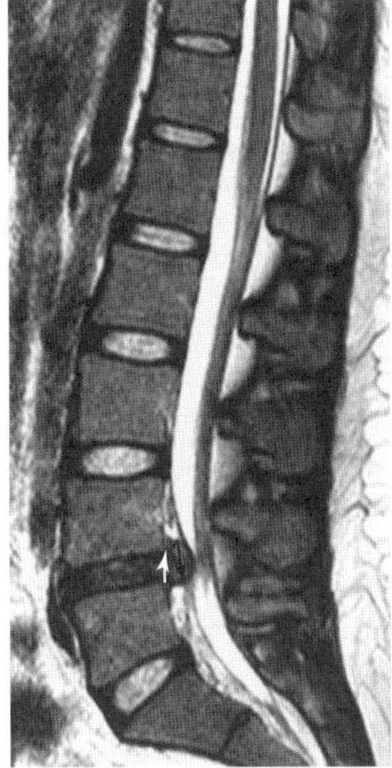

Figure 6-7 T2 MRI demonstrating disk herniation at L4/5.

Neck/Low Back Pain

Among the most common complaints in the physiatrist's office are neck and low back pain. Due to the interplay of multiple musculoskeletal and neurologic structures, many times the pain is multifactorial in origin. Nachemson[3] reported that after approximately 1 month of symptoms, only 15% of patients will have definable disease or injury. *Radiculopathic* (nerve root) pain typically follows a dermatomal/ myotomal distribution and can stem from irritation from disk fragments, bone, and others. In the cervical spine, the most common roots involved are C6 and C7. The most commonly involved levels in the lumbar spine are L5 and S1. Again, a poignant physical exam with tests for root irritation (cervical loading/distraction and straight leg raising) aids in accurate diagnosis.

Spinal Stenosis – Pain typically has a more insidious onset, with the patient complaining of pain that is worse after arising in the morning as well as after ambulating a certain distance. The former is said to be due to the additive compression by engorged epidural veins overnight. The latter is called *neurogenic claudication* (pain worsening when walking down a hill versus up the hill, which is vascular claudication). As in radiculopathic pain, symptoms and findings may have a dermatomal distribution but it tends to be more diffuse. Furthermore, spinal stenosis and degenerative disk disease are not mutually exclusive. More often than not, stenosis results from disk herniation/bulges coupled with spondylytic changes such as facet joint and ligament hypertrophy.

Sacroiliac Joint Pain – The sacrum supports the axial spine and in turn articulates with the iliac wings to form left and right sacroiliac (SI) joints. Myriad ligamentous and muscle attachments contribute to the stability of this joint. Imbalance in the joint can result from repeated lifting and bending, causing a shift on the anteroposterior axis. Repeated forces can cause stress on the myofascial attachments and irritation of the joint lines. The SI joint lines are innervated by L3-S1 root levels and hence may cause radicular-type symptoms when irritated. Common areas of pain in SI joint pathologies include the ipsilateral hip and greater trochanter regions.[4] While evaluating the SI joint as a pain source, one must obtain appropriate history, radiography, and tests for pathologic causes of sacroiliitis (i.e., ankylosing spondylosis). A variety of provocation maneuvers exist (i.e., Faber and Gaenslen tests) to evaluate for SI joint dysfunction.

Treatment

Barring any emergencies, the mainstay of treatment starts with appropriate use of a short period of rest and initiation of PT (i.e., "back school" and McKenzie treatment programs) along with the start of medications including NSAIDs and COX-2 inhibitors. Over the past few years, multiple topical formulations for NSAID delivery have augmented the tools available to the physician. A tapering dose of oral steroid may also be given concomitantly.

Spinal Interventions

Cervical/Lumbar Epidural Nerve Blocks

These injections involve the introduction of local anesthetics, opioids, or steroids that have utility in the management of pain of various etiologies. It is mainly performed in an interlaminar or paramedian approach with a loss-of-resistance technique. This technique involves traversing the supraspinous ligament, interspinous ligament, and then the ligamentum flavum, after which a "sudden loss of resistance" equates entry of the epidural space.

Indications:

- Cervical/lumbar radiculopathy
- Pain from cervical/lumbar spondylosis[5]
- Postlaminectomy syndrome
- Pain from vertebral compression fractures[6]
- Diabetic polyneuropathy
- Phantom limb pain
- Chemotherapy-related neuropathy/plexopathy
- Cancer pain
- Diagnostic neural blockade to aid in differential workup of pain source (i.e., pelvic, back, groin, genital, and lower extremity pain)

Contraindications:

- Local infection
- Patient on anticoagulants
- Coagulopathy
- Sepsis[7]

Complications:

- Dural puncture – reported as 0.5% incidence,[8] may result in CSF loss or introduction of air (pneumocephalus), responsible for significant postprocedure headaches
- Intravenous needle placement given the preponderance of epidural veins/arteries
- Epidural hematoma – usually self-limiting. In setting of anticoagulation, it may cause cord compression, cauda equina syndrome paralysis, apnea, and death
- Infection – high chance of spread given epidural vascularity
- Urinary retention and incontinence[9]
- Direct trauma to spinal cord/nerve roots

Caudal Epidural Nerve Block

Though used relatively infrequently, this injection preceded its lumbar counterpart by nearly 20 years (1901).

Proper technique for the caudal ESI involves the patient positioned in a lateral or prone position. The caudal space is approached through the *sacrococcygeal ligament* that covers the sacral hiatus. The needle is placed over the sacrococcygeal membrane at an angle of about 60° to the coronal plane and perpendicular to the other planes. There is usually a loss of resistance as the membrane is pierced. General indications/contraindications mimic those of the lumbar/cervical approaches where anatomically relevant. There are, however, several key indications where the caudal injection may prevail:

- prior lumbar surgery – can distort anatomy making lumbar approach difficult (i.e., fusion and hardware in place)
- patients on anticoagulation or coagulopathic therapy (since epidural venous plexus usually ends at S4)

Contraindications include infection, sepsis, pilonidal cysts, and congenital anomalies of dural sac and contents.

Complications include dural puncture, needle misplacement, hematoma/ecchymosis, infection, and urinary retention/incontinence.

Facet Joint Injection/Medial Branch Block

The cervical and lumbar facet (zygapophyseal) joints have been considered significant sources of chronic neck and low back pain.[10] The facet joints are diarthrodial, made up of the inferior articular process and the superior articular process of the vertebra one level below. They are also dually innervated, receiving inputs from the medial branch nerves of each level comprising the joint. For example, the L4/5 facet joint is innervated by the medial branches of L4 and L5. Facet blocks are performed by first properly identifying anatomic landmark, which involves oblique images at 10° to 40° from midline for best needle visualization with rotation by another 5° to 10° for joint visualization. Using proper imaging and feel, a mixture of dye, local anesthetic, and steroid is injected.

Indications:

- When making the decision to inject the facet joint or perform a medial branch block, one must identify those with facet syndrome and which levels are symptomatic. Classically, this has been defined by dull, aching pain with tenderness on palpation over the facet joints with occasional overlying muscle spasm. Pain may be unilateral or bilateral with occasional radiation. Definitive diagnosis can be made with pain relief coming from the injection of local anesthetic into the facet joint.

Contraindications:

- Like other injections, these should be avoided in those with medication allergies, systemic or local infection, or coagulopathies.

Complications:

- The most common complication is a transient increase in pain. Other complications include dural penetration, spinal anesthesia, capsule rupture, infection, and vertebral artery puncture (cervical facets).

Selective Nerve Root Blocks (SNRBs)/Transforaminal ESI

Nerve root blocks/transforaminal steroid injections are a useful tool in the workup for back pain, but they are used in a patient subset that differs from that in which facet joint blocks are used. Nerve root blocks attempt to anesthetize the desired nerve for diagnostic and therapeutic purposes. Steroids are used in an attempt to provide long-term relief, primarily in patients with radiculopathy. They can be utilized when physical exam and radiologic findings pinpoint a specific nerve root as cause for pain. Pressure on the nerve may result in an autoimmune response that can elicit pain. Because the venous drainage lies on the outside of the nerve, pressure on the nerve increases the venous pressure. The extrinsic forces on the nerve can lead to resultant ischemia and pain within the nerve root, with pain also being referred down the particular dermatome. Similar to the other injections, the SNRB involves placing a mixture of local anesthetic and steroid in the superior region of the neural foramen where the postganglionic nerve root exits.

Indications:

- After discectomy in patients who have recurrent radiculopathy but no recurrent disk herniation, symptoms are often caused when scar tissue tethers the nerve. Many patients can be treated successfully by using SNRBs.
- In patients with disk herniations, nerve root blocks are helpful. Since the body naturally resolves 90% of disk herniations when given enough time, early pain relief is important to try to avoid surgery. The pain is believed to result from an inflammation of the nerve root more than from direct compression. As a result, potent antiinflammatories (steroid) work well in quelling the process.
  - The injections are also efficacious when facet joint hypertrophy or cysts cause an irritation of the nerve root, though not so much as with discogenic disease.

Contraindications:

- Include a history of allergy to local anesthetics or steroids, systemic or overlying infection, coagulopathy, or, in the case of facet joint injections, severe foraminal stenosis (which can become worse if an injection is made into the joint itself). Severe foraminal stenosis is a relative contraindication to intra-articular facet joint injections. Injections into the facet joints can cause joint swelling, worsening a preexisting foraminal stenosis.

Complications:

- Rare, but can include bleeding, infection, and allergic reactions.
- Intravascular injection may be harmless, but it results in a suboptimal or false-negative result. Furthermore, intravascular injection can be dangerous if the agent is injected into the vertebral artery or radicular branches that enter the neural foramina at various levels.
- Spinal cord infarcts have occurred from both cervical and lumbar SNRBs.
- Direct trauma to the nerve root can occur via the spinal needle, causing increased pain and occasional root avulsion.
- Spinal anesthesia may occur if local anesthetic is inadvertently injected into the nerve root sleeve.
- During cervical procedures, doing so can lead to respiratory arrest. Some patients experience adverse effects from the steroids.
- Consider the total steroid dose when performing injections at multiple levels.

Sacroiliac Joint Injection

- Indicated for sacroiliitis or chronic sacroiliac joint arthropathy. Serves both diagnostic and therapeutic purposes. Under fluoroscopic guidance, the joint space is visualized. A spinal needle is then introduced at the junction of the posterior one-third of the joint line with the middle one-third of the joint. The posterior iliac spine obstructs the superior portion of the joint, making the lower portion of the joint easier to inject. Once the joint space is entered, a small amount of contrast is injected to confirm needle placement. Once the arthrogram is satisfactory, the medication, which is usually a mixture of anesthetic and steroid, is injected.

Other Procedures

RADIOFREQUENCY ABLATION

Involves using a needle (electrode) to deliver a current in either a constant (hot) or a pulsatile (cold) fashion to cause neurolysis of the nerves in the vicinity of the lesion created by the electrode. General indications include failed conservative treatments, transient relief from repeated medial branch blocks, or no indication for surgical intervention. Again, contraindications include coagulopathy, platelet dysfunction, and severe cardiopulmonary disease for procedures involving cervical and thoracic regions.[11] Complications include local postprocedure soreness, sensorimotor deficits from improper needle placement, vascular trauma (cervical region), pneumothorax (thoracic), entry into subarachnoid space via neural foramen (dorsal root ganglion RF), diaphragmatic paralysis and hoarseness (from cervical sympathectomy RF), puncture of abdominal viscera (lumbar sympathectomy RF), or direct disk, cord, and nerve root trauma.

VERTEBROPLASTY/KYPHOPLASTY

A minimally invasive procedure aimed at treating the pain and spinal instability surrounding acute vertebral compression fractures from the age of 2 weeks to 1 year. Anecdotally, many practitioners use a 6 month age limit for compression fractures. Further indications for vertebroplasty include refractory pain from the fracture. Absolute contraindications include diskitis, sepsis, and osteomyelitis. Relative contraindications include significant spinal canal compromise secondary to bone fragments, fractures older than 2 years, >75% collapse of vertebral body, fractures above T5, and traumatic compression fractures or disruption of posterior vertebral body wall. Vertebroplasty focuses on treating pain, while kyphoplasty focuses on restoring stability and vertebral height. Vertebroplasty involves tunneling a large gauge needle into the vertebral body and injecting 3 to 5 mL of methylmethacrylate cement into the vertebral body. Similarly, in kyphoplasty, two balloons are introduced via catheter into the vertebral body. The inflated balloon restores height and then allows for filling with the cement.

Spinal Cord Stimulators – Stimulate dorsal column of the spinal cord to treat patients with chronic intractable pain. Though the exact mechanism is unknown, several theories exist including the "gate" theory and direct inhibition of pain pathways in the spinothalamic tract. The SCS can either be totally implantable or have an external transmitter. SCS placement first involves a trial stage where the lead is placed and managed externally. The latter is internalized pending satisfactory results. Indications for SCS include failed neck/back surgery, peripheral neuropathy, postherpetic neuralgia, CRPS I/II, epidural fibrosis/arachnoiditis causing chronic pain, radiculopathy, phantom limb pain,[12] and ischemic pain from peripheral vascular disease.

Most patients have had chronic pain for greater than 12 months that is refractive to other conservative therapies. Contraindications include coagulopathy, platelet dysfunction, local or systemic infection, and patients with psychological issues (i.e., drug seeking). The most common complications are scar formation, lead migration, and infection.

Neuromodulation has more recently begun to be used for peripheral stimulation in subcutaneous tissue with promising results. It has been used successfully for occipital neuralgia[13] and recalcitrant trigeminal neuralgia,[14] among others.

INTRATHECAL PUMPS

Intrathecal pumps have a place in the management of chronic pain as well as spasticity. A catheter is inserted intrathecally and connected to a pump. Initially, during the trial, the pump is external. If a satisfactory result is achieved, a permanent catheter is placed intrathecally and is tunneled through the subcutaneous tissue to an internal pump that usually sits in a pocket in the anterior abdomen. The pump can then be adjusted to deliver different amounts of medication. Intrathecal infusion bypasses the blood–brain barrier and hence allows a more directed effect on brain and spinal neuroreceptors with less medication. Several medications are used in these pumps, with the two most common ones being preservative-free morphine and baclofen for spasticity management.

REFERENCES

1. Kozin F, Soin JS, Ryan LM, et al. Bone scintigraphy in the reflex sympathetic dystrophy syndrome. *Radiology.* 1981;138(2):437-444.
2. Chelimsky TC, Low PA, Naessens JM, et al. Value of autonomic testing in reflex sympathetic dystrophy. *Mayo Clin Proc.* 1995;70(11):1029-1040.
3. Nachemson A, ed. *Neck and Back Pain: The Scientific Evidence of Causes, Diagnosis, and Treatment.* Philadelphia, PA: Lippincott Williams & Wilkins; 2000.
4. Fortin JD, Aprill CN, Ponthieux B, et al. Sacroiliac joint: pain referral maps upon applying a new injection/arthrography technique. Part I. *Spine.* 1994;19:1475-1482.
5. Pages E. Anestesia metamerica. *Rev Sanid Mil Madr.* 1921;11:351-385.
6. Bromage PR. Identification of the epidural space. In: Bromage PR, ed. *Epidural Analgesia.* Philadelphia, PA: WB Saunders; 1978:178.
7. Cousins MJ, Bromage PR. Epidural neural blockade. In: Cousins MJ, Bridenbaugh DO, eds. *Neural Blockade.* Philadelphia, PA: JB Lippincott; 1988:340-341.
8. Bromage PR. Complications and contraindications. In: Bromage PR, ed. *Epidural Analgesia.* Philadelphia, PA: WB Saunders; 1978:654-711.
9. Armitage EN. Lumbar and thoracic epidural. In: Wildsmith JAW, Armitage EN, eds. *Principles and Practice of Regional Anesthesia.* New York, NY: Churchill Livingstone; 1987:109.
10. Bogduk N, Aprill C. On the nature of neck pain, discography, and cervical zygapophyseal joint blocks. *Pain.* 1993;54:213-217.
11. Falco FJE, Kim D, Zhu J, et al. Interventional pain management procedures. In: Braddom R, ed. *Physical Medicine and Rehabilitation.* 3rd ed. Philadelphia, PA: WB Saunders; 2006:chap 26.

12. Carter ML. Spinal cord stimulation in chronic pain: a review of the evidence. *Anaesth Intensive Care.* 2004;32:11-21.
13. Weiner RL, Reed KL. Peripheral neurostimulation for control of intractable occipital neuralgia. *Neuromodulation.* 1999;2:217-221.
14. Slavin KV, Burchiel KJ. Peripheral nerve stimulation for painful nerve injuries. *Contemp Neurosurg.* 1999;21(19):1-6.

RECOMMENDED READING

Blaes F, Tschernatsch M, Braeu ME, et al. Autoimmunity in complex-regional pain syndrome. *Ann N Y Acad Sci.* 2007;1107:168-173.

Cathelin MF. Une nouvelle voie d'injection rachidenne. Methode des injection epidurales par le procede du canal sacre. *C R Soc Biol Paris.* 1901;53:452.

Coffey RJ, Burchiel K. Inflammatory mass lesions associated with intrathecal drug infusion catheters: report and observations on 41 patients. *Neurosurgery.* 2002;50:78-86.

Gray D, Zahid B, Warfield C. Facet block and neurolysis. In: Waldman S, ed. *Interventional Pain Management.* Philadelphia, PA: WB Saunders; 2001:446-479.

Katz J. Caudal approach – single injection technique. In: Katz J, ed. *Atlas of Regional Anesthesia.* Norwalk, CT: Appleton & Lange; 1994:129.

Kurvers HA, Jacobs MJ, Beuk RJ, et al. The spinal component to skin blood flow abnormalities in reflex sympathetic dystrophy. *Arch Neurol.* 1996;53(1):58-65.

Maleki J, LeBel AA, Bennett GJ, et al. Patterns of spread in complex regional pain syndrome, type I (reflex sympathetic dystrophy). *Pain.* 2000;88(3):259-266.

Paice E. Reflex sympathetic dystrophy. *BMJ.* 1995;310(6995):1645-1648.

Reeves KD. Technique of prolotherapy. In: Lennard TA, ed. *Physiatric Procedures in Clinical Practice.* Philadelphia, PA: Hanley and Belfus; 1995:57-70.

Simon S. Sacroiliac joint injection and low back pain. In: Waldman S, ed. *Interventional Pain Management.* Philadelphia, PA: WB Saunders; 2001:535-539.

Singh V, Piryani C, Liao K, et al. Percutaneous disc decompression, using coblation, in the treatment of discogenic pain. *Pain Physician.* 2002;5:250-259.

Solonen KA. The sacroiliac joint in the light of anatomical, roentological, and clinical studies. *Acta Orthop Scand.* 1957;27(suppl):27.

Uceyler N, Eberle T, Rolke R, et al. Differential expression patterns of cytokines in complex regional pain syndrome. *Pain.* 2007;132:195-205.

Veldman PH, Reynen HM, Arntz IE, et al. Signs and symptoms of reflex sympathetic dystrophy: prospective study of 829 patients. *Lancet.* 1993;342(8878):1012-1016.

Wagner AL. Paraspinal injections: facet joint and nerve root blocks. http://www.emedicine.com/Radio/topic884.htm. Accessed October 7, 2005.

Waldman S. Lumbar epidural nerve block. In: Waldman S, ed. *Interventional Pain Management.* Philadelphia, PA: WB Saunders; 2001:415-422.

Wasner G, Heckmann K, Maier C, et al. Vascular abnormalities in acute reflex sympathetic dystrophy (CRPS I): complete inhibition of sympathetic nerve activity with recovery. *Arch Neurol.* 1999;56(5):613-620.

Chapter 7

MUSCULOSKELETAL/SPORTS/ ORTHOPEDICS

Limb Joint Primary Movers

Motion (ROM in degrees)	Muscles	Nerves	Roots
Shoulder flexion (180)	Anterior deltoid Coracobrachialis	Axillary Musculocutaneous	C5, C6 C6, C7
Shoulder extension (45)	Latissimus dorsi Teres major Posterior deltoid	Thoracodorsal Inferior subscapular Axillary	C6, C7, C8 C5, C6, C7 C5, C6
Shoulder abduction (180)	Middle deltoid Supraspinatus	Axillary Suprascapular	C5, C6 C5, C6
Shoulder adduction (40)	Pectoralis major Latissimus dorsi	Med + lat pectoral Thoracodorsal	C5-T1 C6, C7, C8
Shoulder external rotation (90[a])	Infraspinatus Teres minor	Suprascapular Axillary	C5, C6 C5, C6
Shoulder internal rotation (80[a])	Subscapularis Pectoralis major Latissimus dorsi Teres major	Sup + inf subscapular Med + lat pectoral Thoracodorsal Inferior subscapular	C5, C6 C5-T1 C6, C7, C8 C5, C6, C7
Shoulder shrug	Trapezius Levator scapulae	Spinal accessory (CN XI) C3, C4 ± dorsal scapular (C5)	
Elbow flexion (150)	Biceps brachii Brachialis Brachioradialis	Musculocutaneous Musculocutaneous Radial	C5, C6 C5, C6 C5, C6
Elbow extension	Triceps brachii	Radial	C6, C7, C8
Forearm supination (80)	Supinator Biceps brachii	Posterior interosseous Musculocutaneous	C5, C6, C7 C5, C6
Forearm pronation (80)	Pronator teres Pronator quadratus	Median Anterior interosseous	C6, C7 C8, T1

(Continued)

(Continued)

Motion (ROM in degrees)	Muscles	Nerves	Roots
Wrist flexion (80)	Flexor carpi radialis Flexor carpi ulnaris	Median Ulnar	C6, C7, C8 C7, C8, T1
Wrist extension (70)	Ext carpi rad longus Ext carpi rad brevis Ext carpi ulnaris	Radial Radial Posterior interosseous	C6, C7 C6, C7 C7, C8
MCP flexion (90)	Lumbricals Dors + palm interossei	Median, ulnar Ulnar	C8, T1 C8, T1
PIP flexion (100)	Flexor digitorum sup Flexor digitorum prof	Median Median, ulnar	C7-T1 C7, C8, T1
DIP flexion (90)	Flexor digitorum prof	Median, ulnar	C7, C8, T1
MCP, finger extension	Extensor digitorum Extensor indicis Extensor digiti min	Posterior interosseous Posterior interosseous Posterior interosseous	C7, C8 C7, C8 C7, C8
Finger abduction (20)	Dorsal interossei Abductor digiti min	Ulnar Ulnar	C8, T1 C8, T1
Finger adduction	Palmar interossei	Ulnar	C8, T1
Thumb flexion	Flexor pollicis brevis Flexor pollicis longus	Median, ulnar Anterior interosseus	C8, T1 C7, C8, T1
Thumb extension	EPB Extensor pollicis longus	Posterior interosseous Posterior interosseous	C7, C8 C7, C8
Thumb abduction	Abd pollicis longus Abd pollicis brevis	Posterior interosseous Median	C7, C8 C8, T1
Thumb adduction	Adductor pollicis	Ulnar	C8, T1
Hip flexion (120)	Iliopsoas	Femoral	L2, L3, L4
Hip extension (30)	Gluteus maximus	Inferior gluteal	L5, S1, S2
Hip abduction (40)	Gluteus medius Gluteus minimus	Superior gluteal Superior gluteal	L4, L5, S1 L4, L5, S1

Hip adduction (20)	Adductor longus Adductor magnus	Obturator Obturator, sciatic	L2, L3, L4 L2, L3, L4, L5, S1
Hip external rotation (45)	Obturator int + ext Quadratus femoris Piriformis Sup + inf gemelli Glut max (postfibers)	n. obt int, obturator n. quadratus femoris n. piriformis n. obt int, n. quad fem Inferior gluteal	L3-S2 L2, L3, L4 S1, S2 L4-S2 L5, S1, S2
Hip internal rotation (45)	Gluteus minimus Gluteus medius Tensor fasciae latae	Superior gluteal Superior gluteal Superior gluteal	L4, L5, S1 L4, L5, S1 L4, L5, S1
Knee flexion (135)	Semitendinosus Semimembranosus Biceps femoris	Tibial div. of sciatic Tibial div. of sciatic Tib + per div. sciatic	L5, S1, S2 L4, L5-S2 L5, S1, S2
Knee extension	Quadriceps femoris	Femoral	L2, L3, L4
Ankle dorsiflexion (20)	Tibialis anterior	Deep peroneal	L4, L5, S1
Ankle plantarflexion (45)	Gastrocnemius Soleus	Tibial Tibial	L5, S1, S2 L5, S1, S2
Ankle inversion (35)	Tibialis posterior	Tibial	L4, L5, S1
Ankle eversion (25)	Peroneus longus Peroneus brevis	Superficial peroneal Superficial peroneal	L4, L5, S1 L4, L5, S1
Toe extension	Extensor hallucis longus Extensor digitorum brevis	Deep peroneal Deep peroneal	L4, L5, S1 L5, S1

[a]Shoulder IR/ER varies with elevation of the arm.

CN, cranial nerve; IR, internal rotation; PIP, proximal interphalangeal.

For ROM, 0° is anatomic position. Please note that there is no absolute consensus regarding which muscles are the primary movers of joints or for the root innervations of muscles.

Treatment of Selected MSK Conditions

Upper Limb

AC Sprains/Tears – AC injuries may be seen with falls on the adducted shoulder. A type I (Rockwood classification) injury is a nondisplaced sprain of the AC ligament, manifested by local tenderness w/o anatomic deformity. A type II injury (see Fig. 7-1) involves an AC tear and CC ligament sprain, but the CC interspace is intact. Treatment for type I or II injuries includes an arm sling, ice, analgesics, and progressive ROM exercises. An unstable type II injury may require arm sling use for 2 to 4 weeks. Sports activities can be resumed when full painless ROM is achieved and deltoid strength is near-baseline. Type III to VI lesions involve rupture of the AC *and* CC ligaments with varying displacements of the clavicle. These require orthopedic consultation for potential ORIF, although many separations may be followed conservatively with several weeks of sling-and-swathe immobilization, followed by long-term therapy.

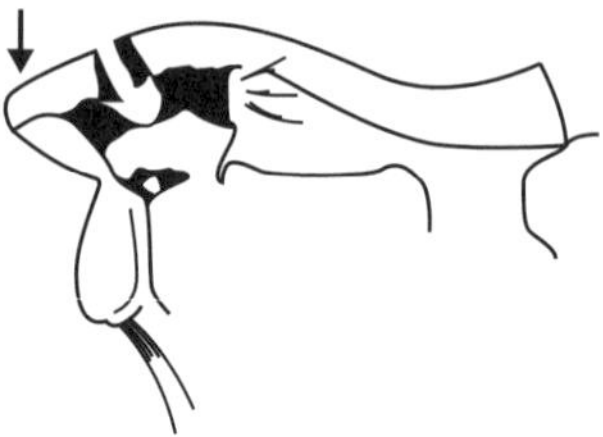

Figure 7-1 Type II injury.

Adapted from Rockwood CA, ed. *Rockwood & Green's Fractures in Adults.* 3rd ed. Philadelphia, PA: JB Lippincott; 1988.

ACJ OA – OA is a very common cause of ACJ pain, especially in the elderly. The presence of ACJ tenderness and pain with cross body abduction suggests ACJ OA. Radiologic studies such as x-rays and US evaluation can help confirm the diagnosis. Treatment includes topical or oral analgesics, PT, injections, and surgery if refractory to conservative care. Traditional injection techniques have proven to be inaccurate; therefore, fluoroscopic or US-guided injections are preferred.[1]

ACJ OA (Rotator Cuff Tendinitis/Shoulder Impingement Syndrome) – Predisposing and causative factors include acromion shape and repetitive overhead activities (i.e., throwing, racquet sports, and swimming). Pain and aches are often worse at night and can be aggravated by overhead activities. Shoulder flexion and abduction may be limited.

A *painful arc* (Fig. 7-2) may be present at about 70° to 110° on passive arm abduction. *Neer's test* (Fig. 7-3) and *Hawkins test* evaluate for shoulder impingement. In Neer's test, the examiner fixes the scapula with one hand and elevates the subject's arm with the other hand. Pain indicates a positive test. Hawkins test is performed by abducting the subject's arm to 90° with the elbow flexed, then internally rotating the shoulder. Hawkins test can also be performed in the

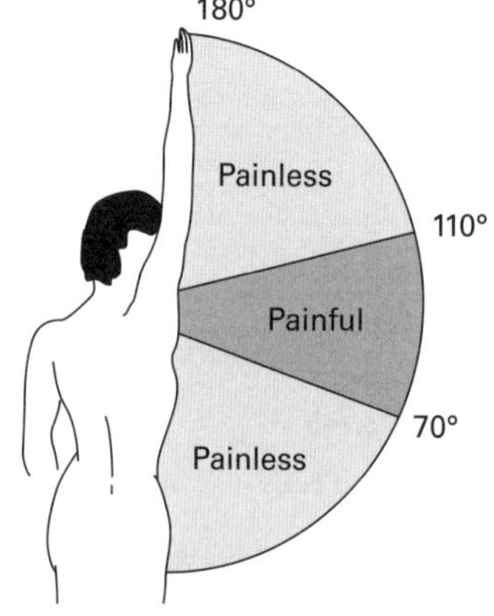

Figure 7-2 Painful arc.

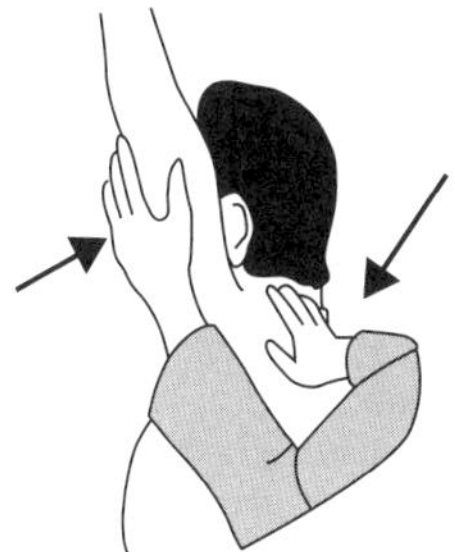

Figure 7-3 Neer's test.

scapular plane. In the *drop arm test,* the arm is passively elevated to 90° in abduction and the patient is asked to hold the arm in position and then slowly lower the arm to the side. The inability to slowly lower the arm or having severe pain when attempting to do so may be indicative of a severe or complete tear of the rotator cuff pathology.

The painful shoulder should initially be *rested* until pain and swelling subside. *Ice* and *NSAIDs* may be helpful. Overhead activities should be avoided. *PT* can institute gentle stretching to preserve ROM and isometric strengthening. A *steroid injection* into the subacromial space may relieve pain and improve motion if the above measures fail. A repeat injection should be avoided in patients with <2 months of pain relief following the first injection. Unless your clinical diagnosis is unchanged, repeat subacromial injection with US guidance to ensure accurate medication placement may be considered for additional diagnostic and therapeutic purposes.[2,3] Exercises should progress until strength and ROM are restored. *Surgery* is an option if several months of conservative treatment/steroid injections fail to resolve the symptoms (or for complete tears). An acromioplasty, the most common procedure, involves acromial shaving to increase the space around the inflamed tendon. The tendon may also be debrided. Several months may be required to regain full strength after surgery.

Anterior Shoulder Dislocation – Anterior dislocations are more common than posterior dislocations. Complications include axillary nerve injury, recurrent dislocations, and rotator cuff tears (especially in older patients). A *Bankart lesion* (Fig. 7-4) is an avulsion of the anteroinferior glenoid labrum and capsule from the glenoid rim and is felt to be a primary etiologic factor in recurrent dislocations. A *Hill-Sachs lesion* is a compression fracture of the humeral head when the posterolateral aspect of the humeral head compresses against the anterior glenoid rim. Age at initial dislocation is prognostic for recurrence: teens/young adults have significantly higher redislocation rates (said to approach 90%) than older patients (said to be ≈10% to 15% for patients >40 years of age).

Various techniques exist for acute reduction, including the modified *Stimson technique,* where the patient lies prone with a wrist weight (i.e., 5 to 10 lbs) on the affected arm as it hangs over the side of the table. Reduction is achieved over 15 to 20 minutes as the shoulder muscles relax.

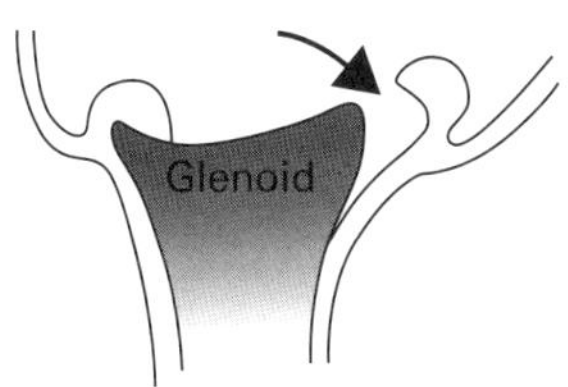

Figure 7-4 Bankart lesion.

A newer technique termed FARES has been published and appears to be superior to the Hippocratic and Kocher methods, but was not compared with the

Stimson technique. This method is performed with the patient supine and longitudinal traction is applied as the shoulder is slowly abducted.[4] Neurovascular status should be checked before and after attempted relocation.

There is no strong evidence to show that immobilization or the duration of immobilization has an effect on the outcome. One option includes bracing in ER, which may reduce the rate of recurrence, though this should be initiated 24 to 48 hours following injury. Early rehabilitation may include icing and sling immobilization for 1 to 3 weeks to allow healing of the capsule. Maintenance of elbow, wrist, and hand ROM is important. Isometric exercises and gentle pendular exercises with the arm in the sling are encouraged, but passive abduction for hygiene is limited to 45° and ER is avoided. The duration of sling use may be shortened in older patients due to the higher risk of frozen shoulder. Once the capsule has healed, shoulder ROM and strengthening are progressed. There is some debate regarding the optimal type and timing of surgery after shoulder dislocation and in shoulder instability.

Adhesive Capsulitis – A syndrome characterized by a progressive painful loss of passive and active glenohumeral ROM that occurs more commonly in females between the ages of 40 and 60 years. Abduction and ER are most affected; internal rotation (IR) is least affected. This condition may be the end result of other conditions that result in prolonged immobility (i.e., bursitis and rotator cuff tendinitis) and has also been associated with other medical conditions (i.e., DM, thyroid dysfunction, and autoimmune diseases). Treatment can consist of an aggressive ROM program, with NSAIDs and heat modalities to improve tolerance. Other techniques include intra-articular steroid injections, brisement (hydrodilation of the capsule), manipulation under anesthesia, and suprascapular nerve blocks. Of these additional options, intra-articular steroid injection has been well studied and appears to improve short-term outcomes. Recovery may take several months to beyond a year.[5]

Bicipital Tendinitis – This overuse injury can be associated with overhead activities or sports and often coexists with the shoulder impingement syndrome, rotator cuff tears, or labral pathology (i.e., SLAP lesions). Examination often reveals a tender bicipital groove. While palpating this structure, assess for instability/subluxation of the bicipital tendon by internally and externally rotating the shoulder. If unstable, the tendon may sublux medially over the lesser tuberosity and a clunk or snap may be appreciated. *Speed's test* (Fig. 7-5) is performed by elevating the subject's arm to 90° with the elbow extended and palm upward, then having the patient attempt forward flexion of the arm against resistance. Pain in the bicipital groove is indicative of a positive test. Treatment includes NSAIDs, activity modification, and progressive exercise

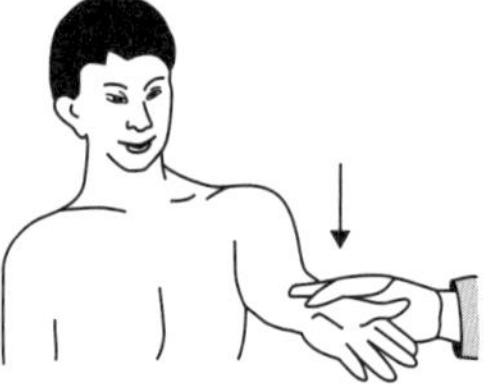

Figure 7-5 Speed's test.

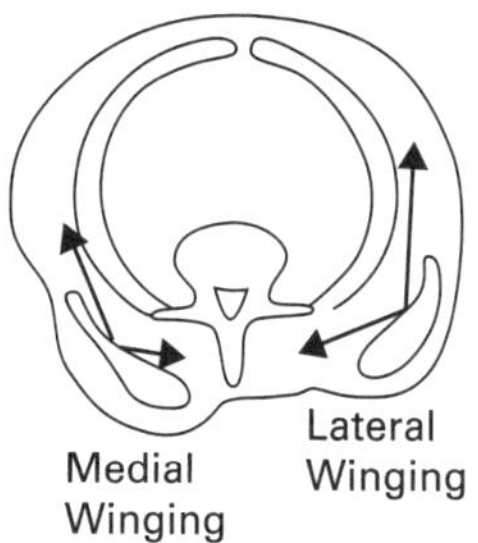

Figure 7-6 Scapular winging.

program, which may include the use of modalities such as heat and postactivity icing. Local corticosteroid injection may be used in refractory cases and US guidance may help increase your accuracy of performing injections into the tendon sheath.[6]

Scapular Winging – Medial scapular winging (Fig. 7-6) is caused by weakness of the serratus anterior (long thoracic nerve). It is elicited by having the patient push against a wall and using resisted forward flexion or resisted scapular protraction.

Lateral winging is caused by weakness of the trapezius muscle (CN XI) and is elicited by shoulder abduction.

Golfer's Elbow (medial epicondylitis) – An overuse syndrome of the tendinous origin of the flexor-pronator mass and medial collateral ligament of the elbow. The initial treatment is *RICE* and *NSAIDs*. Stretching the elbow during the painful period is important. Once pain and inflammation subside, strengthening exercises are started (important groups include the wrist flexors/extensors, wrist radial deviators, forearm pronator/supinators, and elbow flexor/extensors). *Injection of local steroids* into the area of max tenderness can also be considered, with care taken not to injure the ulnar nerve. A *tennis elbow counterforce strap* may be helpful.

Tennis Elbow (lateral epicondylitis) – An extensor tendinopathy, especially of the *ECRB*. The initial treatment is *relative rest, NSAIDs,* and *heat* or *cold* modalities. Wrist extensor *stretching* and *strengthening* should be initiated when tolerated. Conservative measures are usually effective, but recurrences are common. A tennis elbow strap worn circumferentially around the forearm just distal to the elbow may be helpful and a wrist splint may be considered to rest the common wrist extensor tendons. Modifications to the racquet include a *larger racquet grip and head* and *lesser string tension.* A *corticosteroid injection* into the area of max tenderness may be indicated if conservative treatment fails. Treatment with PRP or autologous whole blood has been shown to be more effective than corticosteroids in those patients who have failed conservative treatment.[7,8] No more than three injections should be given at intervals of 5 days to 1 week. Surgical fasciotomy or fixation of the conjoined tendon may be considered if the above measures fail.

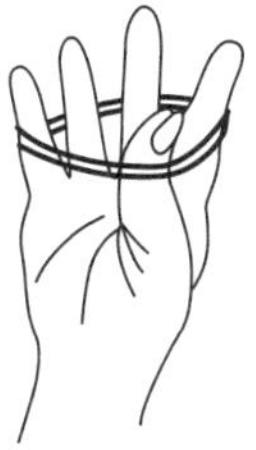

Figure 7-7 Strengthening.

De Quervain's Disease – A tenosynovitis of the first dorsal compartment of the hand, including the APL and EPB tendons. *Finkelstein's test* is positive when pain is elicited in the radial wrist while the wrist is forced into ulnar deviation with the thumb enclosed in a fist. Treatment includes *activity modification* and *NSAIDs* followed by a *stretching* and *strengthening* program (Fig. 7-7). A *thumb spica splint* with the wrist in neutral position and the first MCP immobilized (IP joint is free) is helpful in resting the tendons. *Local* *corticosteroid injections* (maximum of three) into the compartment reduce acute pain and inflammation. US-guided injections have been described and may improve accuracy while decreasing the risk of intratendinous injections.[9] *Surgical decompression* may be curative in severe, refractory cases.

Scaphoid Fracture (most common carpal bone fracture) – Often due to a fall on an outstretched hand. Snuffbox tenderness may be noted. If initial plain films (approximately three to four views) are negative, the wrist should be immobilized (short arm cast or splint with thumb spica) and films repeated in ≈2 weeks (some fractures may not be visible until bone has resorbed around the fracture line). If repeat films are negative and clinical suspicion persists, CT or MRI can be considered.

Because the main blood supply (Fig. 7-8) enters from the distal pole, there is a high incidence of nonunion and AVN in waist and proximal pole fractures. For nondisplaced fractures, a *long arm thumb spica cast* should be used. Isometric muscle contractions can be performed in the cast to counter atrophy. Displaced fractures or nondisplaced fractures with persistent nonunion should be referred for surgical evaluation.

Trigger Finger (digital stenosing tenosynovitis) – Digital tendon sheath inflammation may result in a tendinous knot that gets stuck in the finger pulley system as the finger extends. Patients with DM or rheumatoid arthritis are particularly at risk for developing trigger finger. *NSAIDs* and *steroid injections* help to reduce inflammation and pain. Use of a *volar static hand splint* that immobilizes the MCP but allows full IP flexion rests the flexor tendons and helps break the vicious cycle of inflammation and catching. In some cases, surgery may be necessary to release tendons in fingers that are locked in flexion.

Lower Limb

Greater Trochanteric Pain Syndrome – Classically described as trochanteric bursitis, but improved visualization of the hip via MRI and arthroscopy has proven that other etiologies of lateral hip pain exist (such as gluteus medius or minimus tendinosis or tears and snapping hip syndrome).[10] Pain is noted with walking, running, climbing stairs, sitting, and especially when side-lying on the involved hip. Physical examination often reveals point tenderness over greater trochanter and pain-limited hip abductor strength, and lateral hip pain with Patrick-FAbERE test is noted. Conservative treatment includes *NSAIDs*, an iliotibial band *stretching* program, and hip abductor/extensor strengthening. If refractory to these measures, a *steroid injection* into the bursa (Fig. 7-9) can relieve symptoms in many patients. Various

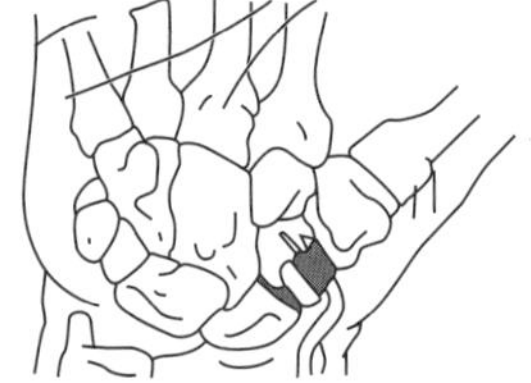

Figure 7-8 Blood supply of the scaphoid.

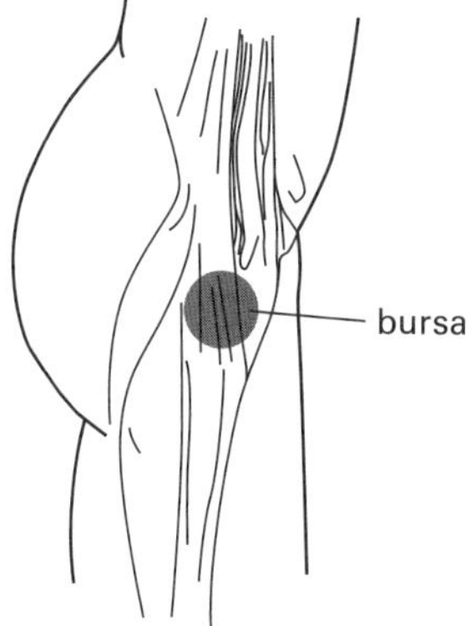

Figure 7-9 Bursa.

etiologies may be responsible for greater trochanteric region pain; therefore, MSK US may become a valuable tool for both diagnostic and therapeutic reasons.[11,12]

Iliotibial Band Syndrome – Potential causes include overtraining or running on uneven surfaces. Lateral knee pain is noted as the ITB slides over the lateral femoral condyle, especially between 20° and 30° of flexion. Predisposing factors include genu varum, tibial varum, varus hindfoot, and foot pronation. Tenderness over the lateral knee and Gerdy's tubercle may be noted on examination. *Ober's test* may be positive. Rehabilitation should be aimed at *stretching* the ITB, hip flexors, and gluteus maximus. Adductors may be strengthened to counteract the tight ITB, and hip abductor strengthening may also be performed to improve dynamic hip stability (Fig. 7-10). Helpful *modalities* include ice, US, and phonophoresis. Foot pronation should be corrected; running only on even surfaces may help. A *steroid injection* into the area of the lateral femoral condyle may relieve pain. Symptoms can generally take 2 to 6 months to improve.

Figure 7-11 illustrates the Ober test for ITB/TFL contraction. The patient lies on the side with the involved side uppermost. The hip is flexed and then abducted as far as possible while stabilizing the pelvis. Next, the hip is brought into extension and the limb is released. The limb will remain abducted if there is tightness at the ITB or TFL.

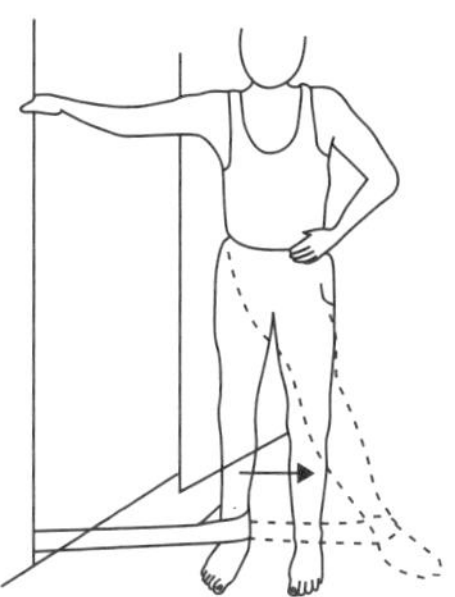

Figure 7-10 Hip adduction strengthening with TheraBand.

Pes Anserine Bursitis (bursa under *S*artorius, *G*racilis, semi*T*endinosis; mnemonic: "*S*ay *G*race before *T*ea") – Pain and tenderness at the insertion of the medial hamstrings at the medial proximal tibia may be noted. The treatment should emphasize *stretching* of the medial hamstrings and improving knee biomechanics. Athletes may wear *protective knee padding*. *Steroid injections* may be very effective, but US guidance should be considered since unguided injections rarely infiltrate the pes anserine bursa.[13]

Anterior Cruciate Ligament – The ACL proceeds superiorly and posteriorly from its anterior medial tibial attachment to attach to the medial aspect of the lateral

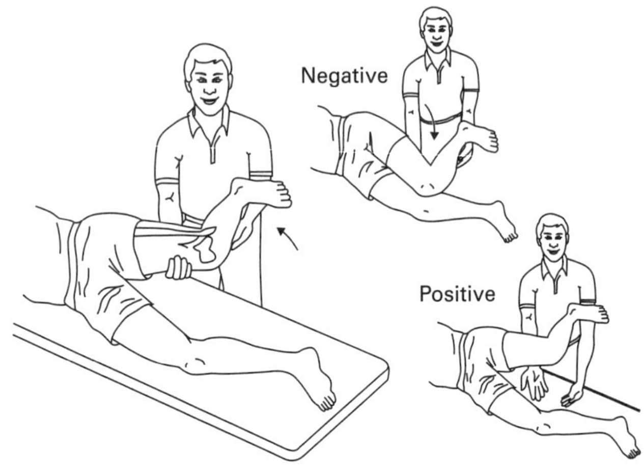

Figure 7-11 Ober test.

femoral condyle (Fig. 7-12). It prevents excessive anterior translation of the tibia and abnormal ER of the tibia on the femur and knee hyperextension. A primary function in the athlete is maintaining joint stability during deceleration.

The most common mechanism of injury is ER of the femur on fixed tibia with a valgus load. Injuries may be due to excessive *pivoting* or *cutting*, as well as hyperextension, hyperflexion, or lateral trauma to the knee. A "pop" is often heard or felt at the time of injury. Immediate swelling due to hemarthrosis and a sense of instability usually follow.

The *Lachman test* (Fig. 7-13) is performed at 20° to 30° of knee flexion and particularly assesses the posterolateral fibers. Some laxity may be normal, so comparison with the contralateral leg is recommended. Sensitivity is higher than the anterior drawer test (99% vs. 54%).[1] The *pivot shift (MacIntosh) test* is performed in the lateral decubitus position with the affected knee extended and the tibia internally rotated. Valgus stress is applied to the knee as it is flexed. A "clunk" felt at 30° of knee flexion is indicative of

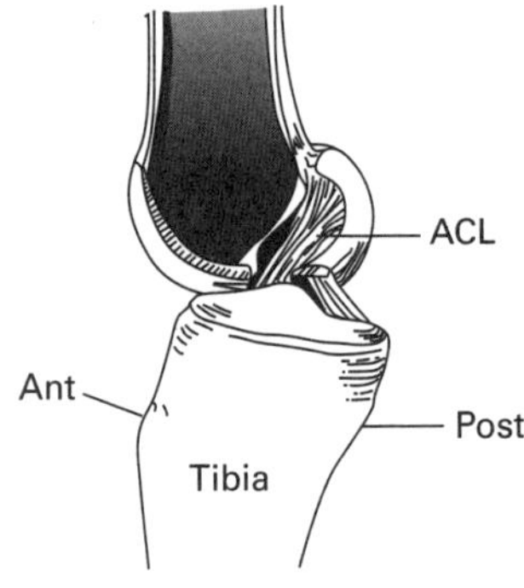

Figure 7-12 The ACL.

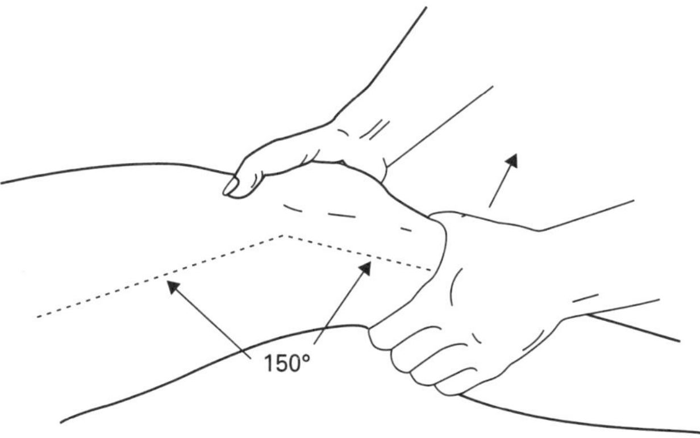

Figure 7-13 The Lachman test.

ACL injury. An *MRI* confirms the diagnosis and may identify other concomitant injuries.

Nonoperative rehabilitation of ACL injury should concentrate on proprioceptive training and strengthening of the hamstrings (i.e., TheraBand; see Fig. 7-14) to prevent anterior subluxation of the tibia. Terminal range squats to strengthen the quads should be encouraged to prevent patellofemoral pain, a frequent occurrence after ACL tears. Bracing should limit terminal extension and rotation. Activity modification (e.g., avoiding cutting and pivoting sports) is extremely important if nonoperative management is given a trial to avoid injury to other intra-articular structures, such as the menisci.

The need for *operative treatment* depends on the amount of damage and degree of laxity and is patient specific as well. A younger, more active patient is more likely to require surgical repair versus the older, sedentary patient. Post-op rehab can last up to 6 to 9 months, although the trend is to shorten this time. Patients are typically WBAT with an extension brace immediately after surgery. As with nonoperative rehab, the emphasis is on strengthening the hamstrings and proprioceptive training. During the first 6 weeks, it is important to regain ROM (can be assisted by CPM) and enhance patellar

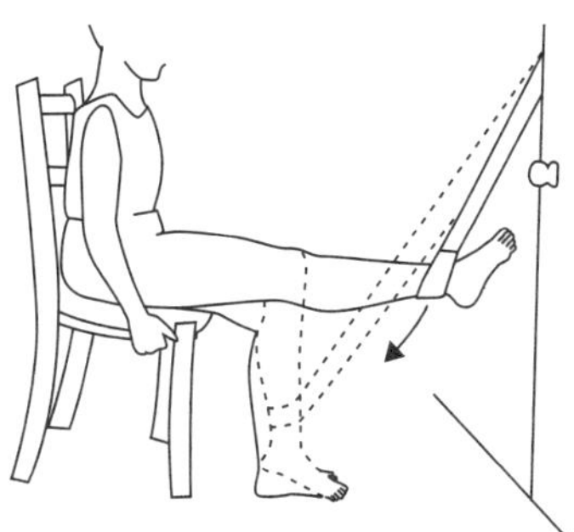

Figure 7-14 Strengthening with TheraBand.

mobility. Intensity and resistance should progressively increase between weeks 6 and 10. By week 10, there should be essentially no limitation in strengthening.

Prevention of these injuries is of utmost importance as well and has been a recent focus of sports medicine research. Young female athletes, especially those that play soccer and basketball, are at a much higher risk of ACL injury than their male peers. ACL injury prevention programs that incorporate proprioceptive and neuromuscular control training may reduce the risk of ACL injuries and, therefore, should be considered in high-risk athletes.[14,15]

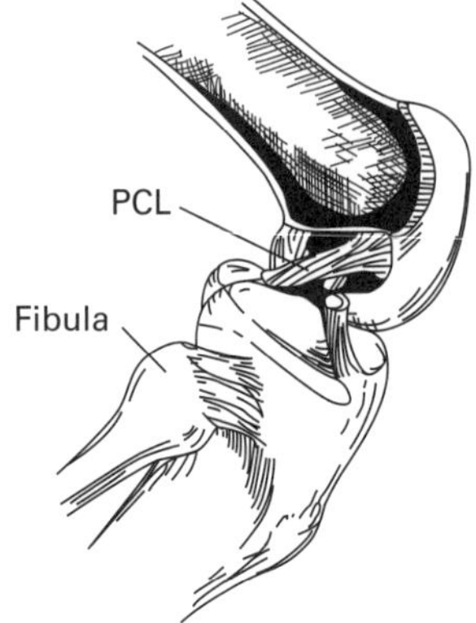

Figure 7-15 The PCL.

From Fu F, Stone D. *Sports Injuries: Mechanisms, Prevention & Treatment.* Baltimore, MD: Williams & Wilkins; 1994.

Posterior Cruciate Ligament – The PCL (Fig. 7-15) arises from the posterior intercondylar tibia and extends anteriorly, superiorly, and medially to attach to the medial femoral condyle. It prevents abnormal IR and posterior translation of the tibia on the femur, which aids knee flexion.

Injury of the PCL classically occurs secondary to an MVA when the tibia strikes the dashboard, forcing the tibia posteriorly. Injury also occurs with high valgus stress or when falling on a flexed knee. Swelling is uncommon. Integrity of the PCL can be tested by the *posterior drawer test* and the *sag test*, where the examiner tries to observe a posterior displacement of the tibial tuberosity (or tibial joint line in relation to the femur) while the patient is supine and the knees are flexed to 90° to allow the quadriceps to relax. After a sag sign is assessed for, the *posterior drawer test* can be used to further test the integrity of the PCL. In addition, a *varus stress* can be applied to an extended knee to assess for concomitant injuries to the PCL and posterolateral corner of the relaxed knee.

Treatment of a mild PCL sprain usually involves quadriceps strengthening without need for bracing. Severe PCL injuries will often need to be repaired arthroscopically.

Meniscal Injury – The menisci (Fig. 7-16) are fibrocartilaginous structures of the intra-articular knee that increase the contact area between the femur and tibia and can act as "shock absorbers" for the knee.

Mechanisms of injury include excessive rotational stresses, typically the result of twisting a flexed knee. The medial meniscus is more often injured than the lateral.

Knee locking, popping, and/or clicking are characteristic complaints. On examination, an effusion, joint line tenderness, and loss of full knee flexion or extension may be noted. *McMurray's test* is performed with the patient supine and hip and knee maximally flexed.

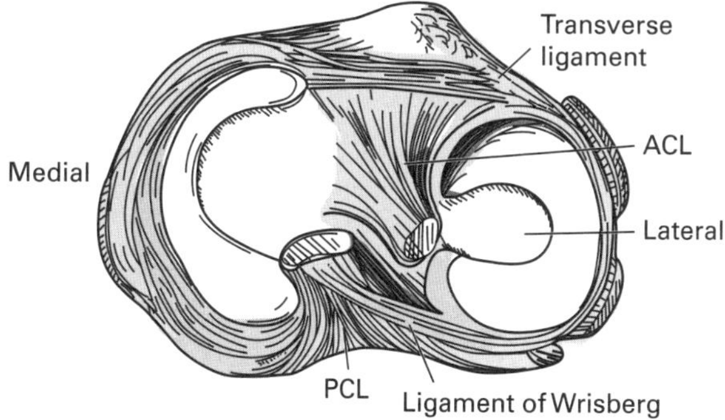

Figure 7-16 The menisci.

From Fu F, Stone D. *Sports Injuries: Mechanisms, Prevention & Treatment.* Baltimore, MD: Williams & Wilkins; 1994.

A valgus-tibial ER force is applied while the knee is extended; a pop or snap suggests a medial meniscus tear. Varus-tibial IR forces are used to evaluate the lateral meniscus. McMurray's test may be poorly tolerated due to pain, and some consider it to be relatively unreliable.[16] Apley's grind test may be positive, but it is avoided by some clinicians for fear of aggravating the injury. *The Thessaly test* has recently been described and validated. It is performed in single leg stance with 20° of knee flexion with assistance from the examiner, who holds the hands while the subject rotates the knee internally and externally.[17] *MRI* may help confirm the clinical diagnosis and identify other injuries. *Arthroscopy* is the gold standard for diagnosis of a tear.

Treatment is dependent on the severity of injury. For the nonsurgically treated patient, early management consists of *RICE*, NSAIDs, hamstring and ITB stretching, and a progressive resistive exercise program for quadriceps/hamstring/hip strengthening. A joint aspiration is sometimes useful to reduce effusion and relieve pain. *Aquatic exercises* and the use of *canes* can unload the affected meniscus. The intensity can be gradually increased with avoidance of activities involving compressive rotational loading. It may be reasonable to gradually resume sports activities once strength in the affected limb approaches 70% to 80% of that of the unaffected limb. Orthopedic referral for possible *arthroscopic surgery* is indicated if the patient is experiencing mechanical symptoms including locking, buckling, or recurrent swelling with pain.

Surgical treatment has been evolving. Total meniscectomy is no longer considered acceptable; efforts are now aimed at preserving as much cartilage as possible in order to prevent degenerative changes. The outer thirds of the menisci are vascular and may be repaired; the inner two-thirds are avascular and may need to be debrided. Following partial meniscectomy, full WB may occur once the patient is pain free. Following meniscal repair, full WB may be delayed for up to 6 weeks. ROM exercise, stretching, and progressive strengthening of the lower limbs are the mainstays of post-op therapy. Deep squatting is discouraged.

Patellofemoral Pain Syndrome – The etiology is postulated to be a combination of overuse, muscular imbalance (i.e., hip abductor and external rotator weakness),[18] and/or biomechanical problems (i.e., pes planus or pes cavus, ↑ Q angle [Fig. 7-17]). Anterior knee pain may occur with activity and worsen with prolonged sitting or descending stairs.

Acute management involves *relative rest, ice,* and *NSAIDs*. Prolonged sitting should be avoided. The mainstay of rehabilitation is to address the biomechanical deficits through a combination of *quadriceps strengthening exercises* with *stretching* of the quadriceps, hamstrings, ITB, and gastroc–soleus complex.

Classically, short arc terminal knee extension (0° to 30°) exercises were utilized, with the belief that they selectively strengthened the VMO. Currently, the idea of VMO selectivity is controversial. In general,

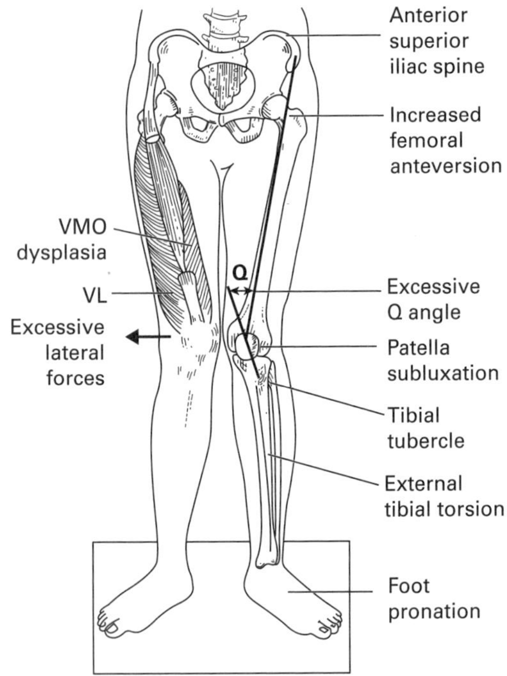

Figure 7-17 Sequelae of an increased Q angle. Normally, the male Q is 13°; the female is 18°.

From Fu F, Stone D. *Sports Injuries: Mechanisms, Prevention & Treatment.* Baltimore, MD: Williams & Wilkins; 1994.

short arc (0° to 45°) closed kinetic chain leg press exercises are recommended to strengthen all four heads of the quads, which are thought to be weakened in aggregate. Full arc and open kinetic chain exercises should be avoided to reduce symptom aggravation.

Taping the patella so that it tracks properly (*McConnell technique*) may improve pain symptoms during exercise. *Orthotics* to correct pes planus or foot pronation and soft braces with patellar cutouts may provide modest symptomatic relief in appropriate cases. Occasionally, *electrical stimulation* and *biofeedback* are useful. Prolonged PT with modalities such as US is generally not helpful or cost-effective. *Surgery* is rarely necessary and is reserved for recalcitrant instability or symptomatic malalignment.

Exercise-Induced Leg Pain – Shin splint, a nonspecific term, refers to exercise-induced tibial pain, without evidence of fracture on x-ray. It is believed to represent periostitis, usually of the posteromedial tibial border (*medial tibial stress syndrome*). Runners, gymnasts, and dancers are at risk, with causes including an increase in exercise intensity, inadequate footwear, hard surface training, or poor biomechanics. Local pain and tenderness are noted along the distal one-third of the tibia. Pain is often quickly relieved by rest and not aggravated by passive stretch. Bone scan may be positive in severe cases. Treatment includes rest, NSAIDs, US, preactivity icing, and correction of aggravating factors.

Causes of TSFs are similar to those of tibial stress syndrome. Stress fractures are also common in the fibula and the metatarsals, especially the second metatarsal. Pain is initially exercise induced only, but progresses to pain with WB or even at rest. There is often exquisite point tenderness along the distal or middle third of the tibia. X-rays may be negative initially, but may show a clear fracture after several weeks (i.e., a positive "dreaded black line" on oblique radiograph, representing an anterior TSF). Bone scans are more sensitive. TSFs can be treated with *relative rest* (i.e., crutches). Medial TSFs can be treated with relative rest for 4 to 6 weeks, NSAIDs, and TENS. Anterior TSFs may require several months of rest from sports activities and ongoing conservative treatment. Recalcitrant cases may eventually require a bone graft.

In *chronic compartment syndrome of the leg*, pain is felt after a specific period of exercise and can be associated with paresthesias, numbness, and weakness in the distribution of the nerve within the compartment. EDx studies are usually normal. Resting and postexercise compartment pressures should be obtained. Resting pressures > 30 mm Hg, 15-second postexercise pressures >60 mm Hg, or 2-minute postexercise pressures >20 mm Hg are all suggestive of chronic compartment syndrome. An initial conservative approach should include NSAIDs, proper footwear selection, and correction of training errors. If symptoms persist 1 to 2 months after a trial of conservative treatment, referral for surgical fasciotomy may be warranted.

Achilles Tendinitis – Overuse, overpronation, heel varus deformity, and poor flexibility of the Achilles tendon/gastroc–soleus/hamstrings may be contributing factors. Basketball players may be particularly susceptible because of the frequent jumping. It is also noted in runners who increase their mileage or hill training. Symptoms include pain and swelling in the tendon during and after activities. On examination, there may be swelling, pain on palpation, a palpable nodule, and inability to stand on tiptoes. Chronic tendinosis may result in tendon weakness, potentially leading to rupture.

There is no consensus on the optimal mode of treatment, but most rehabilitation will likely begin with the PRICE principle. Modalities, especially *US*, may be helpful. Plantarflexor strengthening is important. *Downhill exercises* should be emphasized; uphill running should be discouraged, especially early in rehab. Heel lifts may provide early relief but may lead to heel cord shortening with prolonged use. A properly fitted shoe, often with a stiff heel counter, is important. Injection into the Achilles tendon is not recommended by many sources due to the risk of tendon rupture. For severe or chronic cases, recovery to near-normal strength may take up to 24 months, even with good circulation. For this reason, novel treatments (i.e., PRP) are currently being studied, but results are inconclusive.[19,20] Young, active persons with ruptured tendons are usually operated on; casting is an option for older, sedentary persons.

Ankle Sprains – Lateral ankle sprains are usually due to inversion of a plantarflexed foot. The ATFL is typically the first structure to be involved. With increasing severity of injury, the CFL may be involved next, followed by the PTFL. The anterior drawer test checks ankle ligament stability, primarily the ATFL (displacement ≥ 5 mm is considered positive). The talar tilt test (Fig. 7-18) checks the CFL; it is performed by providing an inversion stress on the talus (a positive test is a marked difference,

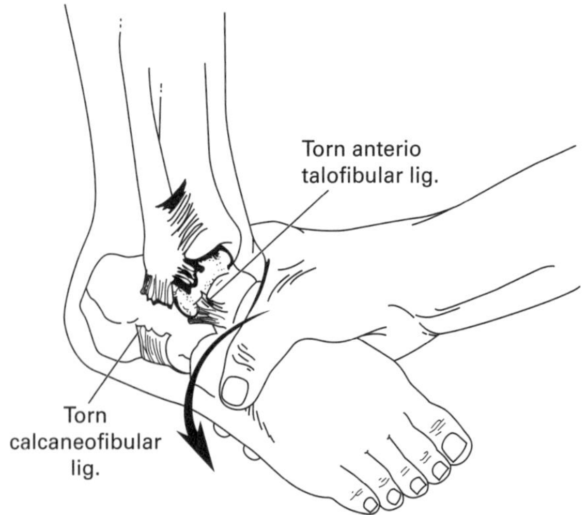

Figure 7-18 Talar tilt test.

Figure Courtesy of Fu F, Stone D. *Sports Injuries: Mechanisms, Prevention & Treatment.* Baltimore, MD: Williams & Wilkins; 1994.

i.e., >10°, in the inversion of the affected vs. the unaffected side). X-rays to check the tibiofibular syndesmosis may be necessary in the event of severe sprains; these require surgical consultation.

Injuries of the medial (deltoid) ankle ligament due to an eversion injury are less common; an associated proximal fibula fracture (Maisonneuve fracture) should be ruled out.

Rehabilitation of ankle sprains involves three phases: *Phase I* normally lasts 1 to 3 days, until the patient is able to bear weight comfortably. This phase involves the *RICE* principle: rest (i.e., crutches), ice 20 minutes 3 to 5×/day, compression with Ace wrap, and elevation of the foot above the heart. Hot showers, EtOH, methyl salicylate counterirritants (i.e., Ben Gay), and other treatments that may increase swelling should be avoided during the initial 24 hours. *Phase II* usually lasts days to weeks. The goals in this phase are to restore ROM, strengthen the ankle stabilizers, and stretch/strengthen the Achilles tendon. *Phase III* is initiated when motion is near normal and pain and swelling are almost absent. Reestablishing motor coordination via proprioceptive exercises and endurance training are emphasized, i.e., balance board, running curves (*figure-of-8*), and zigzag running.

Return to play guidelines vary. Some recommendations may be as follows: Grade I (no laxity and minimal ligamentous tear): 0 to 5 days. Grade II (mild to moderate laxity and functional loss): 7 to 14 days. Grade III (complete ligamentous disruption and cannot bear weight): 21 to 35 days. Syndesmosis injury: 21 to 56 days. Recent literature has demonstrated that an early and accelerated rehabilitation program results in better short-term outcomes for grades I and II lateral ankle sprains.[21]

Plantar Fasciitis – Commonly seen in athletes and in persons whose jobs require much standing or walking. Repetitive microtrauma to the plantar fascia can cause inflammation and pain in the acute phase. In chronic conditions, the fascia is less commonly inflamed; instead, it becomes degenerative and painful and is commonly termed plantar fasciopathy. Biomechanical issues (i.e., an overpronated foot with increased tension on the fascia) are often at fault. The classic symptoms are heel pain with the first few steps in the morning or pain that is worse at the beginning of an activity.

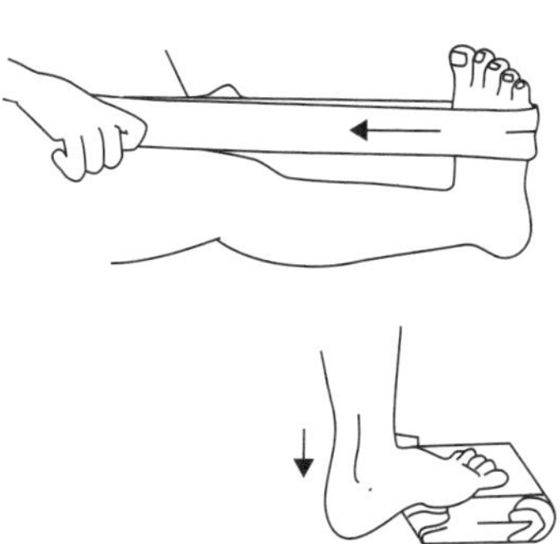

Figure 7-19 Stretching for plantar fasciitis.

Adapted from Rouzier P. *The Sports Medicine Patient Advisor.* Amherst, MA: SportsMed Press; 1999.

The key component of treatment is a home exercise program of *routine, daily stretching* of the plantar fascia (Fig. 7-19) and Achilles tendon, which has proven to be superior to other treatment modalities.[22] Patients should be on *relative rest* from walking, running, and jumping and consider switching to activities such as swimming or cycling to allow for the fascia to heal. *Proper footwear* includes well-cushioned soles, possible use of an extra-deep heel pad/cup insert, and avoiding high heels. *Soft medial arch supports* are generally preferable to rigid orthotics, which can exacerbate symptoms. NSAIDs and ice may help decrease inflammation. For patients not responding to other measures, *splints* may be useful to supply a gentle constant stretch across the sole of the foot and gastrocnemius at night while sleeping. Once the pain resolves, patients should return to increased levels of activity only gradually, while continuing their stretching program.

The majority of cases will improve with conservative measures within 6 to 12 weeks, if faithfully followed. In the rare, persistent case, a *local corticosteroid injection* may be considered. A potential complication is necrosis of the fatty pad of the heel, which cannot be easily reversed or treated. Surgical intervention, which consists of a release of the involved fascia from its attachment to the calcaneus, can be considered if all other measures fail, but is necessary in only very rare cases.

SPORTS/EXERCISE PREPARTICIPATION EVALUATION (PPE)

General Guidelines

Questions about personal and family history of cardiovascular disease are the most important initial component of the H&P. A thorough history of neurologic or MSK problems should also be emphasized. Physical examination should emphasize cardiac auscultation with provocative maneuvers to screen for hypertrophic cardiomyopathy (see below), which is the most common cause of sudden death in young male athletes. The use of ECG in the PPE screen remains controversial.[23] For most young, asymptomatic persons, screening tests such as electrocardiography, treadmill stress testing, and lab tests are not indicated in the absence of symptoms or a significant history of risk factors.[1] For older asymptomatic persons w/o cardiopulmonary risk factors or known metabolic disease, the American College of Sports Medicine recommends exercise stress testing in men ≥ 45 years and women ≥ 55 years before starting a vigorous exercise program (≥60% of Vo_2max).[2] Most older persons can begin a moderate aerobic and resistance training program without stress testing if they begin to slowly and gradually increase their level of activity.[23]

Example of an Appropriate Preparticipation PE

The table below is a guideline for a pre-participation evaluation.

Examination feature	Comments
Blood pressure	Must be assessed in the context of participant's age, height, and gender
General	Measure for excessive height and observe for evidence of excessive long bone growth that suggests Marfan syndrome

Eyes	Important to detect vision defects that leave one of the eyes with worse than 20/40 corrected vision
Cardiovascular	Palpate the point of maximal impulse for increased intensity and displacement that suggest hypertrophy or failure, respectively Perform auscultation with the patient supine and again standing or straining during Valsalva maneuver (a loud systolic murmur that increases with upright posture or Valsalva and decreases with squatting suggests hypertrophic cardiomyopathy) Femoral pulse diminishment suggests aortic coarctation
Respiratory	Observe for accessory muscle use or prolonged expiration and auscultate for wheezing. Exercise-induced asthma will not produce manifestations on resting examination and requires exercise testing for diagnosis
Abdominal	Assess for hepatic or splenic enlargement
GU (males only)	Hernias/varicoceles do not usually preclude sports participation, but it may be appropriate to screen for testicular masses
MSK	The "2 minute orthopedic examination" is a commonly used systematic screen 23 Consider supplemental shoulder, knee, and ankle examinations
Skin	Evidence of molluscum contagiosum, herpes simplex infection, impetigo, tinea corporis, or scabies would temporarily prohibit participation in sports in which direct skin-to-skin competitor contact occurs (i.e., wrestling and martial arts)

Conditions That Contraindicate Sports Participation

The following conditions preclude participation: active myocarditis or pericarditis; hypertrophic cardiomyopathy; uncontrolled severe HTN (static resistance exercises are particularly contraindicated); suspected CAD until fully evaluated; long QT interval syndrome; history of recent concussion and symptoms of postconcussion syndrome (no contact or collision sports); poorly controlled convulsive disorder (no archery, riflery, swimming, weight lifting, strength training, or sports involving heights); recurrent episodes of burning UEx pain or weakness or episodes of transient quadriplegia until stability of cervical spine can be assured (no contact or collision sports); sickle cell disease (no high exertion, contact, or collision sports); mononucleosis with unresolved splenomegaly; eating disorder where athlete is not compliant with treatment or follow-up or where there is evidence of diminished performance or potential injury because of eating disorder.

Rehabilitation after Hip Fracture

The lifetime risk of hip fractures in industrialized countries is 18% for ♀ and 6% for ♂.[24] Osteoporosis and falls are the primary risk factors. Mortality and morbidity following hip fractures are high: 20% are not alive by 1 year postfracture and 33% by 2 years.[25] Nearly one of three survivors is in institutionalized care within a year after the fracture, and as many as two of three survivors never regain their preoperative activity status.[26] Surgery is usually indicated for most hip fractures, unless medically contraindicated or in nonambulatory patients.

Femoral Neck Fracture – Screw fixations (Fig. 7-20) are typical for stable, nondisplaced fractures. Ambulation with WBAT and an appropriate assistive device may be started during the first few days post-op. Bipolar endoprostheses (Fig. 7-21) may be used for unstable, displaced fractures when satisfactory reduction cannot be achieved and the patient is >65 years of age or has preexisting articular pathology (i.e., OA). Patients are usually mobilized quickly and allowed WBAT within the first few days post-op. Abduction pillows and short-term ROM restrictions (no adduction past midline and no IR) may be ordered to reduce the risk of prosthetic displacement.

Intertrochanteric Fractures (Fig. 7-22) – Sliding hip screw fixation allows for early WBAT for stable fractures (intact posteromedial cortex) and provides dynamic compression of the fracture during WB. Intramedullary hip screws are another surgical option. A period of limited WB may be necessary following fixation of unstable fractures. Surgical management for *subtrochanteric fractures* also includes the use of sliding screw fixation

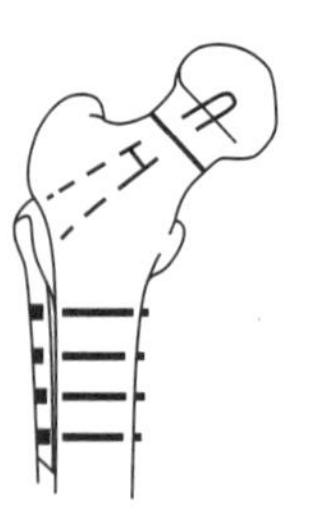

Figure 7-20 Screw fixation.

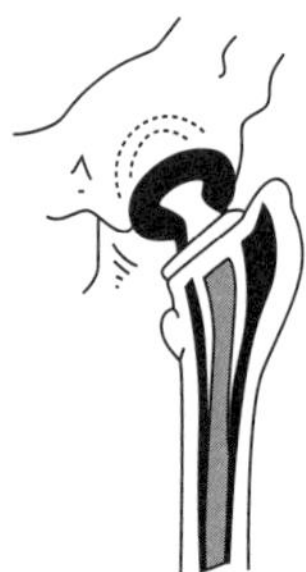

Figure 7-21 Bipolar endoprosthesis.

and intramedullary nails/rods, although initial WB may be more limited.

Complications seen during rehabilitation and convalescence after hip fracture include atelectasis, pneumonia, anemia, fracture nonunion, AVN, surgical site infection, component loosening, leg length discrepancy, HO, DVT, constipation, and skin breakdown.

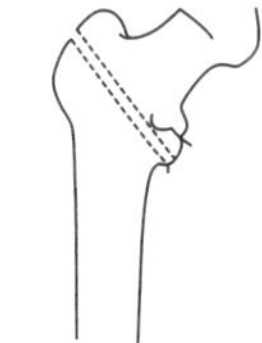

Figure 7-22 Intertrochanteric fracture.

REHABILITATION AFTER JOINT REPLACEMENT

Total Hip Arthroplasty

Biologically fixed or *"cementless" implants* provide a more durable bioprosthetic interface, but require a longer period of protective WB (i.e., touchdown WB to PWB × ≥2 to 3 months) to allow for osseous integration into the porous prosthetic surface. *Cement-fixed implants* are cheaper and may offer immediate WBAT. The cement, however, can be prone to deterioration, which may result in component loosening and ultimately require revision.

Patients may be out of bed to chair with assist on post-op day 1. A triangular hip abduction pillow in bed is highly recommended for the first 6 to 12 weeks. *Hip precautions* generally continue for up to 12 weeks post-op to allow for formation of a pseudocapsule and minimize the chance of dislocation. Patients are allowed flexion up to 90°, passive abduction, and gentle (≤30°) IR while extended. There should be no adduction past midline and no IR while flexed. Active abduction and hyperextension are allowed with a posterior approach (gluteus medius preserved) but avoided after an anterolateral approach (gluteus medius split open). Typical patient instructions are diagrammed in Fig. 7-23.

Other key issues include DVT prophylaxis, monitoring for post-op anemia and infection, and pain control. Patients may often complain about perceived leg length discrepancies during the first several months post-op; PT to address muscle imbalances and tight capsules may be helpful. In general, prognosis following THA is excellent, although being younger, male, obese, and highly active may adversely affect outcomes.[1]

Total Knee Arthroplasty

Cemented fixation may allow immediate WBAT; cementless fixation may require several months of restricted WB for complete stability. Neither addresses the issue of polyethylene liner wear, which may be the key factor in eventual prosthetic failure. Microscopic wear debris can trigger an inflammatory response with ensuing osteolysis and component loosening.

Regaining *knee ROM* (i.e., 0° to 90° before going home) is an important rehabilitation goal for all TKA patients. Pillows under the knee should be avoided. The use of CPM is controversial. Some have argued that it may

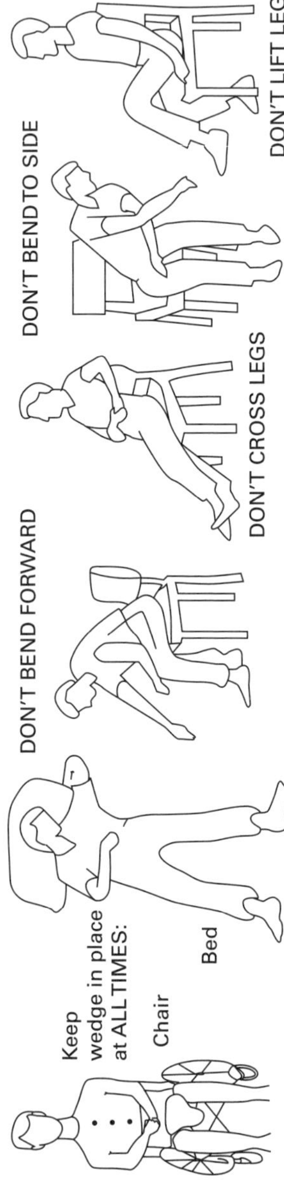

Figure 7-23 Rehabilitation after THA.

decrease length of inpatient rehabilitation stay and improve ROM (by 10°) at 1 year post-op,[2] but most studies have *not* demonstrated long-term benefits in ROM or functional outcome.

REFERENCES

1. Bisbinas I, Belthur M, Said HG, Green M, Learmonth DJ. Accuracy of needle placement in ACJ injections. *Knee Surg Sports Traumatol Arthrosc.* 2006;14(8):762-765.
2. Naredo E, Cabero F, Beneyto P, et al. A randomized comparative study of short term response to blind injection versus sonographic-guided injection of local corticosteroids in patients with painful shoulder. *J Rheumatol.* 2004;31(2):308-314.
3. Panditaratne N, Wilkinson C, Groves C, Chandramohan M. Subacromial impingement syndrome: a prospective comparison of ultrasound-guided versus unguided injection techniques. *Ultrasound.* 2010;18(4):176-181.
4. Sayegh FE, Kenanidis EI, Papavasiliou KA, et al. Reduction of acute anterior dislocations: a prospective randomized study comparing a new technique with the Hippocratic and Kocher methods. *J Bone Joint Surg Am.* 2009;91:2775-2782.
5. Neviaser AS, Hannafin JA. Adhesive capsulitis: a review of current treatment. *Am J Sports Med.* 2010;38(11):2346-2356.
6. Sofka CM, Collins AJ, Adler RS. Use of ultrasonographic guidance in interventional musculoskeletal procedures: a review from a single institution. *J Ultrasound Med.* 2001;20(1):21-26.
7. Mishra A, Collado H, Fredericson M. Platelet-rich plasma compared with corticosteroid injection for chronic lateral elbow tendinosis. *Phys Med Rehabil.* 2009;1(4):366-370.
8. Kazemi M, Azma K, Tavana B, et al. Autologous blood versus corticosteroid local injection in the short-term treatment of lateral elbow tendinopathy: a randomized clinical trial of efficacy. *Am J Phys Med Rehabil.* 2010;89(8):660-667.
9. Jeyapalan K, Choudhary S. Ultrasound-guided injection of triamcinolone and bupivacaine in the management of De Quervain's disease. *Skeletal Radiol.* 2009;38(11):1099-1103.
10. Strauss EJ, Nho SJ, Kelly BT. Greater trochanteric pain syndrome. *Sports Med Arthrosc.* 2010;18(2):113-119.
11. Fearon AM, Scarvell JM, Cook JL, Smith PN. Does ultrasound correlate with surgical or histologic findings in greater trochanteric pain syndrome? A pilot study. *Clin Orthop Relat Res.* 2010;468(7):1838-1844.
12. Labrosse JM, Cardinal E, Leduc BE, et al. Effectiveness of ultrasound-guided corticosteroid injection for the treatment of gluteus medius tendinopathy. *AJR Am J Roentgenol.* 2010;194(1):202-206.
13. Finnoff JT, Nutz DJ, Henning PT, Hollman JH, Smith J. Accuracy of ultrasound-guided versus unguided pes anserinus bursa injections. *Phys Med Rehabil.* 2010;2(8):732-739.
14. Gilchrist J, Mandelbaum BR, Melancon H, et al. A randomized controlled trial to prevent noncontact anterior cruciate ligament injury in female collegiate soccer players. *Am J Sports Med.* 2008;36(8):1476-1483.
15. Torg JS. Clinical diagnosis of ACL instability in the athlete. *Am J Sports Med.* 1976;4:84-93.
16. Karachalios T, Hantes M, Zibis AH, et al. Diagnostic accuracy of a new clinical test (the Thessaly test) for early detection of meniscal tears. *J Bone Joint Surg Am.* 2005;87(5):955-962.
17. Cichanowski HR, Schmitt JS, Johnson RJ, Niemuth PE. Hip strength in collegiate female athletes with patellofemoral pain. *Med Sci Sports Exerc.* 2007;39(8):1227-1232.
18. de Vos RJ, Weir A, van Schie HT, et al. Platelet-rich plasma injection for chronic Achilles tendinopathy: a randomized controlled trial. *JAMA.* 2010;303(2):144-149.

19. Gaweda K, Tarczynska M, Krzyzanowski W. Treatment of Achilles tendinopathy with platelet-rich plasma. *Int J Sports Med.* 2010;31(8):577-583.
20. Bleakley CM, O'Connor SR, Tully MA, et al. Effect of accelerated rehabilitation on function after ankle sprain: randomised controlled trial. *BMJ.* 2010;340:c1964.
21. Rompe JD, Cacchio A, Weil L, et al. Plantar fascia-specific stretching versus radial shock-wave therapy as initial treatment of plantar fasciopathy. *J Bone Joint Surg Am.* 2010;92:2514-2522.
22. Corrado D, Basso C, Schiavon M, et al. Screening for hypertrophic cardiomyopathy in young athletes. *N Engl J Med.* 1998;339:364-369. Baggish A, Hutter AM, Wang F, et al. Cardiovascular screening in college athletes with and without electrocardiography. *Ann Int Med.* 2010;152:269-275.
23. Kurowski K, Chandran S. The preparticipation athletic evaluation. *Am Fam Physician.* 2000;61:2683-2698. ACSM. *Guidelines for Exercise Testing and Prescription.* 6th ed. Baltimore, MD: Lippincott Williams & Wilkins; 2000. Neid RJ. Promoting and prescribing exercise for the elderly. *Am Fam Physician.* 2002;65:419-428.
24. Meunier PJ. Prevention of hip fxs. *Am J Med.* 1993;95(suppl):75-78.
25. Emerson S. 10yr survival after fxs of the proximal end of the femur. *Gerontology.* 1988;34:186-191.
26. Osteoporosis Prevention, Dx, and Therapy. *NIH Consensus Statement* March 27-29. 2000;17:1-36.

RECOMMENDED READING

Scholten RJ. The accuracy of physical dx tests for assessing meniscal lesions of the knee: a metaanalysis. *J Fam Pract.* 2001;50:955-957.

Chapter 8

RHEUMATOLOGY

Osteoarthritis

OA, the most prevalent form of arthritis in the United States, is caused by a disruption of the normal process of degradation and synthesis of articular cartilage and subchondral bone.[1] Biomechanical and biologic factors are implicated. Age, obesity, and female gender are among the risk factors; joint involvement is typically asymmetric. Weight-bearing joints are usually involved.

Characteristically, pain is worsened by joint use (end of day), and stiffness occurs with inactivity (gelling). Classification criteria exist for OA of the hand, hip, and knee and include various combinations of clinical and radiologic features.[2] Generally, evidence of pain at the specified joint, with bony swelling and lack of inflammatory markers (ESR < 20, morning stiffness < 30 minutes, nonerythematous, and cool to touch) in a patient > 50 years, is a consistent feature of the disease. Radiologic confirmation on the basis of joint space narrowing and osteophyte formation can be made.

Nonpharmacologic Management

Strengthening and aerobic exercises (e.g., fitness walking) have been shown in numerous trials to reduce pain and disability while improving quality of life. The FAST confirmed the beneficial effects of quadriceps strengthening and aerobic exercise in patients with knee OA.[3] Felsen reported that a decrease of 2 BMI units (~11.2 lbs) over 10 years in a group of women above median BMI decreased the odds of developing OA by over 50%.[4]

To promote self-efficacy, psychological well-being, and improved pain levels, patients should be encouraged to participate in programs such as the Arthritis Foundation Self-Help Course.[5] For patients who are poorly tolerant of weight-bearing exercises due to their OA, aquatic exercises may be an alternative. (Swimming, however, may worsen lumbar facet arthritis symptoms.) Physical modalities and judicious rest between sessions may also improve tolerance and compliance with exercises.

A cane held in the hand contralateral to a painful hip can help unload the joint and make ambulation more bearable. For a painful knee, the cane can be held in either hand.[6] Knee unloading braces and lateral heel wedges can reduce stress in the medial knee compartment and relieve pain. Environmental adaptations include raising toilet and chair heights.

Pharmacologic Options, per ACR

Pharmaceutical agents are most effective when combined with nonpharmacologic strategies.[7] A trial of acetaminophen is recommended as the initial treatment for mild to moderate hip OA or knee OA without gross inflammation because of its overall cost, efficacy, and toxicity profile.[7] For patients with moderate to severe knee OA and signs of joint inflammation,

IA steroids, COX-2 inhibitors, or NSAIDs (with misoprostol or a proton pump inhibitor if the patient is at risk for adverse upper gastrointestinal events) may be considered as first-line therapy.[7]

Tramadol can be considered in patients with moderate to severe pain with contraindications to NSAIDs/COX-2 agents and/or failing other treatments. The mean effective daily dose for tramadol has generally been ~200 to 300 mg, divided into four doses.[6] More potent opioids can be considered for patients not tolerating or failing tramadol.

Topical analgesics (e.g., methyl salicylate or capsaicin) can be considered in patients with mild to moderate knee OA pain as an adjunctive treatment or as monotherapy. Voltaren (diclofenac) gel is also available to treat the pain of OA of both knees and hands; IA hyaluronan therapy (e.g., Synvisc) is indicated for patients with knee (*not* hip) OA with a poor response to simple analgesics and nonpharmacologic treatment. Studies of IA hyaluronan are somewhat controversial and inconclusive, but generally seem to favor its use in mild to moderate knee OA. Peak effects may be at 8 to 12 weeks; duration of action may be up to 6 months. Limited data are available regarding the efficacy of multiple courses of IA hyaluronan. IA glucocorticoids fluoroscopically guided into the hip joint may be efficacious in some patients.[7]

Alternative and Investigational Treatments

Complementary and alternative medicine treatments abound. Although preliminary studies of glucosamine/chondroitin appeared promising at providing modest short-term symptomatic improvement, a recent NIH-sponsored multicenter trial (GAIT) did not show benefit in pain, function, or radiologic progression in over 1,500 patients with knee OA.[8] Research on the efficacy of acupuncture in OA is likewise promising but qualitatively suboptimal. Other complementary treatments currently under investigation include supplementation with vitamin D and the antioxidant vitamins A, C, E, and coenzyme Q10, and curcumin-phosphatidylcholine.

A recent development in the surgical treatment of knee OA is the UniSpacer, which is FDA approved for isolated, moderate, medial compartment OA. The kidney bean–shaped lightweight metallic alloy device is a self-centering bearing that requires no shaving of bone or screw/cement fixation to the native anatomy. Long-term efficacy is under investigation, though early clinical studies are disappointing with high revision rates and only modest relief of pain.[9]

Greater understanding of chondrocyte biology and the inflammatory mediators of this disease has already led to novel investigational therapeutic targets, known as DMOADs, e.g., iNOS inhibition, pentosan, and IA administration of autologous conditioned serum.

Rheumatoid Arthritis

Rheumatoid arthritis (RA) is a chronic systemic inflammatory disorder affecting women more than men, with ~1% prevalence in the United States. RA can cause an erosive, polyarticular, typically symmetric synovitis with or without extra-articular manifestations (fatigue, anemia, rheumatoid nodules, cardiac valve abnormalities, and pericarditis). Classic late physical examination findings include boutonniere's, swan neck, or mallet finger deformities, symmetric wrist swelling, Baker's cysts, MCP subluxation with ulnar deviation of the fingers, and DIP joint sparing.

Modified ACR/EULAR classification criteria for the diagnosis of RA[10] were introduced in 2010 and focus on early inflammatory disease parameters, rather than late-stage features.[10] As a result, ACPA has been added, as have the acute phase reactants ESR and CRP, while the concept of symmetry has been greatly minimized and erosive disease eliminated from the tree algorithm.

RA Management

RA management must include both early pharmacologic therapy and nonpharmacologic interventions. *ROM exercises* and *stretching* should be regularly practiced. *Isometric* strengthening exercises are preferred to minimize joint inflammation. *Splints*, particularly resting wrist-hand splints and knee or hindfoot splints, are helpful in reducing pain and preventing progression of deformity. A dorsal hand orthosis with an ulnar aspect MCP block and individual finger stops can be useful in the setting of ulnar deviation. Education should emphasize *avoidance of overuse* and *joint protection techniques* (e.g., decreasing activity during flare-ups, modifying activities to reduce joint stress, using splints, and maintaining strength).

Current treatment algorithms involve early institution of DMARDs and/or biologics and have allowed the primary target for treatment of RA to be a state of remission.[11] Although *NSAIDs, COX*-2 inhibitors, and oral steroids may be helpful symptomatically in mild or early disease, they are currently used only as adjunctive therapy. DMARDs offer symptomatic relief, have been shown to modify disease progression, and are currently the first-line therapy in early RA, being initiated within 3 months of disease onset.[12] Examples of currently used DMARDs include MTX, leflunomide, sulfasalazine, and hydroxychloroquine, although MTX is by far the most common and best tolerated.

BIOLOGICS

Biologics (Table 8-1) significantly inhibit joint damage and are often used in combination with DMARDs to offer the most efficient suppression of disease. They include the TNF-α inhibitors, B-cell depletion, IL-6 and IL-1 inhibitors, and CTLA-4Ig. Adverse events, though less common, may be life threatening, and long-term effects are still unclear.

Arthroscopic *synovectomy* can be performed to reduce joint destruction and relieve symptoms not alleviated by conservative management.

Juvenile Idiopathic Arthritis

JIA is a common childhood chronic illness, affecting some 70,000 to 100,000 persons younger than 16 years of age in the United States.[1,13] There are seven subtypes: systemic, polyarthritis RF positive,

TABLE 8-1 Biologics

Biologic class	Generic name	Trade name
TNF-α inhibitor	Etanercept	Enbrel
	Infliximab	Remicade
	Adalimumab	Humira
	Certolizumab	Cimzia
	Golimumab	Simponi
CTLA-4Ig	Abatacept	Orencia
B-cell depletion	Rituximab	Rituxan
IL-6 inhibitor	Tocilizumab	Actemra
IL-1 inhibitor	Anakinra	Kineret

polyarthritis RF negative, oligoarthritis (persistent and extended), enthesitis-related arthritis, psoriatic, and undifferentiated. Girls are more frequently affected than boys, although this may vary with JIA subtype. Diagnosis requires onset prior to age 16 years, persistent arthritis in one or more joints for 6 or more weeks, and exclusion of other childhood arthritides. RF-positive subtype I is relatively less frequent, occurring in up to 10% of the JIA population. Oligoarticular JIA is characteristically seen in young girls (ages 1 to 5 years), is ANA positive, and is notable for its often asymptomatic uveitis (30% to 50%), which can lead to blindness. Other subtypes may also be complicated by ocular involvement. There is significant lifelong functional limitations in >30% of JIA patients after ≥10 years of follow-up. Many children do not reach the expected adult height. Ocular outcomes have improved, although they still represent a significant cause of blindness. Mortality rates are 3 to 14 times greater than expected. Unlike previously thought, many patients with JIA will continue to have active inflammatory arthritis in adulthood.

Treatment: Similar to adults, treatment of JIA involves DMARD and biologic therapy with NSAIDs and systemic steroids as bridge therapy for symptomatic control. IA steroids (i.e., for acutely inflamed joints) can be used for pain control. Cyclosporine is used for JIA that is complicated by the macrophage activation syndrome and anakinra for the systemic subtype, which tends to be less responsive to MTX and TNF inhibition. *Prone lying* and *splints* may prevent/correct contractures. *Heat* for nonacutely inflamed joints may help reduce stiffness. Physical therapy for flexibility and muscle strengthening is fundamental. Swimming, cycling, and isometric exercises are relatively less stressful to the joints.

Ankylosing Spondylitis

AS is one of the classic seronegative spondyloarthropathies. Risk factors include HLA-B27 and male gender (male to female incidence is 2:1).[1] Onset is typically in late adolescence or early adulthood. Initial symptoms include pain and stiffness in the buttock or lumbar area, which are worse with inactivity and improve with exercise or hot showers. B/l, symmetric *sacroiliitis* is a characteristic early X-ray finding. Inflammation of the spine can lead to syndesmophyte formation and then ultimately to a kyphotic bony ankylosis ("*bamboo spine*"). Progression of spinal inflexibility can be followed by Schober's test. Although the course of AS is variable, the majority of patients have mild disease and normal longevity.[1] Extra-articular manifestations include peripheral large joint arthritis, uveitis, cardiac conduction abnormalities, aortic regurgitation, and pulmonary fibrosis of the upper lobes. *Uveitis* typically is painful, monoarticular, and acute. It is associated with redness and photophobia and may progress to blindness.

Treatment includes *spinal extension exercises* (e.g., swimming and push-ups), expansive chest breathing, pectoral and hip flexor stretching, and prone lying. A *hard mattress*, preferably w/o pillows behind the head, should be recommended. NSAIDs (e.g., naproxen and indomethacin) may reduce pain and symptoms of spinal stiffness. Sulfasalazine is useful in cases of significant peripheral arthritis. TNF-α inhibitors should be used for patients with axial manifestations. Often hip replacement surgery is required.[14]

Fibromyalgia

FM is an incompletely understood clinical syndrome affecting women much more frequently than men. It is characterized by widespread, chronic pain and systemic symptoms (e.g., fatigue, sleep disturbance, and depression).

The ACR criteria[15] include (1) *pain and tenderness lasting for 3 months* or longer (involving bilateral sides, plus above and below the waist; in addition, axial skeletal pain must be present) and (2) *pain in 11 or more of 18 predetermined tender points on examination* (see below), elicited by applying approximately 4 kg/cm pressure (enough to blanch a fingernail). More recently, a nontender point diagnostic criterion has been introduced for use by primary care providers and underscores the chronic widespread nature of this pain syndrome.[16] The SS score, with an emphasis on fatigue, nonrestorative sleep patterns, and cognitive abnormalities, is part of the diagnostic tool, but is envisioned to be useful in following the disease longitudinally (Fig. 8-1).[16]

Treatment should include education (e.g., FM typically has a nonprogressive course), low-impact aerobic activities, and analgesia. Recently, tai chi has been demonstrated to have a positive effect on pain and function in FM.[17] Pharmaceutical options include low-dose tricyclic antidepressants at bedtime, SSRIs, NSAIDs, tramadol, pregabalin,

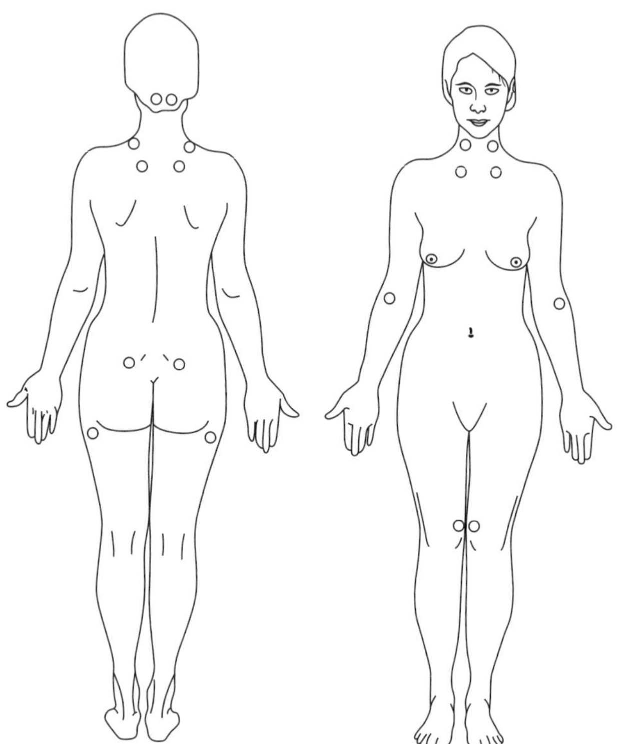

Figure 8-1 FM test areas.

duloxetine, and tender point injections. TENS, acupuncture, massage, and relaxation therapy are other options. The underlying depression should be addressed.

REFERENCES

1. Klippel J, ed. *Primer on the Rheumatic Diseases.* 13th ed. Atlanta, GA: Arthritis Foundation; 2008.
2. American College of Rheumatology. Criteria for Rheumatic Diseases. http://www.rheumatology.org/practice/clinical/classification/index.asp. Accessed January 7, 2011.
3. Ettinger WH. A randomized trial comparing aerobic exercise and resistance exercise with a health education program in older adults with knee OA [FAST]. *JAMA.* 1997;277:25-31.

4. Felsen DT, Zhang Y, Anthony JM, et al. Weight loss reduces the risk for symptomatic knee OA in women. The Framingham Study. *Ann Intern Med.* 1992;116:598-599.
5. Arthritis Foundation. Arthritis Foundation Self Help Program. http://www.arthritis.org/self-help-program.php. Accessed January 7, 2011.
6. Vargo MM. Contralateral vs. ipsilateral cane use. Effects on muscles crossing the knee joint. *Am J Phys Med Rehabil.* 1992;71:170-176.
7. ACR guidelines. Recommendations for the medical management of OA of the hip and knee: 2000 update. *Arthritis Rheum.* 2000;43:1905-1915.
8. Sawitzke AD, Shih H, Finco MF, et al. Clinical efficacy and safety of glucosamine, chondroitin sulphate, their combination, celecoxib or placebo taken to treat osteoarthritis of the knee: 2-year results from GAIT. *Ann Rheum Dis.* 2010;69(8):1459-1464.
9. Bailie AG, Lewis PL, Brumby SA, et al. The Unispacer knee implant: early clinical results. *J Bone Joint Surg Br.* 2008;90(4):446-450.
10. Aletaha D. 2010 rheumatoid arthritis classification criteria. *Arthritis Rheum.* 2010;62:2569-2581.
11. Smolen JS, Aletaha D, Bijlsma JWJ, et al. Treating rheumatoid arthritis to target: recommendation of an international task force. *Ann Rheum Dis.* 2010;69:631-637.
12. Saag KG, Teng GG, Patkar NM, et al. ACR 2008 recommendations for the use of nonbiologic and biologic disease modifying antirheumatic drugs in RA. *Arthritis Rheum.* 2008;59:762-784.
13. Molnar G, ed. *Pediatric Rehabilitation.* 3rd ed. Philadelphia, PA: Hanley & Belfus; 1999.
14. Gorman JD. Treatment of AS by inhibition of TNF-α. *N Engl J Med.* 2002;246:1349-1356.
15. Wolfe F, Smythe HA, Yunus MB, et al. The ACR 1990 criteria for the classification of fibromyalgia. *Arthritis Rheum.* 1990;33:160-172.
16. Wolfe F, Clauw DJ, Fitzcharles MA, et al. The American College of Rheumatology preliminary diagnostic criteria for fibromyalgia and measurement of symptom severity. *Arthritis Care Res.* 2010;62:600-610.
17. Wang C. A randomized trial of tai chi for fibromyalgia. *N Engl J Med.* 2010;365:743-754.

Chapter 9

OSTEOPOROSIS

OP is a systemic skeletal disease characterized by low bone mass, caused by an imbalance between bone resorption and bone formation, and microarchitectural deterioration of bone tissue, with a consequent increase in bone fragility.

The *WHO definition of OP* is a *t*-score (measured using DXA scan) of ≥2.5 SDs below the mean BMD value for young, healthy, white women (or *t*-score of ≤–2.5).[1] Patients who have already experienced ≥1 fracture are considered to have severe or "established" OP. *Osteopenia* is defined as a *t*-score between –1 and –2.5.[2] The WHO diagnostic classification should not be applied to premenopausal women, men younger than 50 years, or children. Instead of a *t*-score, the ISCD recommends using ethnic or race-adjusted *z*-scores, with *z*-scores of ≤–2.0 defined as either "low bone mineral density for chronological age" or "below the expected range for age" and those ≥–2.0 being "within the expected range for age."[3]

Risk factors for OP include advanced age (>50 years); female gender; Caucasian race; positive family history; smoking; immobilization; calcium deficiency; history of prior fractures; decreased estrogen, weight (<127 lbs), or BMI; alcohol use; and smoking.[2] Secondary causes of OP include disuse, hyperthyroidism, steroids, and heparin. Muscle pull is more important than weight bearing in disuse OP prevention.[4]

Supplements and Pharmacotherapy

The NOF guidelines recommend a *calcium* intake of ≥1,200 mg/day for all patients (including supplements if necessary) and 400 to 800 IU/day of *vitamin D*.[2] The NOF recommends pharmacotherapy in postmenopausal women and men over 50 years with the following: (1) *t*-score ≤–2.5 at the femoral neck or spine; (2) a hip/vertebral fracture; (3) *t*-score between –1.0 and –2.5 at the femoral neck or spine, a 10-year probability of a hip fracture ≥3%, or a 10-year probability of a major OP-related fracture ≥20% based on the US-adapted WHO algorithm.[2]

Estrogen is effective in studies with BMD and vertebral fractures as the primary outcome.[1] Hip and vertebral fracture risk is reduced with estrogen use in observational studies.[1] A *bisphosphonate* (ones that are FDA approved include alendronate, ibandronate, risedronate, and zoledronic acid) is recommended if HRT fails or is contraindicated/refused: there is a dose-dependent increase in spine and hip BMD; vertebral fracture risk is reduced by 30% to 50%.[1] The goal of *selective estrogen receptor modulators* (raloxifene) is to maximize the beneficial effect of estrogen on bone while minimizing the deleterious effects on breast and endometrium. Raloxifene has reduced vertebral fracture risk by 36% in large clinical trials.[1] *Salmon calcitonin* (100 IU IM/SQ qd) improves BMD and reduces vertebral fracture risk at the lumbar spine, but not at the hip.[5]

Nasal calcitonin (200 IU qd) has similar benefits, but is not as effective in treating bone pain as the injectable.[1]

Exercise and Rehabilitation

The NOF recommends an exercise prevention program, emphasizing weight bearing, of 45 to 60 minutes per day, four times per week.[2] Interventions to reduce the risk and/or impact of falls (e.g., appropriate assistive mobility devices, exercise programs, hip padding, and avoidance of medications affecting the CNS) may reduce hip fracture incidence. Poor back extensor strength correlates with a higher incidence of vertebral fractures.[6]

Acute vertebral fractures can be painful and are often managed with *bed rest, orthotic immobilization,* and *analgesics* (e.g., narcotics). NSAIDs should be used with caution. Spine surgery is reserved for rare cases involving neurologic deficits or an unstable spine. Vertebral injection of polymethyl methacrylate (i.e., *vertebroplasty*) anecdotally improves acute pain; it is unknown, however, if this rigid vertebral reinforcement increases the long-term risk of fracture of adjacent vertebrae.[1] *Postural training, back extensor exercises, pectoral stretching, walking,* or other weight-bearing exercises are key to rehabilitation. Rigid orthoses to limit spinal flexion (e.g., cruciform anterior spinal hyperextension [CASH] and Jewett) may reduce the risk of additional vertebral body fractures.

REFERENCES

1. Osteoporosis Prevention, Diagnosis, and Therapy. *NIH Consensus Statement* March 27-29. 2000;17:1-36.
2. Dawson-Hughes B, Looker AC, Tosteson AN, et al. The potential impact of new National Osteoporosis Foundation guidance on treatment patterns. *Osteoporos Int.* 2010;21:41-52.
3. International Society for Clinical Densitometry Official Positions. www.iscd.org.
4. Abramson AS. Influence of weight-bearing and muscle contraction in disuse OP. *Arch Phys Med Rehabil.* 1961;42:147-151.
5. Ahmed SF, Elmantaser M. Secondary osteoporosis. *Endocr Dev.* 2009;16:170-190.
6. Sinaki M. Can strong back extensors prevent vertebral fractures in women with osteoporosis? *Mayo Clin Proc.* 1996;71:951-956.

Chapter 10

THERAPEUTIC EXERCISE

Muscle Fiber Characteristics

Type I muscle fibers are "slow-twitch," highly fatigue-resistant, grossly dark fibers ("dark meat") that appear light on myosin ATPase (at pH 9.4) or PAS staining. *Type II* fibers comprise the "white meat" but are dark histologically with these stains (see Table 10-1 for characteristics of each type/subtype).

All fibers in a given motor unit are of the same type. According to the *Henneman size principle*, smaller motor units are recruited first and then progressively larger units are sequentially recruited as the strength of contraction increases.

EMG predominately records type I fiber activity. FES preferentially recruits type II fibers but may turn type IIs into type Is after long-term use. Steroids predominately cause type IIb fiber atrophy. Both types decrease with aging.

Strength Training

Isometric Strengthening – Tension is generated without visible joint motion or appreciable change in muscle length (e.g., pushing against a wall). This is most efficient when the exertion occurs at the resting length of the muscle and most useful when joint motion is contraindicated (e.g., s/p tendon repair) or in the setting of pain or inflammation (e.g., rheumatoid arthritis). Chance of injury is minimized. Isometric exercise should be avoided in the elderly and in patients with HTN due to its tendency to elevate BP.

Isotonic Strengthening – This is characterized by constant external resistance, but variable speed of movement. Examples include free weights,

TABLE 10-1 Characteristics of Skeletal Muscle Fiber Subtypes

	Type I: Slow oxidative	**Type IIa: Fast, oxidative glycolytic**	**Type IIb: Fast glycolytic**
Motor unit type	Slow fatigue resistant	Fast fatigue resistant	Fast fatigable
Oxidative capacity	High	Moderately high	Low
Glycolytic capacity	Low	High	Highest
Contractile speed	Slow	Fast	Fast
Fatigue resistance	High	Moderate	Low
Motor unit strength	Low	High	High

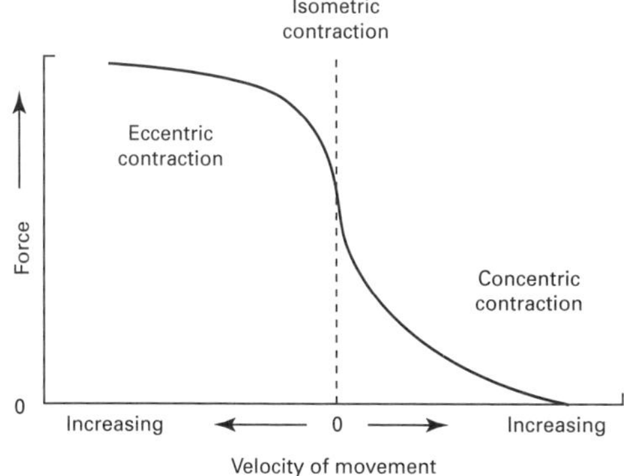

Figure 10-1 Forces are greatest with high-velocity eccentric contractions.

weight machines (e.g., Nautilus), calisthenics (e.g., pull-ups, push-ups, and sit-ups), and TheraBand. The equipment is readily available, but there is potential for injury with this type of exercise (Fig. 10-1).

Isokinetic Strengthening – This is characterized by a relatively constant angular joint speed, but variable external resistance. (Special equipment is required, e.g., Cybex and Biodex.) If the user pushes harder, the speed of the manipulated piece of equipment will *not* increase, but the resistance supplied by the machine will. This maximizes resistance throughout the length–tension curve of the exercised muscles and is beneficial in the early phases of rehabilitation. The chance of injury is relatively low (Fig. 10-2).

Progressive Resistive Exercise – In the *DeLorme method*, a 10-repetition maximum (RM) is first determined. Ten reps of the exercise are performed in sets of 50%, 75%, and 100% of the 10 RM. The sessions are performed

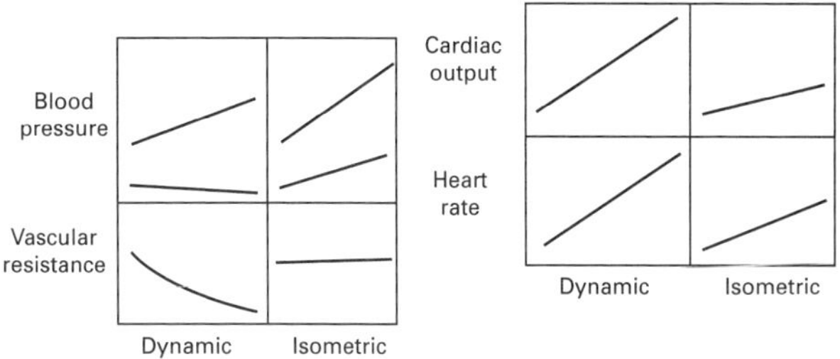

Figure 10-2 Acute hemodynamic responses to dynamic (isotonic) vs. isometric exercise.

≈3 to 5×/week and the 10 RM is redetermined ≈qwk. In the *Oxford technique*, the order of the sets is reversed, so that 10 reps at 100% of the 10 RM are performed first, followed by sets of 75% and 50%.

The *DeLorme axiom* posits that high-resistance, low-rep exercise builds strength, while low-resistance, high-rep exercise improves endurance.[1] deLateur[2] later demonstrated that for the most part, strength and endurance gains are equivalent for the two types of exercise as long as muscles are exercised to fatigue. High-resistance, low-rep exercise, however, achieves its results more efficiently (fewer reps/less time).

Moritani and de Vries[3] demonstrated that gains in the first few weeks of strength training were mostly due to neural factors (e.g., improved coordination of muscle firing) and not muscle hypertrophy.

Aerobic Exercise

Regular aerobic exercise increases Vo_2max and decreases resting BP, whereas strength training does *not* have an effect on either of these. Other long-term cardiovascular adaptations/benefits of aerobic exercise include *increased* stroke volume (SV), cardiac output (CO), work capacity, and HDL; and *decreased* resting HR, HR response to submaximal workloads, and triglyceride levels. Diabetic patients benefit from reduced obesity and insulin requirements. Improvements in mood, sleep, immune function, and bone density, among others, are also reported in the literature (Table 10-2).

Anaerobic threshold signifies the onset of metabolic acidosis during exercise, traditionally determined by serial measurements of blood lactate. It is noninvasively determined by assessment of expired gases during exercise testing, specifically pulmonary ventilation (VE) and carbon dioxide production (Vco_2). The anaerobic threshold signifies the peak work rate or oxygen consumption at which energy demands exceed circulatory ability to sustain aerobic metabolism.[4]

TABLE 10-2 Example of an Aerobic Exercise Program for a Presumably Healthy Individual[5]

Program phase	Week no.	Exercise dur/freq (per week)	Intensity (%Vo_2max)	Program phase	Week #	Exercise dur/ freq (per week)	Intensity (%Vo_2max)
Initial	1	12 min/3×	40–50	Improvement	6–9	21 min/3–4×	70–80
	2	14 min/3×	50		10–16	24 min/3–4×	70–80
	3	16 min/3×	60		17–23	28–30 min/4–5×	70–80
	4	18 min/3×	60–70		24–27	30 min/4–5×	70–85
	5	20 min/3×	60–70	Maintenance	28+	30–45 min/3×	70–85

Vo_2 is the body's rate of O_2 utilization (mL O_2/kg/min). Once Vo_2max is reached, further increases in work rate are powered by anaerobic (glycolytic) metabolism. Vo_2max can be calculated by the *Fick equation*: Vo_2max = max CO × (a-v O_2 difference), where CO = SV × HR.

The Exercise Prescription

Preexercise Evaluation – Physician evaluation should be comprehensive and include key elements of patient history, such as current and previous exercise patterns, motivations/barriers to exercise, discussion of risks/benefits of exercise, preferred types of activity, social support, and time and scheduling considerations. Special attention must be given to physical limitations, current and past medical problems, current medications, history of exercise-induced symptoms (shortness of breath, asthma, hives, and chest pain), and a thorough review of heart disease risk factors. These include family history of heart disease before age 50 years, DM, HTN, smoking, hyperlipidemia, sedentary lifestyle, and obesity.[4] Identify those in need of exercise stress testing as per AHA/ACSM guidelines.

Components of an Exercise Prescription – These five essential components apply when developing exercise prescriptions for persons of all ages and fitness levels. Careful consideration should be given to the individual's health status, medications, risk factors, behavioral characteristics, personal goals, and exercise preferences.

Mode is the particular form or type of exercise. The selection of mode should be based on the desired outcomes, focusing on exercises that are most likely to sustain participation and enjoyment.

Intensity is the relative physiologic difficulty of the exercise. Intensity and duration of exercise interact and are inversely related.

Duration (time) is the length of an exercise session.

Frequency refers to the number of exercise sessions per day and per week.

Progression (overload) is the increase in activity during exercise training, which, over time, stimulates adaptation.[4]

REFERENCES

1. DeLorme TL. Restoration of muscle power by heavy-resistance exercises. *J Bone Joint Surg Am.* 1945;27:645-667.
2. deLateur BJ. A test of the DeLorme axiom. *Arch Phys Med Rehabil.* 1968;49:245-248.
3. Moritani T, de Vries HA. Neural factors vs. hypertrophy in the time course of muscle strength gain. *Am J Phys Med Rehabil.* 1979;58:115-130.
4. Braddom RL, ed. *Physical Medicine and Rehabilitation.* 3rd ed. Philadelphia, PA: Elsevier; 2007.
5. American College of Sports Medicine. *ACSM's Guidelines for Exercise Testing and Prescriptions.* Baltimore, MD: Williams & Wilkins; 1995.

Chapter 11

MODALITIES

Essential Points of Prescription of Modalities

- Diagnosis
- Impairments/disabilities
- Precautions
- Modality
- Area to be treated
- Intensity/settings/temperature range
- Frequency of treatment
- Duration of treatment
- Goals/objectives of treatment
- Date of reevaluation

Selected Modalities

Heat – The therapeutic temperature range is 40° to 45° C. Heat should be maintained for 5 to 30 minutes. Superficial heat is considered to penetrate 1 to 2 cm; deep heat, 3.5 to 8 cm.

Conduction is transfer of heat by contact, for instance, paraffin baths and hot packs (e.g., Hydrocollator packs). Although paraffin bath temperatures are ≈52° to 54° C, poor heat conductivity allows tolerance. *Convection* involves the flow of heat, e.g., fluidotherapy, whirlpool, and moist air. Examples of conversion (where nonthermal energy is converted to heat) include infrared, US, SWD, and MWD. Infrared has a 2-cm depth penetration. US penetrates 3.5 to 8 cm; the greatest heating is at the bone–tissue interface. US parameters include a frequency of 0.8 to 1.1 MHz; intensity of 0.5 to 4 W/cm^2; treatment area of 100 cm^2; and duration of 5 to 8 minutes. SWD penetrates 4 to 5 cm; fat is heated more than muscle; the most commonly used frequency is 27.12 MHz. MWD is rarely used. Penetration is not as deep as SWD; the 915 MHz frequency penetrates deeper than 2,450 MHz.

Contraindications to heat therapy include acute hemorrhage or bleeding dyscrasia, inflammation, malignancy, insensate skin, inability to respond to pain, atrophic skin, and ischemia. Contraindications for *US* also include treatment over fluid-filled cavities (e.g., eyes and uterus) or near a pacemaker, laminectomy site, or joint prostheses. *SWD* should not be used in children (immature epiphyses) and persons with metallic implants, contact lenses, or menstruating/pregnant uteri. *MWD* should not be used over the eyes due to the risk of developing cataracts.

Cryotherapy – Cold, unlike heat, is limited to superficial applications only. The physiological effects of cold include hemodynamic vasoconstriction and slowing of NCV (via conduction block, i.e., C and A-δ fibers). Group

Ia firing rates are likewise decreased, reducing the muscle stretch reflex (and thereby reducing spasticity). Cold is *contraindicated* in the setting of ischemia, insensate skin, severe HTN, or cold sensitivity syndromes (i.e., Raynaud's syndrome, cryoglobulinemia, and cold allergy).

Traction

Cervical traction – About 25 to 30 lbs of force is recommended for cervical traction (of this, about 10 lbs is used to overcome the effects of gravity, i.e., the weight of the head). The intervertebral space is greatest at 30° of flexion; extension is not recommended due to vertebrobasilar insufficiency.

Lumbar traction – A force of 26% of the body weight is needed to overcome the effects of friction when lying supine with the hips and knees flexed.[1] An additional 25% of body weight is needed to achieve vertebral separation. A split lumbar traction table can essentially eliminate the frictional component. Although often prescribed for back pain (e.g., herniated disks and radiculopathy), the efficacy of this modality is not clear.

General *contraindications* for spinal traction include ligamentous instability, osteomyelitis, discitis, bone malignancy, spinal cord tumor, severe osteoporosis, and untreated HTN. Contraindications specific to *C-spine* traction include vertebrobasilar artery insufficiency, rheumatoid arthritis, midline herniated disk, and acute torticollis. Contraindications specific to *L-spine* traction include restrictive lung disease, pregnancy, active peptic ulcers, aortic aneurysm, gross hemorrhoids, and cauda equina syndrome.

TENS – Several theories explaining the mechanism of action of TENS exist. In the "gate theory" introduced by Melzack and Wall,[2] stimulation of large myelinated fibers (A-β and A-γ) excites interneurons in the substantia gelatinosa, which in turn exerts an inhibitory influence on lamina V, where the small unmyelinated A-δ and C pain fibers synapse with spinal neurons.

"Conventional" or high-frequency (50 to 100 Hz) TENS uses barely perceptible, low-amplitude, short-duration signals. Periodic adjustments to the pulse width and frequency may be necessary due to accommodations to the settings. *"Acupuncturelike"* TENS uses larger amplitude, low-frequency (1 to 4 Hz) signals that may be uncomfortable. β-Endorphin release may play a role in the analgesic effects. *Contraindications* to TENS include using near pacemakers (controversial), gravid uteri, and carotid sinuses.

Massage – Classic Western techniques include *effleurage* (stroking), *petrissage* (kneading), *tapotement* (percussion), and *Swedish* (tapotement + petrissage + deep tissue massage). *Deep friction massage* is used to break up adhesions in chronic muscle injuries. *Myofascial release* attempts to release soft tissue entrapped in tight fascia through the prolonged application of light pressure in specific directions. *Eastern techniques* include acupressure and Shiatsu massage.

Absolute contraindications to massage include malignancy, DVT, atherosclerotic plaques, and infected tissues. *Relative contraindications* include incompletely healed scar tissue, anticoagulation, calcified soft tissues, and skin grafts.

Phonophoresis – Topical medications (e.g., steroids and anesthetics) are mixed with an acoustic coupling medium, which are then driven into the tissue by US. Common uses include osteoarthritis, bursitis, capsulitis, tendonitis, strains, contractures, scar tissue, and neuromas.

Iontophoresis – Electrical currents are used to drive medications across biological membranes into the symptomatic areas, while theoretically avoiding the systemic side effects of the medications.

REFERENCES

1. Judovich BD. Lumbar traction therapy: elimination of physical factors that prevent lumbar stretch. *JAMA*. 1955;159:549-550.
2. Melzack R, Wall PD. Pain mechanisms: a new theory. *Science*. 1965;150:971-979.

Chapter 12

CONCUSSION

The term *mild traumatic brain injury* has generally been used synonymously with the word "concussion"; however, at the Third International Conference on Concussion in Sport, held in Zurich in 2008, "[the panel of experts] acknowledged that the terms refer to different injury constructs and should not be used interchangeably."[1] *Concussion* is defined as a complex pathophysiological process affecting the brain, induced by traumatic biochemical forces.[1] It may be caused by a direct blow to the head or any other part of the body that leads to impulsive forces transmitted to the head, causing the rapid onset of short-lived neurologic impairment, which may or may not involve the loss of consciousness.[1] Acute symptoms result from a functional disturbance rather than a structural brain injury, which is further supported by the absence of abnormalities on standard neuroimaging.

Concussions are metabolic injuries with cellular dysfunction as the culprit for the acute and subacute symptoms. Immediately after a concussion, there are multiple cascades of ionic, metabolic, and physiologic events. The earliest changes involve the release of excitatory amino acids and a large efflux of potassium causing hyperglycolysis. This is followed by persistent calcium influx thought to cause neurovascular contriction which protects the brain from massive swelling. These events result in an increase in energy demand but a decrease in energy supply, which leads to a cellular energy crisis.[2,3] It is this crisis that is thought to be the mechanism for postconcussive vulnerability because the brain is thought to be less equipped to respond to a second head injury leading to long-lasting effects. After hyperglycolysis, the brain experiences depressed metabolism, complicated by the persistent and elevated calcium levels, which may impair oxidative metabolism and activate pathways leading to cell death.[3] Animal models have shown that the metabolic dysfunction lasts up to 2 weeks; it is postulated that the period of derangement is longer in humans.[4]

Symptoms of concussion can be somatic, cognitive, and/or emotional. Headache is the most common symptom of concussion[5] and may develop immediately or minutes to hours after injury.[2] Loss of consciousness can occur but is relatively uncommon and, contrary to prior practice, is not a necessary sign for the diagnosis of concussion. In fact, confusion and retrograde and/or anterograde amnesia are the more common forms of altered mental status after a concussion,[2] with one study suggesting that amnesia is most predictive of postinjury difficulties and those with persistent memory deficits were more likely to have more symptoms, longer duration of symptoms, and poorer performance on neurocognitive tests.[6] One or more of the following additional symptoms and signs can be experienced or observed with a concussion: loss of consciousness, immediate motor phenomena, dizziness, blurry vision, poor balance, tinnitus, confusion, sleep disturbances, fatigue, slow mental processing, and mood disturbances.[7]

Resolution of symptoms, clinical and cognitive, occurs in a sequential order, with most adult concussions resolving in 7 to 10 days, and it is considered within normal limitations for symptoms to last up to 3 months postinjury.[8] Multiple studies have revealed that younger athletes are more likely to have a longer recovery time when compared with college and professional athletes.[9,10] There is also evidence suggesting that athletes with a history of multiple concussions may take longer to recover from a concussion.[11]

Postconcussion syndrome is a controversial term, lacking a generalized consensus among medical professionals on a universally accepted definition; it is a collection of symptoms occurring within the initial week of an injury and lasting up to 3 months or more. Signs and symptoms are the same as those associated with a concussion and cause social and vocational difficulties requiring a multidisciplinary team approach for testing and treatment. The team may consist of a neuropsychologist, physiatrist, neurologist, psychiatrist, and/or primary care physician providing the following resources: cognitive rehabilitation, psychotherapy, stress management, vocational counseling, and medications.[12]

Second impact syndrome (SIS), a term coined in 1984 by Saunders and Harbaugh,[13] is a rare occurrence where an athlete, still suffering from postconcussive symptoms from an initial head injury, sustains a second head injury that results in a loss of autoregulation of cerebral vasculature, leading to vascular engorgement, cerebral swelling, and brain herniation that is usually fatal. Other than boxers, reports of SIS have never been described in anyone older than 19 years of age. There is controversy over the actual incidence of SIS and little epidemiologic data about supporting the existence of SIS.[14] The United States has a higher incidence of cases among football players as compared with Australia. In Australia, the injury rate is higher but reported less.[14]

When evaluating an injured player, one must recognize the symptoms and signs of a concussion, which can be delayed for hours postinjury. Once a player shows any features of a concussion, they should be either medically evaluated on-site by a health care provider or removed from the game with urgent physician referral. Once first aid issues have been addressed on field and the player had been ruled out for more serious medical conditions, sideline evaluation of cognitive function should be assessed with the use of brief neuropsychological tests. There are many accepted neuropsychological assessment tools used in the acute and subacute settings; however, details of such studies are beyond the scope of this chapter. Further investigation of concussion does not involve neuroimaging unless there is a high suspicion for structural intracerebral injury, including, but not limited to, subdural or epidural hematomas.[1]

The essentials of *concussion management* are physical and cognitive rest until the symptoms resolve. During the period of recovery while the patient is still symptomatic, physical activity as well as activities requiring concentration and attention should be avoided because they may exacerbate symptoms and delay recovery.[1] No further intervention is required during this time of rest; however, pharmacological therapy is applicable when managing specific prolonged symptoms, commonly associated with cognition and mood; drug therapy may also be initiated to modify the underlying pathophysiological process of a concussion, although studies supporting this approach of treatment are based on severe brain injury and have not been established in mild traumatic brain injuries.[15]

There are factors, such as loss of consciousness, that are symptom modifiers, indicating additional cognitive and physical investigations and contributing to a more comprehensive management strategy. Age is a considerable modifying factor, as well as the loss of consciousness. Although it is not an appropriate measure of injury severity, prolonged loss of consciousness of more than 1 minute is a factor that may modify management.[1,16] Although not an exhaustive list, the following are additional modifying factors: number, duration, and severity of symptoms; concussive convulsions; frequency and timing between prior and current concussion, if applicable; age; comorbidities; behavior; medications; and type of sport or activity.[1]

There are numerous grading scales or guidelines for concussion management in athletes that are widely used by medical professionals, although only one scale is evidence based.[17] Most studies differ greatly in the relative importance of loss of consciousness. To date, no study has been evaluated by a double-blinded prospective study testing the validity of these numerous grading scales.[18] A correct assessment of the level of severity after concussion can only be made when symptoms have disappeared. Despite the controversies, the grading scales are still widely used to assist in acute management of the athlete, especially the Colorado and Cantu Guidelines (Table 12-1).[19,20]

TABLE 12-1 Concussion Grading Scales

Guidelines	Grade 1	Grade 2	Grade 3
Colorado	Confusion without amnesia No loss of consciousness	Confusion with amnesia No loss of consciousness	Loss of consciousness (of any duration)
Cantu	No loss of consciousness or Posttraumatic amnesia lasts longer than 30 min	Loss of consciousness lasts less than 1 min or Posttraumatic amnesia lasts longer than 30 min but less than 24 h	Loss of consciousness lasts more than 1 min or Posttraumatic amnesia lasts longer than 24 h or Postconcussion signs/ symptoms last longer than 7 days

Adapted from Lovell MR, Collins MW, Bradley J. Return to play following sports-related concussion. *Clin Sports Med.* 2004;23:421-441.

TABLE 12-2 Graduated RTP Protocol

Rehabilitation stage	Functional exercise at each stage of rehabilitation	Objective of each stage
1. No activity	Complete physical and cognitive rest	Recovery
2. Light aerobic exercise	Walking, swimming, or stationary cycling keeping intensity <70% MPHR No resistance training	Increased HR
3. Sport-specific exercise	Skating drills in ice hockey and running drills in soccer No head impact activities	Add movement
4. Noncontact training drills	Progression to more complex training drills (e.g., passing drills in football and ice hockey). May start progressive resistance training	Exercise, coordination, and cognitive load
5. Full contact practice	Following medical clearance, participate in normal training activities	Restore confidence and assessment of functional skills by coaching staff
6. RTP	Normal game play	—

HR, heart rate; MPHR, maximum predicted heart rate.

Adapted from McCroy P, Meeuwisse W, Johnston K, et al. Consensus statement on concussion in sport – the 3rd International Conference on Concussion in Sport, held in Zurich, November 2008. *J Clin Neurosci.* 2009;16:755-763.

At the Zurich Conference in 2008, the most recent "Return to Play" (RTP) protocol was established; it is a graded program of exertion that an athlete follows once they are symptom free. Each step is approximately 24 hours and the athlete progresses to the next level if they are asymptomatic, unless they develop postconcussive symptoms or signs that would then push them back to the previous asymptomatic level. In certain circumstances, adult athletes may RTP more rapidly, including same day of injury without risk of sequela, when assessment is performed by an experienced physician with appropriate and available resources.[21] It was only at the collegiate and high school levels where athletes were documented to have delayed onset of symptoms and neuropsychological deficits after injury (Table 12-2).[22,23]

REFERENCES

1. McCroy P, Meeuwisse W, Johnston K, et al. Consensus statement on concussion in sport – the 3rd International Conference on Concussion in Sport, held in Zurich, November 2008. *J Clin Neurosci.* 2009;16:755-763.
2. Lovell MR, Collins MW, Bradley J. Return to play following sports-related concussion. *Clin Sports Med.* 2004;23:421-441.

3. Giza CG, Hovda DA. The neurometabolic cascade of concussion. *J Athl Train.* 2001;36(3):228-235.
4. Hovda DA, Prins M, Becker DP. Neurobiology of concussion. In: Bailes JE, Lovell MR, Maroon JC, eds. *Sports-Related Concussion.* St. Louis, MO: Quality Medical Publishing; 1999:12-51.
5. Collins MW, Field M, Lovell MR, et al. Relationship between post-concussion headache and neuropsychological test performance in high school athletes. *Am J Sports Med.* 2003;31:168-173.
6. Collins MW, Iverson GL, Lovell MR, et al. On-field predictors of neuropsychological and symptom deficit following sports-related concussion. *Clin J Sport Med.* 2003;13:222-229.
7. Erlanger D, Kausik T, Cantu R, et al. Symptom-based assessment of the severity of concussion. *J Neurosurg.* 2003;98:34-39.
8. McCroy P, Johnston K, Meeuwisse W, et al. Summary and agreement statement of the 2nd International Conference on Concussion in Sport, Prague 2004. *Br J Sports Med.* 2005;39:196-204.
9. Field M, Collins MW, Lovell MR, et al. Does age play a role in recovery from sports-related concussion? A comparison of high school and collegiate athletes. *J Pediatr.* 2003;142(5):546-553.
10. Lovell MR, Collins MW, Iverson GL, et al. Recovery from mild concussion in high school athletes. *J Neurosurg.* 2003;98(2):296-301.
11. Moser RS, Schatz P, Jordan BD. Prolonged effects of concussion in high school athletes. *Neurosurgery.* 2005;57:300-306.
12. Legome EL. Postconcussive syndrome in emergency management. http://emedicine.medscape.com/article/828904-treatment. Accessed March 15, 2012.
13. Saunders R, Harbaugh R. The second impact in catastrophic contact-sports head trauma. *JAMA.* 1984;252:538-539.
14. Bey T, Ostick B. Second impact syndrome. *West J Emerg Med.* 2009;10(1):6-10.
15. McCroy P. Should we treat concussion pharmacologically? The need for evidence based pharmacological treatment for the concussed athlete. *Br J Sports Med.* 2002;36:3-5.
16. Lovell M, Iverson G, Collins M, et al. Does loss of consciousness predict neuropsychological decrements after concussion? *Clin J Sport Med.* 1999;9:193-199.
17. Cantu RC. Posttraumatic retrograde and anterograde amnesia: pathophysiology and implications in grading and safe return to play. *J Athl Train.* 2001;36:244-248.
18. Standaert CJ, Herring SA, Cantu RC. Expert opinion and controversies in sports and musculoskeletal medicine: concussion in the young athlete. *Arch Phys Med Rehabil.* 2007;88:1077-1079.
19. Colorado Medical Society School and Sports Medicine Committee. Guidelines for the management of concussion in sports. *Colo Med.* 1990;87:4.
20. Cantu RC. Guidelines for return to contact sports after a cerebral concussion. *Phys Sports Med.* 1986;14(10):75-83.
21. Pellman EJ, Viano DC, Casson IR, et al. Concussion in professional football: players returning to the same game – part 7. *Neurosurgery.* 2005;56:79-92.
22. Collins MW, Lovell MR, Iverson GL. Cumulative effects of concussion in high school athletes. *Neurosurgery.* 2002;51:175-181.
23. McCrea M, Guskiewicz KM, Marshall SW, et al. Acute effects and recovery time following concussion in collegiate football players. *JAMA.* 2003;290:2556-2563.

Chapter 13

CARDIAC REHABILITATION

INTRODUCTION

Under the broadened scope of the recent AHRQ guidelines, CR may include exercise programs, education and risk factor modification for secondary prevention, and psychosocial counseling.[1] CR is indicated after acute MI, coronary revascularization, and cardiac transplantation or in patients with CHF or chronic stable angina. CR improves Vo_2max, peripheral O_2 extraction, ST depression, exercise tolerance, subjective sense of well-being, and return to work rates. It also lowers BP, resting HR, and myocardial O_2 demand. In addition, CR has been shown to improve glycemic control and cause favorable lipoprotein changes (reducing TG and elevating HDL levels). Long-term moderate exercise in CR has been demonstrated to increase the quantity of mitochondrial enzymes in "slow twitch" muscle fibers and development of new muscle capillaries. Angiographic studies have shown reduced atherosclerotic lesions in stable angina patients undergoing intensive physical exercise and on low-fat diet over 1 year without lipid-lowering agents[2] (It should be noted that it has been traditionally stated that CR does *not* raise [improve] anginal threshold, whereas angioplasty and CABG can.) (Fig. 13-1).

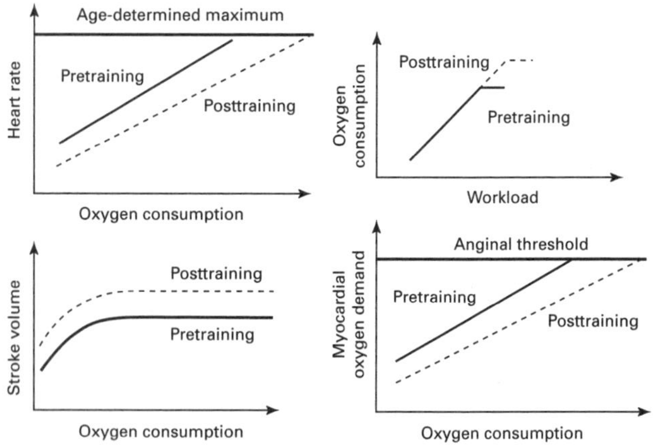

Figure 13-1 Benefits of CR. Compare pretraining (*solid lines*) with posttraining (*dashed lines*).

Adapted from Braddom RL, ed. *Physical Medicine and Rehabilitation.* Philadelphia, PA: WB Saunders; 1996.

Individual trials of CR after MI have *not* shown a statistically significant lower mortality rate in the CR groups, but a meta-analysis of 22 randomized trials (n = 4,554) has shown a benefit in overall mortality in the CR group (0.80 odds ratio vs. no CR) during a 3-year average post-MI period.[3]

Epidemiology

In 1997, 1.1 million Americans were diagnosed with acute MI, and 800,000 patients underwent coronary revascularization.[4] Limited data suggest that CR is a cost-effective use of medical care resources[1]; however, only 10% to 20% of appropriate candidates are thought to participate in formal CR programs.[4] In the Medicare claims analysis for hospitalizations during 1997 of over 250,000 persons older than 65 years, CR use was only 13.9% in patients hospitalized for acute MI and 31% in those who underwent CABG. Women, the very elderly, nonwhites, and patients with multiple comorbidities were even less likely to receive CR.[5] Low participation may be due to geographic factors and a failure of physicians to refer patients, particularly the elderly and women.

Phases of CR

Phase I – *The inpatient training phase* can begin from days 2 to 4 of hospitalization and typically lasts ≈1 to 2 weeks. Goals include prevention of the sequelae of immobilization, education and risk factor modification, independent self-care activities, and household distance ambulation on level surfaces. Protocol-limited submaximal stress testing is often done in uncomplicated patients prior to d/c as a guideline for outpatient ADLs and simple household activities.

Phase II – *The output training phase* starts 2 to 4 weeks post-d/c and typically lasts 8 to 12 weeks. Goals include increasing cardiac volume (CV) capacity and gradually returning to normal activity levels. A functional exercise tolerance (ECG stress) test is typically done 6 to 8 weeks of the postcardiac event (which allows time for the formation of a stable scar over the infarcted area) to guide the exercise prescription and determine eligibility for resuming work and sex.

Phase III – *The maintenance phase* is ideally a lifelong program of home- or gym-based exercise, aimed at maintaining or adding onto benefits obtained during phases I and II, generally under minimal or no clinical supervision.

Absolute contraindications for functional stress testing include recent change in resting ECG or serious cardiac arrhythmias, unstable angina, acute or worsening LV dysfunction, uncontrolled HTN, systemic illness, severe aortic stenosis, or severe physical disability precluding treadmill or arm ergometry use. *Relative contraindications* include hypertrophic cardiomyopathy, electrolyte abnormalities, moderate valvular disease, or significant arterial or pulmonary HTN.

Note: These contraindications for exercise stress testing are similar to the contraindications for CR in general.

The 2006 Centers for Medicare & Medicaid Services' expanded coverage for outpatient CR indications include the following:

- Acute MI within the preceding 12 months
- CABG
- Stable angina pectoris
- Heart valve repair/replacement
- PCI with or w/o stenting
- Heart or lung transplant

Note: Heart failure is currently not covered by most insurers, although it is recommended in the ACC/AHA Heart Failure Guidelines.

Exercise Prescription

The exercise prescription should address the type, intensity, content, and duration and frequency of exercise. *Isotonic, aerobic,* and rhythmic exercises involving large muscle groups should be emphasized. Isometrics and resistive exercise are relatively safe in patients with good LV function, but are contraindicated with CHF, severe valvular disease, uncontrolled arrhythmias, or peak exercise capacity <5 METs. (One MET is the metabolic equivalent of a unit of resting O_2 uptake, quantitated as 3.5 mL O_2 uptake/kg/min.) Maximum values of MET usually occur between the ages of 15 and 30 years and progressively decrease with age. However, they can be increased with conditioning and aerobic exercise. Twelve METs is seen in maximal exercise in young men; distance runners can average 18 to 24 METs, while 10 METs is generally equated with nonathletic, healthy middle-aged men.

The exercise content should include three phases. The first phase should involve a 5- to 10-minute warm-up. The warm-up should consist of flexible movement and stretching that gradually increase HR to target range. The subtle increase in O_2 demand minimizes exercise-related CV complications. The second phase is the conditioning or training phase and should be a minimum of 20 minutes up to the recommended 30 to 45 minutes of aerobic activity. Finally, the third phase is cooling down and should last anywhere from 5 to 10 minutes. This period involves low-intensity exercise allowing for recovery and dissipation of the heat load. Omitting this phase can result in decrease in venous return, reducing coronary blood flow while myocardial oxygen consumption remains elevated and can cause such complications as hypotension, angina, and ventricular arrhythmias.

Exercise intensity can be determined by a variety of methods, usually by calculating a "target" HR. The AHA method uses 70% to 85% of the maximum attained by stress testing. For young, healthy adults not undergoing formal exercise stress testing, 70% to 85% of (220 – age) can also be used for general exercise prescriptions, which is based on the assumption that 220 is the appropriate maximum for a newborn and that the maximum decreases ≈1 bpm/year. This latter formula, however, does *not* apply after MI.

The standard deviation for this equation is 10 to 15 bpm. Since this formula was derived from studies of men, it may overestimate the HR in women. Therefore, it may be more appropriate to measure the *peak exercise capacity* or the maximum ability of the CV system to deliver O_2 to exercising skeletal muscle and its ability to extract O_2 from the blood. Peak exercise capacity can be measured clinically by O_2 uptake (Vo_2), CO_2 production (Vco_2), and minute ventilation via gas analyzers during exercise. Maximal O_2 uptake eventually reaches a plateaulike effect despite increasing workload. *AT* is another index used to estimate exercise capacity. AT is defined as the point at which minute ventilation increases disproportionately relative to Vo_2 (often seen at 60% to 70% of Vo_2max). AT is an indicator of increase in lactic acid produced by working muscles and can be used to distinguish cardiac and noncardiac (pulmonary or musculoskeletal) causes of exercise limitation.

The *Karvonen formula* calculates a "heart rate zone," which is the resting HR in the sitting position *plus* 40% to 85% of (max HR determined by exercise tolerance testing minus resting HR). For deconditioned patients, the exercise program should begin at the lower end of the spectrum (i.e., 40% to 60%) and then increase as fitness improves.

Borg's RPE scale is particularly useful for cardiac transplant patients since denervation of the orthotopic heart makes HR parameters unreliable. The traditional Borg RPE scale is scored from 6 to 20, where 13 is rated as "somewhat hard" and corresponds with an exercise intensity sufficient to provide training benefits but still allow conversation during exercise. A score of 12 to 13 corresponds to about 60% of max HR; 15 corresponds to 85% of max HR. The Borg scale is probably more psychologic than physiologic, but encourages independence in exercise (i.e., phase III CR) as external monitoring devices are weaned off.

For patients on *β-blockers*, training at 85% of symptom-limited HR or 70% to 90% of the max workload determined by exercise testing is recommended.[6] Pacemakers do not necessarily preclude exercise training in a CR program.

Usual exercise duration/frequency is 20 to 30 minutes tiw × 12 weeks or more when training at 70% of the max HR. Shorter durations of training on a daily basis for very deconditioned individuals may also be helpful. In general, there is no contraindication to exercising everyday, but the likelihood of musculoskeletal injury increases.

The following risk stratification was developed by the AHA and is useful in determining the extent of medical supervision necessary for exercise training.

- Class A individuals are apparently healthy and have no evidence of CV risk with exercise.
- Class B individuals have established CHD that is clinically stable. They have low risk of CV complications with vigorous exercise.
- Class C individuals are at moderate risk of cardiac complications during exercise by virtue of history of multiple MIs or arrest, NYHA class III or IV CHF, <6 METs, or significant ischemia on exercise test.

- Class D individuals have unstable cardiac disease and require restriction of activity; exercise is contraindicated.

Note: Patients referred for cardiac rehab typically belong to classes B or C.

Postcardiac Event Sexual Counseling

Typical criteria for safe resumption of sexual activity after a cardiac event (i.e., MI or CABG) include a stable, asymptomatic patient and tolerance of exercise at 5 to 7 METs without abnormal ECG, BP, or HR changes. The time required is variable but is usually about 6 weeks postevent for sex with established partners in familiar positions. A useful clinical test is the *two-flight stair-climbing test*: walking for 10 minutes at 120 paces/min (≈3 m/h or 4.3 METs) and then climbing two flights of stairs (≈22 steps) in 10 seconds.

Sexual activities associated with sudden death in a cardiac patient include illicit affairs and sex after heavy meals and alcohol intake.

Miscellaneous

Sternal Precautions – Following sternotomy, typical instructions include no pushing, pulling, or lifting objects heavier than 5 to 10 lbs for 6 to 8 weeks. A "side-rolling" maneuver for getting out of bed is typically taught, and manual wheelchair propulsion is usually prohibited during this time as well.

Cardiac Precautions for Persons with CAD in Nonacute Inpatient Settings – Activity should be terminated if any of the following develops: new-onset cardiopulmonary symptoms; HR decreases >20% of baseline; HR increases >50% of baseline; SBP increases to 240 mm Hg; SBP decreases ≥30 mm Hg from baseline or to <90 mm Hg; DBP increases to 120 mm Hg.[7] These guidelines were developed by studying 64 physically disabled male patients with CAD using arm ergometers.[7] Individualized parameters for maximum or minimum HR and BP are also frequently used.

NYHA Classification (for CHF and angina)

I. >7 METs tolerated asymptomatically, without functional limitation.
II. <6 METs tolerated, but higher levels of activities cause symptoms.
III. Asymptomatic at rest and with most ADLs; >4 METs not tolerated.
IV. Symptomatic at rest and with minimal physical activities.

Considerations for CR Exercise in the Elderly

- Greater emphasis on warm-up activities including flexibility and ROM exercises, which help enable musculoskeletal and CV readiness.
- Cooldown activities are also of vital importance for the gradual decrease in peripheral vasodilation that can lead to hypotension, especially seen in the delayed baroreceptor responsiveness associated with aging.
- The elderly require a longer rest period in between exercises because of the slower return of exercise HR to resting HR.

– Aging is associated with decrease in skin blood perfusion, lowering the efficiency to sweat and regulate heat dissipation (temp. regulate) during exercise. Thus, a low-intensity exercise would be warranted for the elderly in hot/humid environments.

REFERENCES

1. Wenger NK. Clinical Guideline No. 17, AHCPR Publication No. 96-0672, 1995 (reviewed by the AHRQ, 2000).
2. Schuler G. Regular physical exercise and low-fat diet: effects on progression of CAD. *Circulation.* 1992;86:1-11.
3. O'Connor GT. An overview of randomized trials of rehabilitation with exercise after MI. *Circulation.* 1989;80:234-244.
4. Ades PA. Cardiac rehabilitation and 2° prevention of coronary heart disease. *N Engl J Med.* 2001;345:892-902.
5. Suaya JA, Shepherd DS, Normand SL, et al. Use of cardiac rehabilitation by Medicare beneficiaries after myocardial infarction or coronary bypass surgery. *Circulation.* 2007;116:1653.
6. Flores AM, Zohman LR. Rehab of the cardiac patient. In: DeLisa J, ed. *Rehabilitation Medicine: Principles and Practice.* 3rd ed. Philadelphia, PA: Lippincott-Raven; 1998:1347-1349.
7. Fletcher BJ. Cardiac precautions for non-acute inpatient settings. *Am J Phys Med Rehabil.* 1993;72:140-143.

Chapter 14

PULMONARY REHABILITATION

PR is a multidisciplinary program that provides persons with the ability to adapt to chronic lung disease.[1] Rehabilitation for patients with chronic lung conditions is well established and widely accepted as a means of alleviating symptoms and optimizing function.[2] In COPD, PR has been shown to improve dyspnea, exercise capacity, and health-related quality of life, while reducing health care utilization.[2] When considering PR interventions, the respiratory disorders can be generally characterized as *ventilatory* disorders (CO_2 retention) or *obstructive* disorders (oxygen impairment).[3]

The characteristics of obstructive and restrictive disorders are shown in Table 14-1.

VENTILATORY DISORDERS (RESTRICTIVE OR MECHANICAL DISORDERS)

Caused by

- neuromuscular disorders or skeletal disorders
- respiratory muscle function decreasing with a decrease in VC, RV, FRC, and TLC (e.g., myopathy, motor neuron disease, myelopathy, MS, and chest wall deformity)[4]

Keys to clinical monitoring include spirometry for VC and max insufflation capacity, peak cough flows, and noninvasive CO_2 monitoring. Expiratory flow should exceed 160 L/min ($\approx$3 L/s) for secretions to be adequately cleared from the airways.[3] If these flows cannot be achieved naturally, insufflation followed by a caregiver-provided abdominal thrust ("quad cough") or use of an *insufflator–exsufflator device* (CoughAssist,

TABLE 14-1 Characteristic Physiologic Changes Associated with Pulmonary Disorders

Measure	Obstructive disorders	Restrictive disorders	Mixed disorders
FEV_1/FVC	Decreased	Normal or increased	Decreased
FEV_1	Decreased	Decreased, normal, or increased	Decreased
FVC	Decreased or normal	Decreased	Decreased or normal
TLC	Normal or increased	Decreased	Decreased, normal, or increased
RV	Normal or increased	Decreased	Decreased, normal, or increased

From *The Merck Manual for Healthcare Professionals*, The Merck Manuals Online Medical Library.

Respironics) may be beneficial. Invasive suctioning is a less ideal alternative and must be used with caution.[4] With paralyzed abdominal muscles due to a UMN lesion, cough can be produced by FES.[4] Positive expiratory pressure mask therapy and autogenic drainage are additional methods to mobilize secretions.[4] *Glossopharyngeal breathing* can be used to maximize insufflation and can serve as a backup in the event of ventilator failure.[3]

Respiratory muscles can be aided by devices such as mouthpiece or nasal IPPV and intermittent IAPV. The latter can augment TV by 250 to 1200 mL. CPAP and BiPAP can be useful at night in patients with obstructive sleep apnea by keeping airways patent. Intubation, tracheostomy, and supplemental oxygen therapy are probably overutilized in patients with ventilatory disorders, whereas noninvasive assisted ventilation and assisted cough are probably underutilized.

Obstructive Disorders (Intrinsic Disorders)

These include COPD, asthmatic bronchitis, and cystic fibrosis, characterized by a decrease in VC, FEV_1, and MVV and an increase in RV, FRC, and TLC.[4] A PR program includes evaluating the nutritional state, optimizing pharmacologic management (e.g., anticholinergics, bronchodilators, steroid inhalers, and expectorants), supplemental O_2 use, controlled breathing methods (e.g., *pursed lip breathing* to help manage dyspnea), airway secretion management techniques, and an exercise program.[5]

Lower limb exercises and ambulation programs can greatly improve exercise tolerance and are strongly recommended for patients with COPD.[2] Additionally, high- and low-intensity programs, strength training, and endurance training are all considered clinically beneficial for patients with COPD.[2] Long-term psychological interventions, e.g., relaxation therapy, are yet to be proven beneficial in randomized controlled trials, but are supported by expert opinion.[2]

Supplemental home O_2 may be indicated when Po_2 is consistently ≤55 to 60 mm Hg. Medicare guidelines[6] for coverage of home O_2 generally require documentation of resting, sleep, or exercise Po_2 ≤55 mm Hg or Sao_2 ≤ 88% (on room air). Patients with Po_2 of 56% to 59% or Sao_2 of 89% may be eligible with concomitant CHF, pulmonary HTN, or other criteria. Long-term oxygen therapy has been shown to improve survival and quality of life in COPD.

Surgical options:

1. Lung volume reduction surgery
   a. Patients with advanced emphysema
   b. 20% to 30% of one or both lungs removed
   c. Found to reduce hyperinflation, improve FEV_1 and forced vital capacity (FVC), and improve quality of life[3]
   d. Suggested that patients first enroll in trial of PR
2. Lung transplant
   a. Used in children with cystic fibrosis and primary pulmonary HTN and adults with COPD, pulmonary HTN, and pulmonary fibrosis
   b. Smoking is an absolute contraindication

c. History of cancer, psychiatric diagnoses, obesity, and correctable coronary artery disease are relative contraindications.
d. Majority of the programs require some baseline functional exercise capacity – 600 feet by some patients and 250 feet by some other patients in the 6-minute walk test.[2]

REFERENCES

1. Ries AL. Pulmonary rehabilitation: Joint American College of Chest Physicians/ American Association of Cardiovascular and Pulmonary Rehabilitation evidence-based guidelines. *Chest.* 2007;131:4S-42S.
2. Braddom RL. *Physical Medicine and Rehabilitation.* 4th ed. Philadelphia, PA: Saunders; 2011.
3. Bach JR. Pulmonary rehabilitation. In: O'Young BJ, ed. *Physical Medicine and Rehabilitation Secrets.* 2nd ed. Philadelphia, PA: Hanley & Belfus; 2002;1359-1385.
4. Alba A, Chan L. Pulmonary rehabilitation. In: Braddom R, ed. *Physical Medicine and Rehabilitation.* 3rd ed. Philadelphia, PA: Saunders Elsevier; 2007;739-753.
5. Gonzalez P, Cuccurullo S. Pulmonary rehab. In: Cuccurullo, ed. *Physical Medicine and Rehabilitation Board Review.* New York, NY: Demos Medical Publishing; 2004; 535-608.
6. Medicare Carriers Manual, Claim Processing, Part 3. HCFA Publication 14-3: PB 94-954799; 1994.

Chapter 15

BURN REHABILITATION

- Secondary to external agents (heat, cold, chemicals, electricity, and radiation)
- #1 cause of accidental deaths in children under 2 years[1]
- Leads to hypermetabolic state

Depth/Degree

1. Superficial thickness (first degree): epidermis only
   - red and painful, heals spontaneously in 3 to 7 days
2. Partial thickness (second degree): 7 to 21 days to heal
   a. superficial: epidermis with blistering; basal layer remains intact
   b. deep: dermis involved with blistering
3. Full thickness (third degree): full epidermis and dermis involvement, with possible fat, muscle, or bone affected
   - eschar forms and requires debridement with grafting

Rule of 9's

	Adult TBSA (%)	Infant TBSA (%)
Head	9	18
Each upper extremity	9	9
Each lower extremity	18	14
Anterior trunk	18	18
Posterior trunk	18	18
Perineum	1	—

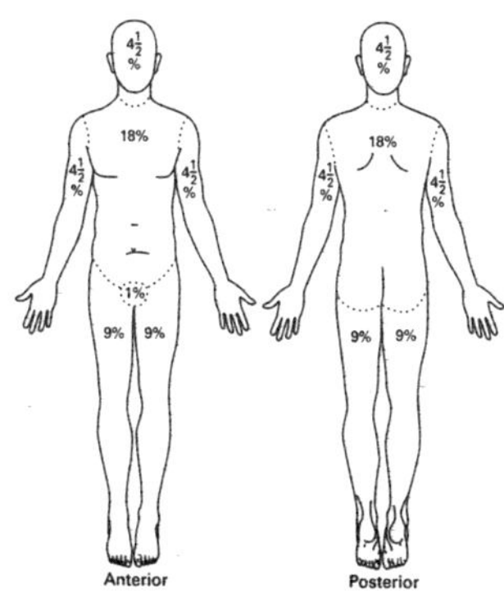

Figure 15-1 Diagram of the rule of 9's

Parkland Formula = 4 mL lactated Ringer's solution × body weight in kg × TBSA% burned

- Administer ½ the 24-hour total over the first 8 hours, ¼ over the next 8 hours, and the remaining ¼ over the last 8 hours

American Burn Association Classification

BSA	Partial thickness (%)	Full thickness (%)
Minor	<15	<2
Moderate	15–20	2–10
Major	>25	>10

Major burn also involves any insult to the eye, face, ear, or perineum or any electrical or inhalation injury.

Rehabilitation Goals

1. Limit loss of ROM
2. Reduce edema
3. Prevent contractures with positioning/splinting
   - including capsular contractions or shortening of tendons and muscles which cross joints
4. Scar management
   - hypertrophic scarring: present at ≥3 months after burn injury with ≥2 mm in thickness
   - more likely to occur if wounds take >2 weeks to heal
   - usually matures at 1½ years
   - need 25 mm of pressure to counteract the contraction of a scar

Positioning to Prevent Contracture

- Extension and abduction
- Prevent dependent edema
- Special beds (Kin Air, Roho)

Splinting – must be done in conjunction with mobilization

- examples: resting hand splint, knee extension with dorsiflexion of lower extremity, and elbow extension

Compression Garments

- decrease hypertrophic scarring
- blood flow reduced with pressure on capillaries, causing reduced scar formation
- 23 hours/day wearing schedule

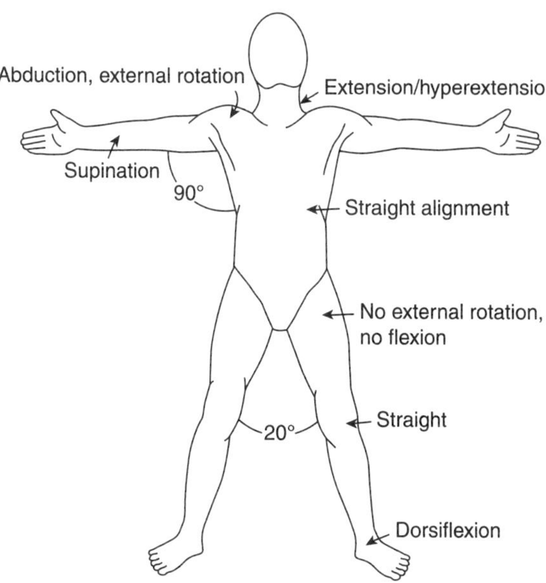

Figure 15-2 Proper positioning for patient with a burn injury.[2]

Nutrition

- 2,000 to 2,200 calories/day
- Supplements: Vit C, Vit A, zinc, copper, and manganese

Complications[3]

- peripheral neuropathy and multiple mononeuropathy
- bone/joint changes and osteophytes
- heterotopic ossification: elbow is the #1 site
- scoliosis/kyphosis
- subluxation/dislocation

REFERENCES

1. Esselman PC, Thombs BD, Magyar-Russell G, et al. Burn rehabilitation: state of the science. *Am J Phys Med Rehabil.* 2006;85:383-413.
2. Cuccurullo SJ, ed. Rehabilitation of burn issues. In: *Physical Medicine and Rehabilitation Board Review.* New York, NY: Demos Medical Publishing; 2002:791-800.
3. Esselman PC, Moore ML. Issues in burn rehabilitation. In: Braddom, RL, ed. *Physical Medicine and Rehabilitation.* 3rd ed. New York, NY: W.B. Saunders; 2006: 1399-1413.

Chapter 16

PHYSIOLOGICAL CHANGES WITH AGING

Muscle

- *Aging:* Muscle power decreases by 3.5% per year and muscle strength decreases by 1.4% to 2.5% per year after the age of 60 years
- *Immobility:* Loss of 1% to 3% strength per day

Gait (Decline in speed)

- Decline of 0.2% per year up to age 63 years and 1.6% per year after 63 years
- Typically increased double limb support, slower speed, shorter stride length, and broader base of support

Bone

- Age plays a role in the rate of bone turnover
- Osteoporosis: *t*-score < –2.5
- Osteopenia: *t*-score between –1.0 and –2.5

Cardiovascular

- With aging
  - Left ventricular hypertrophy
  - Increased systolic blood pressure
  - Decreased
    - Arterial compliance
    - Baroreceptor sensitivity
    - Sinoatrial node automaticity
- With immobility
  - Resting tachycardia (HR increases ≈1 bpm q2d)
  - Inordinate HR responses to submaximal exercise
  - Decreased
    - Stroke volume
    - Cardiac output
    - Vo_2max
    - Postural hypotension (HR ↑ by ≥20 bpm and SBP ↑ ≥20 mm Hg upon rising)

Pulmonary

- Decreased lung compliance
- Decreased vital capacity

Genitourinary

- Decreased
  - Renal blood flow
  - GFR
  - Bladder distensibility

Gastrointestinal

- Decreased food intake due to
  - Diminished taste odor
  - Slow gastric emptying
  - Diminished central feeding drive
  - Dysphagia
- Change in hepatic metabolism, which changes drug clearance

RECOMMENDED READING

Braddom RL. *Physical Medicine and Rehabilitation*. Philadelphia, PA: Elsevier-Saunders; 2011.

Chapter 17

ELECTRODIAGNOSTIC STUDIES

Electrodiagnostic studies (also known as NCS/EMG or sometimes just EMG) include nerve conduction studies (NCSs or NCVs) and EMG. Other less commonly performed electrodiagnostic tests include somatosensory evoked potentials, brainstem auditory evoked potentials or responses, single-fiber EMG (SFEMG), repetitive stimulation studies, and sympathetic skin response. This discussion is limited to the most commonly used studies, NCS and EMG. As they are usually performed together and reported as one comprehensive report, they will be referred to as a single test (NCS/EMG). This test provides physiologic information about nerves and muscles in real time. It gives information about muscle and nerve function, unlike most radiologic studies, which give a static picture of anatomy and do not directly assess function.

Indications for electrodiagnostic testing include numbness, tingling/paresthesias, pain, weakness, atrophy, depressed deep tendon reflexes, and/or fatigue. EMG/NCS can serve as an important part of a patient's clinical picture. Electrodiagnostic tests are used to (1) establish a correct diagnosis, (2) localize a lesion, (3) determine the treatment when a diagnosis is already known, and (4) provide information about the prognosis.[1] NCS/EMG should be considered an extension of a good history and physical examination.

Initial Settings for NCS

Sweep speed is the horizontal axis on the recording in units of time (milliseconds [ms]). *Gain* is the vertical axis on the graph in units of voltage (millivolts [mV] for motor studies or microvolts [μV] for sensory studies).

Motor settings: sweep – 2 ms/division, gain – 5 mV/division.
Sensory settings: sweep – 2 ms/division, gain – 20 μV/division.[1]

Initial settings for EMG

Sweep speed: 10 ms/division
Low-frequency filter: 10 to 30 Hz
High-frequency filter: 10,000 to 20,000 Hz
Amplifier sensitivity: 50 to 100 μV[1]

Introduction to NCS

NCS is the recording of an electrical response of a nerve (via an electrode over that nerve or a muscle) that is stimulated (electrically depolarized using a probe) at one or more sites along its course. The action potential (AP) that is propagated is the summative response of many individual axons or muscle fibers. For motor nerves, this response is called a compound motor action potential (CMAP) and represents the summative response of motor units (MUs) that are firing. CMAPs are usually recorded in mV. For sensory nerves, the response is called an SNAP and represents the summation of individual sensory nerve fibers. SNAPs are very small-amplitude potentials that are usually recorded in μV. Late responses (evoked potentials that record over a very long pathway) include F waves and H-reflexes. *Orthodromic* refers to conduction in the same direction as occurs physiologically (i.e., a sensory fiber conducts from the extremity toward the spine). *Antidromic* refers to conduction in the opposite direction to the physiological direction.

Components of the AP

Latency is the time it takes from stimulation to the beginning of the AP (the speed of transmission). The latency of a sensory nerve is dependent on the conduction speed of the fastest fibers and the distance it travels. The latency of a motor nerve also includes the time it takes for the AP to synapse at the NMJ and the speed of conduction of the electrical potential through the muscle. Since there is no myoneural junction of sensory nerves, the latency of a sensory nerve is directly related to the conduction velocity (CV). Latency measurement requires standardized and accurately recorded distance or else the results are meaningless.

Conduction velocity reflects how fast the nerve AP is propagating. In sensory studies, the velocity is measured directly from the time it takes the AP to travel the measured distance (distance/latency). In a motor nerve, two different sites have to be stimulated to calculate the velocity (velocity = change in distance/change in time) and account for the myoneural junction. The presence of a myelin covering speeds up NCV via a process known as saltatory conduction. Myelinated nerves conduct impulses approximately 50 times faster than unmyelinated nerves. In myelinated nerves, the CV is primarily dependent on the integrity of the myelin covering. Slowing or latency prolongation usually implies demyelination.

Amplitude correlates with axonal integrity. Decreased amplitude could indicate an axonal lesion (if the amplitude is decreased both distally and proximally) or it can indicate a conduction block across the site of injury (if the amplitude is low distally and not proximally).[2,3]

TYPES OF NERVE INJURIES

Nerve injuries can be classified depending on whether there is injury to the axon, the myelin, or both. Often, especially with trauma, the affected structures do not always fit into one category. It is the job of the electromyographer to diagnose and communicate the type of injury that exists, the severity, and the location. Seddon proposed a classification of nerve injuries in 1943 that is still commonly used as it correlates well with electrophysiology:

1. **Neurapraxia** – defined as conduction block. This type of nerve injury occurs in the peripheral nerve with minor contusion or compression. There is preservation of the axon; only the myelin is affected. The transmission of APs is interrupted for a brief period, but recovery is usually complete in days to weeks.
2. **Axonotmesis** – more significant injury: breakdown of axon with accompanying Wallerian degeneration distal to the lesion. There is preservation

of some of the supporting connective tissue stroma (Schwann cells and endoneurial tubes). Regeneration of axons (through collateral sprouting or axonal growth) can occur with good functional recovery, depending on the amount of axonal loss.

3. **Neurotmesis** – severe injury with complete severance of the nerve and its supporting structures; extensive avulsing or crush injury. The myelin, axon, perineurium, and epineurium are all disrupted. Spontaneous recovery is not expected.

Injury to the myelin can be focal (local), uniform (throughout the nerve), or segmental (affecting some parts of the nerve but not others):

1. *Uniform demyelination* – slowing of CV along the entire nerve (e.g., Charcot-Marie-Tooth disease).
2. *Segmental demyelination* – uneven degree of demyelination in different areas along the course of the nerve; may have variable slowing (temporal dispersion).
3. *Focal nerve slowing* – localized area of demyelination causing nerve slowing; decreased CV is noted across the lesion.
4. *Conduction block* – severe focal demyelination that prevents propagation of the AP through the area. There will be more than 20% amplitude decrement when the nerve is stimulated proximal to the lesion. The distal CMAP amplitude remains intact. Clinically, conduction block presents as weakness.

Axonal injuries will lead to Wallerian degeneration distal to the lesion. Low-amplitude CMAPs will be noted with both proximal and distal stimulation. On EMG, abnormal spontaneous potentials (fibrillations [fibs] and positive sharp waves [PSWs]) are seen. The MU recruitment will be decreased (increased firing frequency of existing MUs). With reinnervation, MUs may become polyphasic with high amplitude and long duration.[4,5]

H-Reflex

The *H-reflex* (Hoffmann reflex) is a true reflex and is the electrical equivalent of the monosynaptic or oligosynaptic stretch reflex. It is a sensitive but nonspecific tool for possible S1 radiculopathy, especially when clinical, radiologic, and electrophysiologic signs of motor root involvement are lacking. In some cases, it may be the only abnormal study. The H-reflex is usually elicited by submaximally stimulating the tibial nerve in the popliteal fossa. Such stimulation can be initiated by using slow (less than 1 pulse/s), long-duration (0.5 to 1 ms) stimuli with gradually increasing stimulation strength. The stimulus will travel along the most excitable Ia afferent nerve fibers, through the dorsal root ganglion (DRG). It then gets transmitted across the central synapse to the anterior horn cell, which then sends it down along the alpha motor axon to the muscle. Hence, the H-reflex is a measure of the time it takes for the orthodromic sensory response to get to the spinal cord proximally and the orthodromic motor response to reach the muscle distally (on which the recording electrode is placed). A generally acceptable result would be a motor response usually between 0.5 and 5 mV in amplitude and a latency of 28 to 30 ms. H-reflex studies are usually performed bilaterally because asymmetry of responses is an important criterion for abnormality. An abnormal latency greater than 0.5 to 1.0 ms (as compared with the other side) or H-reflex absence in patients under 60 years may suggest a lesion along the H-reflex pathway (afferent and/or efferent fibers). This may be due to an S1 radiculopathy. The standard formula for calculating the H-reflex is 9.14 + 0.46 (leg length in cm from the medial malleolus to the popliteal fossa) + 0.1 (age). For a patient older than 60 years, 1.8 ms will be added to the total calculated value.

In normal infants or adults with UMN (corticospinal tract) lesions, the H-reflex may be elicited in muscles other than the gastrocnemius/soleus muscles or flexor carpi radialis. It is often absent in patients older than 60 years. The reflex can be potentially inhibited by antagonist muscle contractions and initiated by agonist muscle contractions.

The H-reflex does have some limitations. It is unable to distinguish between acute and chronic lesions, may be normal with incomplete lesions, is diluted by focal lesions, and is nonspecific in terms of injury location. Once the H-reflex is found to be abnormal, it will usually remain so, even with resolution of symptoms.

F Waves

F wave or F response is a small-amplitude, variable-latency late motor response that occurs following the activation of motor nerves. It derives its name from the word "foot" because it was first recorded from the intrinsic foot muscles. Unlike the H-reflex, the F wave does not represent a true reflex because there is no synapse from an afferent impulse to a motor nerve. Depolarizing peripheral nerves with external stimuli evokes potentials propagating both proximally and distally. Electrical stimulation of a peripheral nerve results in an orthodromic CMAP. In addition, the proximally (antidromically) propagating potential activates a small percentage of anterior horn motor neurons. In turn, this generates an orthodromic motor response (the F wave) along the same axon that activates a few muscle fibers picked up by the recording electrode.[6,7]

F waves can be obtained from any muscle by a supramaximal stimulus. Because of their variability (as opposed to H-reflexes), multiple stimulations must be used to obtain the shortest latency. F waves may be useful in the evaluation of peripheral neuropathies with predominantly proximal involvement, such as Guillain-Barré syndrome and chronic inflammatory demyelinating polyneuropathies, in which distal conduction velocities may be normal early in the disease. However, the value of the F wave in evaluating focal nerve lesions, such as radiculopathy or peripheral nerve entrapment, is extremely limited largely due to the variability of F-wave responses. In addition, most muscles receive innervation from multiple roots, so the fastest (nonaffected) fibers will be normal, as well as the fact that the results are nonspecific. It is a pure motor response, and its long neural pathway dilutes focal lesions and hinders the specificity of injury location. F waves are also generally not seen in nerves where the CMAP amplitude is severely reduced, such as severe axonal loss, since the F-wave amplitude is only 1% to 5% of the amplitude of the CMAP.

Normal latency of F wave: upper limb: 28 ms; lower limb: 56 ms. Side-to-side difference: <2.0 ms for upper limbs; <4.0 ms for lower limbs.

Blink Reflex

The most complicated of the late responses is the blink reflex. It is the electrophysiologic correlate of the corneal reflex. The sensory afferent limb of the reflex is the supraorbital nerve, a branch of the ophthalmic division of the trigeminal nerve (CN V_1). Intervening synapses (pons and medulla) are stimulated. The motor efferent limb is the facial nerve (CN VII), which innervates the orbicularis oculi muscle. As with the corneal reflex, stimulation of one side of the supraorbital branch of the trigeminal nerve elicits a motor response (eye blink) bilaterally through the facial nerves. Abnormalities anywhere along the reflex arc (central or peripheral) can be detected.

There is an early response (R1) due to a disynaptic reflex arc from the ipsilateral sensory nucleus of V to the ipsilateral facial nerve. There is also a late response (R2) due to multiple interneurons connecting the ipsilateral sensory nucleus of V to the ipsilateral spinal motor nucleus of V and then to the bilateral facial nuclei.

Recording electrodes are placed below and slightly lateral to the pupils bilaterally. Reference electrodes are placed just lateral to the lateral canthus bilaterally. The ground can be placed on the chin. The stimulator is placed over the medial supraorbital ridge of the eyebrow. The sweep speed should be 5 or 10 ms with initial sensitivity of 100 or 200 μV.

Normal latency for R1 response is <13 ms. Normal latency for ipsilateral R2 is <41 ms. Normal latency for contralateral R2 is 44 ms. Acceptable normal bilateral variation for R1 is <1.2 ms, for ipsilateral R2 is <5 ms, and for contralateral R2 is <7 ms (Table 17-1).

TABLE 17-1 Basic Abnormal Patterns[a]

Lesion	Electrodiagnostic pattern if affected side stimulated	Electrodiagnostic pattern if unaffected side stimulated
Unilateral CN V	Delayed (partial injury) or absent (complete injury) R1 and bilateral R2	Normal R1 and bilateral R2
Unilateral CN VII	Delayed or absent R1 and ipsilateral R2	Delayed or absent contralateral R2
Unilateral midpontine	Delayed R1 and normal bilateral R2	Normal R1 and bilateral R2
Unilateral medullary	Delayed ipsilateral R2	Delayed contralateral R2
Demyelinating peripheral neuropathy	Possible delay or absence of R1 and bilateral R2	Possible delay or absence of R1 and bilateral R2

[a]Using the anatomy outlined above and these basic patterns, complex and bilateral lesions can be extrapolated.

Preston DC, Shapiro BE. Blink reflex. In: *Electromyography and Neuromuscular Disorders.* 2nd ed. Philadelphia, PA: Elsevier; 2005:59-64.

EMG Including Monopolar versus Concentric Needle

EMG testing involves evaluation of the electrical activity of skeletal or voluntary muscles. Muscles contract and produce movement through the orderly recruitment of MUs. An MU is defined as one anterior horn cell, its axon, and all the muscle fibers innervated by that motor neuron. An MU is the fundamental structure that is assessed in EMG testing. EMG requires a thorough knowledge of the anatomy of the muscle being tested in order to place the needle electrode in the appropriate muscle.

Monopolar needles are 22G to 30G Teflon-coated stainless steel needles with an exposed tip of 0.15 to 0.2 mm^2 (Fig. 17-1A). They require a surface electrode or a second needle as a reference lead. Another surface electrode serves as a ground. A monopolar needle records the voltage changes between the tip of the electrode and the reference. Since it picks up from a full 360° field around the needle, it registers larger amplitude and has increased polyphasicity when compared with the concentric needle. The smaller diameter and the Teflon coat make the monopolar needle less uncomfortable. This, combined with its cost advantage over the concentric, has led to its preferential clinical use.

Concentric needles are 24G to 26G stainless steel needles (Fig. 17-1B). The needle comprises a reference (cannula) electrode with a bare inner

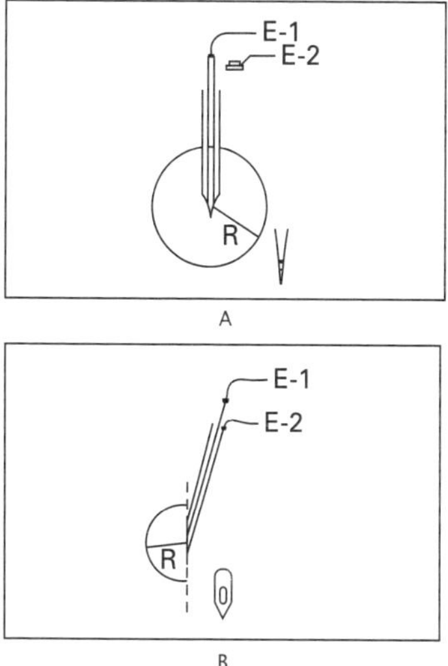

Figure 17-1 Needle electrodes. **A.** Monopolar needle. **B.** Concentric needle.

Adapted from Dumitru D, ed. *Electrodiagnostic Medicine.* 2nd ed. Philadelphia, PA: Hanley & Belfus; 2002.

wire in the center of the shaft that is the recording electrode. The concentric needle can register the voltage changes between the wire and the shaft. The pointed tip of the needle has an oval (beveled) shape. Since the exposed active recording electrode is on the beveled portion of the cannula, the concentric needle picks up from a 180° field. Therefore, it registers smaller amplitude (since it has a smaller recording area). A separate surface electrode serves as the ground.

Effects of Temperature and Age on NCS

Cooling is thought to prolong the opening of Na^+ channels.[8,9] Decreasing the temperature of a limb affects SNAPs and CMAPs by prolonging latency, decreasing CV, and increasing amplitude and duration. CV decreases 2.4 m/s per 1° C decrease. Correction formulas exist but the best approach is to warm the limb prior to the NCS (32° in the upper limbs and 30° in the lower limbs).

As patients age, SNAP and CMAP amplitudes decrease and latencies increase. Motor NCSs for newborns are 50% of adult values since myelination is incomplete. Normal adult values are attained by age 5 years. After age 60 years, there is a progressive decline of 1 to 2 m/s per decade in the NCS of the fastest motor fibers.

The Needle EMG Examination

The EMG evaluation typically has four components:

1. Insertional activity
2. Activity at rest
3. MU analysis
4. Recruitment

Insertional Activity

Healthy muscle is electrically silent at rest. Insertional activity[8,9] refers to the brief electrical activity associated with the needle entering the sarcolemma, which causes muscle fiber injury. The associated sound should be crisp. Insertional activity is classified in three ways:

1. *Normal insertional activity* only lasts a few hundred milliseconds and is due to muscle depolarization.
2. *Increased insertional activity* occurs due to denervation or cell membrane irritability and lasts >300 ms. There may be evidence of initially positive deflection waveforms that do not persist. If these positive waveforms are sustained and fire regularly, they are considered abnormal spontaneous potentials (see below).
3. *Decreased insertional activity* occurs when the needle is placed into atrophied muscle, fat, or edema and lasts <300 m/s.

Activity at Rest

NORMAL SPONTANEOUS ACTIVITY

A needle should be inserted into a muscle at three to four different depths and in three to four different directions (examining three or four electrically discrete areas of muscle) for insertional activity and activity at rest. The needle can be withdrawn almost to the skin and then redirected in a different direction, again stopping at three or four different depths. This can be repeated so that the needle examines about 12 to 16 discrete areas of the muscle (depending on the patient's tolerance).

- After insertion of the needle into normal muscle at rest, there should be electrical silence (Fig. 17-2A).
- Normal muscle may also display end plate activity. This occurs after a needle is placed in the region of the NMJ or end plate. The needle should be moved out of the end plate, as the clinician cannot get reliable information about the muscle. Either of two waveforms may occur: miniature end plate potentials (MEPPs) or end plate potentials (EPPs). The patient may complain of increased pain. It is important to recognize these potentials so that they are not misinterpreted as abnormal spontaneous potentials.
  - MEPPs – Represent spontaneous release of single quantum of acetylcholine (ACh) at the presynaptic terminal that manifests as end plate noise (Fig. 17-2B).
  - EPPs or "end plate spikes" – Represent single muscle fiber depolarizations at the presynaptic terminal with resultant release of large amounts of ACh (Fig. 17-2C).
- MEPPs and EPPs may or may not be present together (Fig. 17-2D).

ABNORMAL SPONTANEOUS ACTIVITY

- Usually represents pathology (injury or denervation) that stems from a muscle or nerve. These spontaneous depolarizations have an abnormal morphology and firing pattern.
- Examples of *muscle fiber*–generated spontaneous potentials: Fibs triphasic with initial positive (downward) deflection, PSWs biphasic with positive deflection, myotonic discharges, and complex repetitive discharges (CRDs).

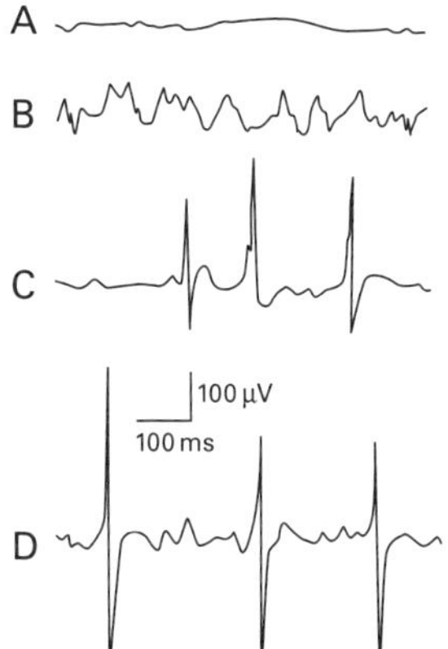

Figure 17-2 End plate activity.

Adapted from Dumitru D, ed. *Electrodiagnostic Medicine.* 2nd ed. Philadelphia, PA: Hanley & Belfus; 2002.

Courtesy of DeLisa JA, ed. *Manual of Nerve Conduction Velocity and Clinical Neurophysiology.* 3rd ed. New York, NY: Raven Press; 1994.

- Examples of *neural*-generated spontaneous potentials: Myokymic discharges, cramps, neuromyotonic discharges, tremors, fasciculations, and multiple MU potentials.
- Fibs and PSWs appear 3 weeks or more after injury.
- Abnormal spontaneous potentials are usually of small amplitude. Therefore, the gain on the EMG machine should be set to 50 to 100 μV for the best visualization (Fig. 17-3).

Grading of fibs and PSWs is from 0 to 4+, with a sweep of 10 ms/division

(0) no fibs or PSWs present
(1+) one fib/PSW per screen persistent within two areas
(2+) fibs/PSWs in *greater than two areas,* about two per screen
(3+) fibs/PSWs in most muscle regions, greater than half of the screen
(4+) fibs/PSWs in all areas of the muscle and fill the entire screen

Fasciculation potentials originate from a single MU and may have an intermittent or a normal firing pattern. When associated with PSWs or fibs, they suggest pathology. In the absence of fibs or PSWs, they may be due to stress, fatigue, or caffeine (Fig. 17-4).

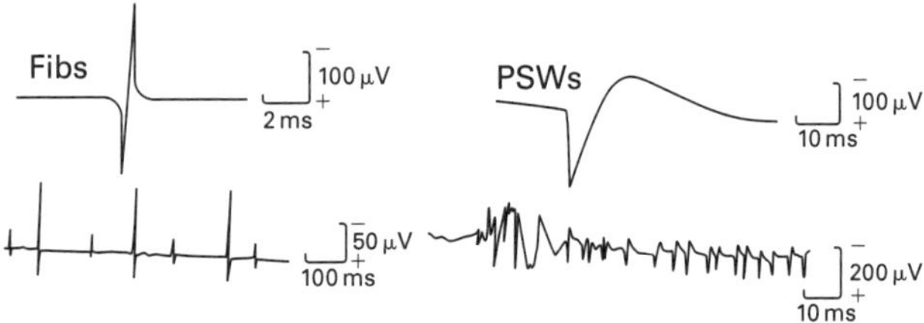

Figure 17-3 Fibs and PSWs.

Adapted from DeLisa JA, ed. *Manual of Nerve Conduction Velocity and Clinical Neurophysiology.* 3rd ed. Baltimore, MD: Raven Press; 1994.

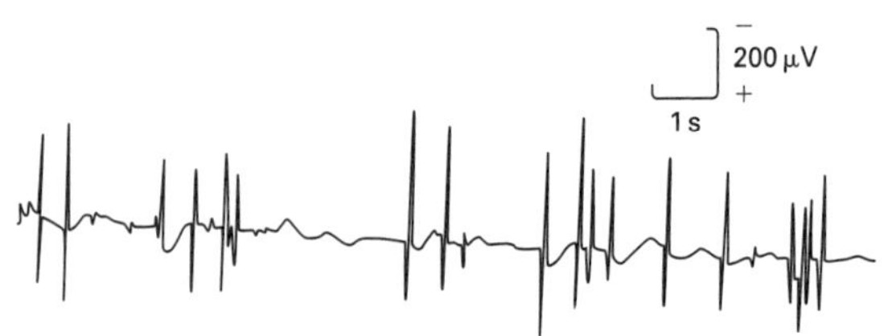

Figure 17-4 Fasciculation potentials.

Adapted from DeLisa JA, ed. *Manual of Nerve Conduction Velocity and Clinical Neurophysiology.* 3rd ed. Baltimore, MD: Raven Press; 1994.

CRDs frequently result from denervation and reinnervation through collateral sprouting. Their presence suggests a chronic process such as chronic radiculopathy, peripheral neuropathy, anterior horn disease, polymyositis, or myxedema (Fig. 17-5).

Myotonic discharges (Fig. 17-6) originate in the muscle due to membrane instability. They have a characteristic waxing and waning character and have been compared with a dive-bomber sound. They are commonly seen in myotonic dystrophy, myotonia congenita, polymyositis, chronic radiculopathy, peripheral neuropathy, maltase deficiency, and hyperkalemic periodic paralysis (Table 17-2).

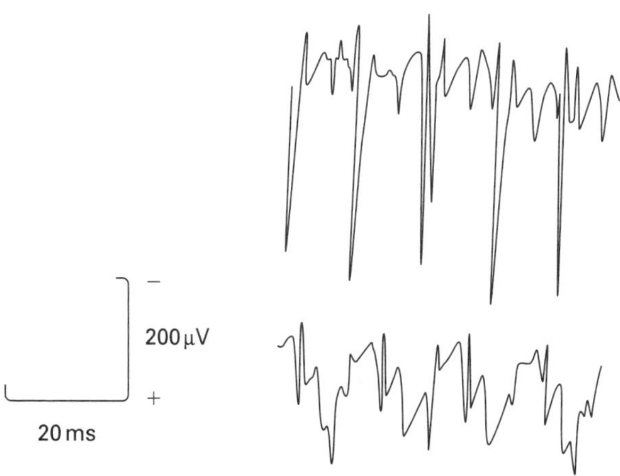

Figure 17-5 CRDs.

Adapted from DeLisa JA, ed. *Manual of Nerve Conduction Velocity and Clinical Neurophysiology.* 3rd ed. Baltimore, MD: Raven Press; 1994.

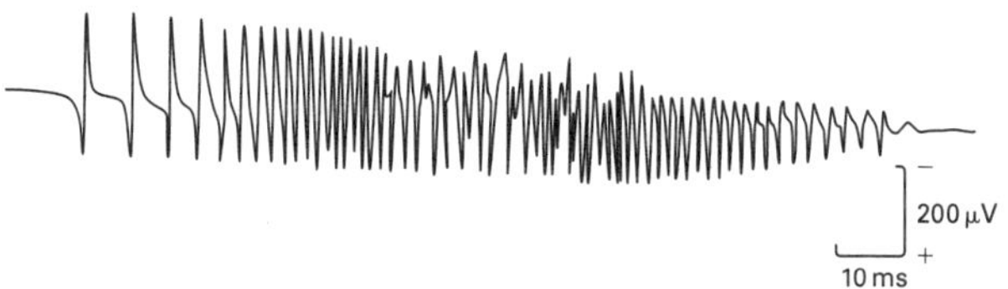

Figure 17-6 Myotonic discharges.

Adapted from Goodgold J. *Electrodiagnosis of Neuromuscular Diseases.* 2nd ed. Baltimore, MD: Williams & Wilkins; 1977.

TABLE 17-2 Abnormal Spontaneous Potentials

	MMEPs	EPPs	Fib potentials	Positive sharp waves	Fasciculation potentials	Complex repetitive discharge	Myotonic discharges
Sound	Sea shells	Sputtering fat in a hot pan	Drops of rain on a tin roof	Dull thud	Varies	Misfired motor boat	Dive bomber
Firing pattern	Irregular	Irregular	Regular	Regular	Irregular	Regular/starts and stops abruptly	Waxes and wanes
Duration (ms)	1–2	3–5	1–5	10–30	5–15	Variable	>5–20
Amplitude (μV)	10–20	100–200	20–1,000	20–1,000	>300 m	50–500	20–300
Rate (Hz)	150	50–100	0.5–15	0.5–15	0.1–10	10–100	20–100
Waveform/deflection	Monophasic negative (upward)	Biphasic negative (upward)	Triphasic with initial positive (downward) deflection	Biphasic with initial positive (downward) deflection	Similar to motor unit action potential (MUAP)	Similar to MUAP, fibs, and PSWs	Similar to EPP, fibs, and PSWs
Cause	MEPPs	Irregularly firing muscle fiber APs	Spontaneous depolarization of a muscle fiber	Spontaneous depolarization of a muscle fiber	Spontaneous involuntary discharge of single MU	Depolarization of single muscle fiber with ephaptic spread to adjacent denervated fibers	Spontaneous discharge of a muscle fiber
Seen in	Needle in the end plate	Needle in the end plate	Denervation (may be due to neurogenic muscle disorder or disorders of the NMJ)	Denervation (may be due to neurogenic, muscle disorder or disorders of the NMJ)	Processes that affect the lower motor neuron (LMN). Also seen in benign fasciculations	Chronic neuropathic and myopathic disorders	Myotonic dystrophy, myotonia congenita and paramyotonia, some myopathies, hyperkalemic periodic paralysis, and rarely in denervation

Other potentials that are nerve generated include cramp potentials, myokymia, and neuromyotonia. These are beyond the scope of our discussion here.
Adapted from Preston DC, Barbara ES. *Electromyography and Neuromuscular Disorders: Clinical-Electrophysiologic Correlations.* Philadelphia, PA: Butterworth-Heinemann; 2005:215-225.

MU Analysis

After analysis of insertional activity and spontaneous activity, the next step is to analyze the motor unit action potentials (MUAPs). First assess the morphology (duration, amplitude, phases, and rise time). This should be done during a minimal contraction (sometimes positioning changes can bring this on). A trigger and delay line can be helpful in assessing MU stability.

An MU is defined as an individual motor neuron, the muscle fibers it innervates (ranging from five to hundreds), and the NMJs between these two components. MUAP morphology varies depending on the age of the patient and the muscle being tested.

Duration is measured from the initial deflection from the baseline to the return to baseline (typically 5 to 15 ms) and reflects the synchrony of muscle fibers firing. The duration is increased with asynchronous firing of the fibers of an MU (as in reinnervation or other neuropathic processes) and is decreased in myopathic processes (fewer fibers contribute to the MU). *When listening to the MUs, duration correlates with pitch; thus, long duration is dull and thuddy and short duration is crisp and staticlike.*

Amplitude is measured from the most positive to the most negative peak of the MU and reflects fiber density. The criteria for normal amplitude depend on the type of needle used (several hundred microvolts to a few millivolts for concentric needles, 1 to 7 μV for a monopolar needle). Amplitude increases (1) as the needle approximates the MU, (2) as the number of muscle fibers of the MU is increased, (3) with increasing diameter of the muscle fibers (muscle fiber hypertrophy), and (4) with more synchronous firing of the muscle fibers. Also, amplitude may be increased after reinnervation (neuropathic injuries) and may be decreased in myopathies. *When listening to the MUs, amplitude correlates with volume (not pitch).*

Phases are determined by counting the number of baseline crossings and adding one. Polyphasia implies asynchronous firing of muscle fibers within an MU. Polyphasia is nonspecific and can be seen in both neuropathic and myopathic lesions. The MUAP is generally 2 to 4 phases. All muscles will normally exhibit about 10% polyphasia except the deltoid (up to 25% is normal). *When listening to the MUs, polyphasia results in a clicking sound.*

Serrations (or turns) are defined as changes in the direction of a potential that do not cross baseline. Serrations also imply asynchronous firing of muscle fibers within an MU. Often serrations will become phases with a slight movement of the needle.

Satellite potentials are seen only after denervation has occurred. Satellite potentials appear after collateral sprouting from adjacent intact MUs. The new sprouts are unmyelinated and conduct slower than the original MU. As the reinnervation matures and myelinates, the satellite potential moves toward the MUAP until it eventually becomes an additional phase of the MUAP (these may require a trigger and delay line to be appreciated).

Rise time is measured from the initial positive deflection to the first negative peak. It correlates with the proximity of the recording electrode to the MUAP being measured; thus, *as the discharging MU is approached, the sound will become sharper.* The electromyographer's qualitative analysis will be more accurate the closer they are to the MU. An acceptable rise time is 0.5 ms or less.

Stability – the morphology of an MU is stable in normal MUAPs. Unstable MUAP morphology (changes in amplitude or number of phases) occurs in primary NMJ disorders and disorders associated with new or immature NMJs (reinnervation). A trigger and delay function on the EMG machine may be helpful here.

Recruitment

MUAPs normally fire in a semirhythmic pattern with a slight variation in the time between each MUAP. There are two ways to increase force during a muscle contraction: *increase the MU firing rate* or *recruit more MUs.* Normally, one MU fires semirhythmically around 5 Hz. If more force is needed, that unit increases its firing rate (activation) and a second unit is recruited. Most MUs will fire at about 10 Hz before recruiting a second MU. *Decreased recruitment* usually occurs in neuropathic disorders where the nerve is damaged. There are therefore fewer MUs available to fire. In order to increase the strength of a contraction, these MUs fire at a higher frequency. This is also described more accurately as an increase in MU firing frequency. *Early or increased recruitment* usually occurs in myopathic processes with a loss of muscle fibers. In order to increase the strength of a contraction, the remaining muscle fibers are quickly recruited. Many MUAPs are activated with minimal contraction. It is important not to confuse decreased recruitment (increased firing frequency of the MUs as seen in a neuropathic process) with early recruitment (recruitment of many MUAPs with slight contraction as seen in a myopathic process).

As a rule of thumb, myopathic MUAPs have early recruitment of short duration with low amplitude and an increased firing rate. Neuropathic MUAPs have late recruitment of increased duration and increased amplitude. MUAPs of CNS disorders have normal morphology, but may have a decreased activation.[10,11]

Specific Disorders

Median Neuropathy at the Wrist (Carpal Tunnel Syndrome)

Median neuropathy at the wrist presents with a combination of signs/symptoms known as carpal tunnel syndrome (CTS) – the most common entrapment neuropathy. Etiologies are multifactorial with varying contributions of local and systemic factors. The initial presentation is usually due to a demyelinating lesion of the median nerve sensory fibers. Demyelination may also affect the motor fibers early on. This may progress to axonal loss of both sensory and motor fibers.

Patient presentation is the most important aspect of the clinical diagnosis of CTS. The symptoms include numbness, tingling, and pain along the median nerve distribution (palmar surface of the first 3½ digits). Symptoms may be worst or most prevalent at night and may wake the patient from sleep. Weakness of grip strength (inability to open jars or dropping objects) may occur as symptoms progress and median motor fibers become involved. CTS can be bilateral, but the dominant hand is usually affected first. Physical examination involves sensory test (pin prick, 2-point discrimination, and/or *Semmes-Weinstein* pressure monofilaments) and motor test/inspection for abductor pollicis brevis (APB) atrophy and weakness. The special/provocative tests may assist in diagnosis (Table 17-3). The affected side should always be compared with the nonaffected side.

Electrodiagnostic studies are helpful in confirming the diagnosis of CTS (85% to 90% sensitivity) and determining the type of lesion (demyelinating, axonal, or both). However, one must keep in mind that all those with abnormal studies do not necessarily have CTS and all those with CTS do not necessarily have abnormal studies. Classic evaluation of CTS includes motor and sensory NCS of median nerve and its comparison with the ulnar nerve (ipsilaterally) and median nerve (contralaterally). A needle study may be helpful to assess for axonal damage or reinnervation and to rule out radiculopathy or other nerve lesions. Antidromic SNAPs are recorded with the active electrode over the proximal interphalangeal (PIP) joint of the second or third digit and stimulating the mid-palm (7 cm from electrode) and across the carpal tunnel (14 cm from electrode). *Note*: larger/smaller distances can be used depending on the size of the patient's hand – it is important to change the distance in your recordings, as this will affect the velocity.

TABLE 17-3 Provocative Tests and Their Descriptions

Provocative tests	Description
Carpal compression test	Direct application of pressure (150 mm Hg) on the patient's wrist for 30 s. Positive if pain, numbness, or paresthesia develops in a median distribution
Flick test	The patient shakes down their hands (like a thermometer) to relieve the pain
Phalen's test	Reproduction of symptoms in a median distribution with prolonged (30 s to 1 min) wrist flexion
Tinel's test	Pain, numbness, or paresthesia in a median nerve distribution elicited by mild taps along the course of median nerve at the wrist
Reverse Phalen's test	Reproduction of symptoms in a median distribution with prolonged (30 s to 1 min) wrist extension

The electrodiagnostic analysis of CTS depends upon evidence of median nerve slowing, conduction block, or axon loss in the carpal tunnel. Commonly used criteria include prolonged absolute motor or sensory latency, sensory slowing across the carpal tunnel (or relatively prolonged or slowed in comparison with other nerves or the contralateral median nerve) as well as amplitude changes that would indicate axonal loss or a conduction block.

Sensory changes that may indicate CTS (note that all findings must be taken in the context of the global findings in all nerves):

- CV <44 m/s (median nerve across the carpal tunnel)
- latency of >0.5 ms compared with the ipsilateral ulnar nerve
- amplitude of the median response across the carpal tunnel <50% of the distal amplitude or the contralateral amplitude

Motor changes that may indicate CTS (sensory fibers are usually affected first):

- latency of >4.2 ms at a distance of 8 cm from the active electrode
- latency of >1 ms greater than the ipsilateral ulnar motor nerve latency

The EMG test should include the APB muscle. If the APB is abnormal (PSW/fibs), more proximal median as well as nonmedian innervated muscles should be tested to rule out a more proximal median neuropathy, peripheral neuropathy, plexopathy, radiculopathy, or a lesion of the anterior horn cell.

A possible source of confusion in median nerve electrodiagnostic studies is a *Martin-Gruber anastomosis.* This relatively common anastomosis (found in 15% to 20% of population) occurs when ulnar fibers (destined for ulnar innervated muscles) travel with the median nerve at the elbow. In the forearm, the nerve fibers travel with the anterior interosseous nerve and cross over to join the ulnar nerve (median to ulnar anastamoses). There are three classic electrodiagnostic findings:

1. The median CMAP has a positive (downward) initial deflection after median nerve stimulation at the elbow that is not seen with wrist stimulation. This deflection occurs because ulnar fibers (traveling at the elbow with median nerve fibers, before joining the ulnar nerve in the forearm) arrive first and stimulate the adductor muscle of the thumb causing downward deflection to be recorded over the APB.
2. The CMAP amplitude of median nerve stimulation at the elbow will be larger compared with the wrist stimulation. This can occur without median nerve entrapment. The amplitude is increased because at the elbow the ulnar nerve hitchhiking fibers are stimulated and added to the median CMAP, whereas at the wrist only median nerve fibers are stimulated and recorded.
3. There may be a false increase in median NCV in the forearm based on proximal (at the elbow) stimulation calculations. This is more prevalent in patients with CTS. Ulnar fibers stimulated with the median nerve at the elbow do not have to traverse the carpal tunnel and will therefore result in a faster proximal latency than normal.

Ulnar Neuropathy at the Elbow

Ulnar neuropathy at the elbow (*cubital tunnel syndrome*) is the second most common mononeuropathy of the upper extremity (second only to CTS). Patients usually complain of sensory changes in the fourth and fifth digits and/or weakness of the hand. Physical examination must include inspection for deformity and signs of muscle atrophy (first dorsal interosseous and abductor digiti minimi [ADM]), individual muscle strength testing, thorough sensory examination (including the dorsal ulnar cutaneous nerve), and special tests. Tinel's sign occurs when mild taps at the ulnar groove or cubital tunnel cause numbness or paresthesia in the hand along the ulnar nerve distribution. Froment's sign occurs when the patient is asked to hold a piece of paper between thumb and index finger and there is flexion of the thumb at the IP joint. The patient will substitute the flexor pollicis longus muscle (innervated by the median nerve) for the adductor pollicis muscle (innervated by the ulnar nerve).

Electrodiagnostic studies may help pinpoint the site of compression of the ulnar nerve, prognosticate, and distinguish ulnar neuropathy at the elbow from other pathologies. Depending on the severity, SNAPs may be affected, resulting in decreased amplitude. A side-to-side difference of more than 50% is considered significant. The dorsal ulnar cutaneous nerve should be tested in suspected ulnar neuropathy at the elbow. This cutaneous nerve takes off just before the ulnar nerve enters Guyon's canal, which helps distinguish between ulnar neuropathy at Guyon's canal (the dorsal ulnar cutaneous response will be normal) and that more proximally. If CMAPs are decreased and the SNAPs are normal, consider cervical radiculopathy.

Slowing of the ulnar motor response across the elbow may be noted. Slowing of more than 10 m/s (compared with distal CV) is considered significant. If the elbow is not flexed (90° to 135°), the CV may be falsely decreased. The length of the segment should be measured by following the path of the nerve with the elbow bent. An amplitude drop of more than 20% to 30% compared with the distal segment may indicate conduction block. The "inching technique" (stimulating at 1-cm intervals and assessing for a drop in amplitude or excessive latency) can further help localize the site of entrapment.

Needle EMG testing can be difficult to interpret. Because the innervation of the flexor carpi ulnaris (FCU) sometimes occurs proximal and sometimes distal to the elbow, it is frequently spared in ulnar neuropathy at the elbow. NCS (including evaluation of the dorsal ulnar cutaneous nerve) must be taken into consideration when making a diagnosis.

Peroneal Neuropathy

The common peroneal nerve (also known as the fibular nerve) gives off a branch to the short head of biceps femoris that then proceeds to wind around the fibular head/neck where it becomes very superficial. This is the main site of entrapment of the common peroneal nerve, which then courses into the fibular tunnel and divides into superficial and deep peroneal nerves. The etiology of compression is usually trauma, habituation, iatrogenic, or work related. The pathophysiology can present as myelin, axon, or mixed damage, based on severity and etiology of compression. The clinical presentation is usually foot drop (steppage gait with inability to dorsiflex) and paresthesia/numbness on the dorsum of the foot and lateral leg.

The electrodiagnostic study remains the best test to assess the degree of nerve damage and pinpoint the location of entrapment. The classic NCS includes a sensory study of the bilateral superficial peroneal nerves and a motor study of the peroneal nerves with recording electrode at extensor digitorum brevis (EDB; tibialis anterior muscle can be used as the recording electrode if the EDB is atrophied). The motor studies are performed with stimulation at the ankle, below the fibular head, and in the lateral popliteal fossa. These findings should be compared with the contralateral side. In general, a lower extremity motor CV of <40 m/s is considered abnormal. The proximal segment velocity should be greater than distal velocity due to greater axonal diameter in the proximal segment of the nerve. An accessory peroneal nerve should be suspected if the peroneal CMAP is larger on proximal (fibular head) stimulation than on distal (ankle) stimulation. This anomalous innervation can be found by stimulating posterior to the lateral malleolus. The amplitude of the CMAP stimulating at the ankle plus the amplitude of the CMAP stimulating posterior to the lateral malleolus will approximate the CMAP amplitude stimulating over the fibular head. Needle EMG helps confirm axonal loss, assess the degree of involvement of the muscles innervated by the peroneal nerve, localize the lesion, and rule out L5 radiculopathy/plexopathy. The examination of the short head of the biceps femoris muscle is very important, as this is the only peroneal nerve–innervated muscle above the knee. If this muscle demonstrates abnormality, the lesion is proximal to the fibular head.

Peripheral Neuropathy

Peripheral neuropathy is a generalized dysfunction of the peripheral nerves. The distal segments of the nerves are usually more affected than the proximal segments. Thus, the longer the nerve, the more it is usually affected. Peripheral neuropathies typically occur in a "stocking and glove" distribution, affecting the feet and hands with numbness, pain, or paresthesias. Electrodiagnostic studies (NCS/EMG) are used to determine the presence of peripheral neuropathy and can help to identify its characteristics and severity. Peripheral neuropathy is classified based on the types of fibers involved (sensory or motor), the primary pathology affecting the component of the nerve (axonal or demyelinating), and its extent (segmental or uniform). When performing electrodiagnostic testing, both sensory and motor nerves must be tested in at least three extremities to differentiate between single entrapment neuropathy and a generalized process. Relevant findings must be found in at least three extremities to be diagnosed as a peripheral neuropathy. Early in the progression of peripheral neuropathy, changes may not be seen in the upper extremity.

Nerve Conduction Studies

1. *Sensory NCS*: SNAPs may be reduced
   a. If *axonal*: amplitude of SNAP will be reduced or unobtainable
   b. If *demyelinating*: SNAP can have an increased latency (decreased CV); demyelination may result in loss of SNAP through conduction block (neurapraxia).
2. *Motor NCS*:
   a. If *axonal*: amplitude of CMAP may be affected or unobtainable.
   b. If *demyelinating*: CMAP may have increased distal latency or slowing CV. (CV less than 80% of the lower limit of normal suggests a demyelinating neuropathy.) Conduction block may also cause decreased CMAP.
3. *Uniform versus segmental*: Assessed by location of slowing CV. If segmental, some fibers will travel slower than others and the CMAP will be dispersed, with a longer duration and lower amplitude (temporal dispersion). If uniform, all fibers are slowed, which will result in a uniform slowing of CV, prolonged latencies, and normal duration and amplitude NCS.

Note that late responses (F waves and H-reflexes) assess both the proximal and distal segments of a peripheral nerve and therefore may also be affected. However, findings are nonspecific.

EMG – Test proximal and distal muscles to assess for axonal neuropathy and rule out additional or concomitant pathology. Findings are usually negative in peripheral neuropathy except in a few cases:

1. *Axonal motor neuropathy*: affected muscles (usually distal) may demonstrate spontaneous activity (fibs and PSW). If an axonal lesion is present, the duration of the disease can be assessed by evaluating chronic changes in MUAPs (increased duration, polyphasicity, or large amplitude reveals reinnervation and reorganization).
2. *Chronic neurogenic disorders:* may see CRDs.

There are many causes for peripheral neuropathy, including genetic and acquired disorders. These disorders are further typified based on separate classifications of peripheral neuropathy that can be derived using electrodiagnostic studies (Table 17-4).[12,13]

Plexopathy – The functional anatomy of the brachial plexus can be divided into supraclavicular (roots and trunks) and infraclavicular (cords and peripheral nerves or branches) (Fig. 17-7). The pattern of findings will help to localize the lesion. In general, infraclavicular lesions will cause weakness in a muscle group without affecting the antagonist muscles of that group, whereas supraclavicular lesions will affect both. Electrodiagnostic testing is a physiological examination, which can help to localize the site of a plexus lesion and provide an evaluation of the prognosis. The unaffected limb should be used as a control to compare nerve responses from the two sides tested.

TABLE 17-4 Common Disorders of Polyneuropathy

EMG finding	Uniform demyelinating mixed sensorimotor	Segmental demyelinating	Axonal loss: motor > sensory	Axonal loss: sensory only	Axonal loss: mixed sensorimotor	Mixed axonal/ demyelinating sensorimotor
Common diseases	1. HMSN I, III, and IV 2. Metachromatic leukodystrophy 3. Krabbe's leukodystrophy 4. Adrenomyeloneuropathy 5. Congenital hypomyelinating neuropathy 6. Tangier disease 7. Cackayne's syndrome 8. Cerebrotendinous xanthomatosis	1. AIDP: Guillain-Barré syndrome 2. CIDP 3. Leprosy (Hansen's disease) 4. Diphtheria 5. Lyme disease 6. Monoclonal gammopathy 7. Osteosclerotic myeloma 8. Carcinoma 9. AIDS 10. Acute arsenic polyneuropathy 11. Pharmaceuticals (amiodarone, perhexiline, and high-dose Ara-C)	1. Acute intermittent porphyria 2. Axonal Guillain-Barré syndrome 3. HMSN II and V 4. Paraneoplastic motor neuronopathy 5. Hypoglycemia 6. Lead neuropathy 7. Dapsone neuropathy 8. Vincristine neuropathy	1. Sjogren's syndrome 2. Fisher variant Guillain-Barré syndrome 3. HMSN I–IV 4. HSAN 5. Friedreich's ataxia 6. Chronic idiopathic ataxic neuropathy 7. Amyloidosis 8. Paraneoplastic sensory neuronopathy 9. Lymphomatous sensory neuronopathy 10. Spinocerebellar degeneration 11. Abetalipoproteinemia (Bassen-Kornzweig disease) 12. Paraproteinemias 13. Primary biliary cirrhosis 14. Crohn's disease 15. Acute sensory neuronopathy (*cis*-platinum toxicity) 16. Pyridoxine toxicity	1. Alcoholic polyneuropathy 2. Vitamin deficiency (B_{12} and folate) 3. Sarcoidosis 4. Multiple myeloma 5. Paraneoplastic syndrome 6. Gouty neuropathy 7. Connective tissue disorders (RA, SLE, and amyloidosis) 8. Myotonic dystrophy 9. Post gastrectomy and gastric bypass 10. Chronic liver disease 11. Hypothyroidism 12. Lyme disease 13. HIV 14. Critical illness neuropathy 15. Metal neuropathy (mercury, thallium, gold, etc.) 16. Vincristine neuropathy 17. Toxic neuropathy (acrylamide, carbon disulfide, and carbon monoxide)	1. Diabetic polyneuropathy 2. Uremia

CIDP, chronic inflammatory demyelinating polyneuropathy; HMSN, hereditary motor sensory neuropathy; HSAN, hereditary sensory and autonomic neuropathy; RA, rheumatoid arthritis; SLE, systemic lupus erythematosus.

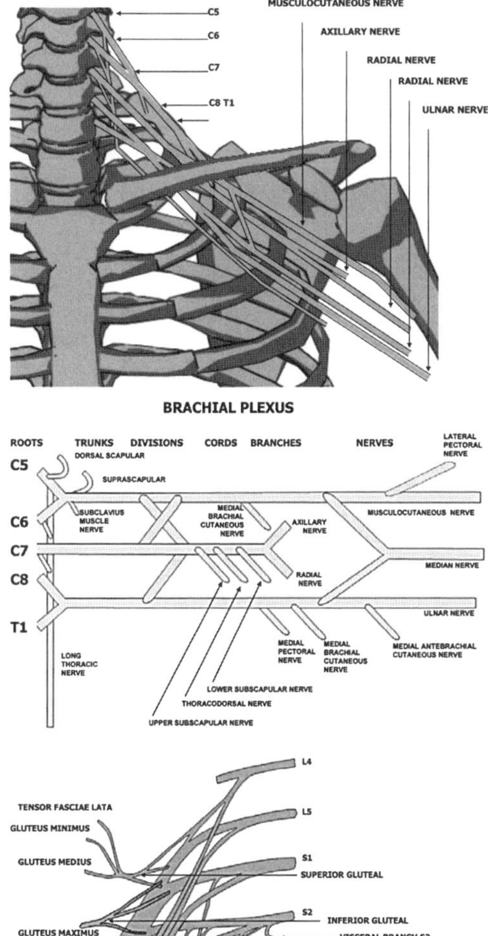

Figure 17-7 Brachial and lumbosacral plexus anatomy.
Illustrations courtesy of Dennis J. Dowling, D.O., F.A.A.O.

Sensory Studies – Sensory NCSs are usually a more sensitive indicator of injury to the plexus than the motor nerve response. The distal latency and CV are usually normal. SNAP amplitude reflects the number of functioning axons in continuity with the sensory root cell body. Lesions proximal to the DRG, such as radiculopathy and nerve root avulsions, have normal SNAPs even though sensation may be affected clinically. Lesions distal to the DRG disconnect the sensory nerve cell body from its axons, resulting in decrement or absence of the SNAP. Therefore, differentiation between pre- and postganglionic lesions is extremely important.

Motor Studies – CMAPs are usually not affected unless the injury is severe. Motor latencies and conduction velocities are usually unaffected. Stimulation at Erb's point may reveal slowing if there is a demyelinating lesion in the brachial plexus. CMAP amplitudes may be decreased if there is severe axonal damage. In plexopathies, side-to-side amplitude differences can give an approximation of the degree of axonal injury during the first few months. A 70% decrement in CMAP amplitude correlates to 70% axon loss. Amplitude differences of less than 50% may not be significant.

Late Response – Most lesions are incomplete and the effect is diluted along the neural path of transmission of the F wave. Therefore, F-wave prolongation is a nonspecific finding and F wave and H-reflexes are usually not helpful in the diagnosis of plexopathies.

EMG – Acute plexopathies usually show fibs and PSWs in the distribution of the nerve segment involved (see Tables 17-5 and 17-6). In chronic lesions where reinnervation has occurred, long-duration, high-amplitude, or polyphasic MUAPs may be noted. It may take up to 3 weeks for electrodiagnostic abnormalities to develop. The paraspinal muscles, as well as muscles not in the distribution of the nerve segment involved, are expected to be normal.

TABLE 17-5 Localization of Lesions in the Brachial Plexus

Area of injury	Affected sensory NCS	Affected motor NCS	Positive finding EMG
Root (radiculopathy)	Normal	CMAPs decreased	Cervical paraspinals and myotome pattern
Upper trunk	Lateral antebrachial cutaneous nerve Median nerve first digit Radial	Musculocutaneous nerve to biceps, suprascapular nerve to supraspinatus, and axillary nerve to deltoid Radial nerve to extensor digitorum communis	Supraspinatus, biceps, pronator teres, deltoid, brachioradialis, and extensor carpi radialis

Area of injury	Affected sensory NCS	Affected motor NCS	Positive finding EMG
Middle trunk	Median nerve to third and fourth digits		Latissimus dorsi, teres major, extensor digitorum communis, pronator teres, and flexor carpi radialis
Lower trunk	Ulnar nerve to fifth digit Medial antebrachial cutaneous nerve	Ulnar nerve to ADM and median nerve to APB	APB, flexor digitorum superficialis, ADM, FCU, and flexor digitorum profundus
Lateral cord	Lateral antebrachial cutaneous nerve and median nerve to first digit	Musculocutaneous nerve to biceps	Biceps, pronator teres, and flexor carpi radialis
Posterior cord	Radial	Axillary nerve to deltoid and radial nerve to extensor carpi ulnaris	Latissimus dorsi, teres major, deltoid, and radial muscles
Medial cord	Ulnar nerve to fifth digit and medial antebrachial cutaneous nerve	Ulnar nerve to ADM and median nerve to APB	Ulnar muscles, flexor digitorum superficialis, flexor pollicis longus, and APB

RADICULOPATHY

Radiculopathy is a lesion of a specific nerve root that is generally caused by compression of that root. Electrodiagnostic studies aid in the diagnosis of radiculopathy, but they must be done in conjunction with a thorough history and physical examination. Imaging studies may be complementary, but they do not give information about nerve function. Physical examination findings suggestive of radiculopathy can include decreased reflexes, weakness in myotomal distribution, and/or decreased sensation in a dermatomal distribution. Despite the fact that sensory complaints are common in patients with suspected/diagnosed radiculopathy, the SNAPs will be normal in amplitude and latency as the lesion is proximal to the DRGs. If there are abnormal SNAP findings, a different (or coexisting) lesion distal to the DRG should be considered.

CMAPs reflect the number of motor fibers activated upon stimulation. In most cases, the CMAP will also be normal in a radiculopathy. In a

TABLE 17-6 Localization of Lesions in the Lumbosacral Plexus

Nerve	Division	Roots	Affected sensory NCS	Affected motor NCS	Positive finding EMG
Iliohypogastric	Posterior	L1,2	None	None	Transversus abdominis and external and internal oblique
Lateral femoral cutaneous	Posterior	L2,3	Lateral femoral cutaneous nerve	None	None
Femoral	Posterior	L2,3,4	Saphenous nerve	Femoral nerve	Iliopsoas, pectineus, sartorius, and quadriceps
Obturator	Anterior	L2,3,4	None	Obturator nerve	Adductor longus, brevis, and magnus; gracillis; and obturator internus
Superior gluteal	Posterior	L4,5,S1	None	Superior gluteal nerve	Gluteus minimus and medius, TFL
Inferior gluteal	Posterior	L5,S1,2	None	Inferior gluteal nerve	Gluteus maximus
Sciatic (peroneal division)	Posterior	L4,5,S1,2	Superficial peroneal (and sural nerve)	Peroneal nerve	Short head of biceps femoris, tibialis anterior, EDB, peroneus tertius, and peroneus brevis and longus (brevis and longus are from the superficial branch)
Sciatic (tibial division)	Anterior	L4,5,S1,2,3	Sural nerve	Tibial nerve	Long head of biceps femoris, semimembranosus, semitendinosus, adductor magnus, plantaris, popliteus, gastrocnemius, tibialis posterior, soleus, flexor digitorum longus, and flexor hallucis longus
Sural (contains branches from the tibial and peroneal nerves)	Anterior and posterior	Mostly S1	Sural nerve	None	None

severe, multilevel radiculopathy, the CMAP amplitude may be reduced as a result of Wallerian degeneration distal to the lesion.

The H-reflex can be used to assess the afferent and efferent S1 fibers and can be helpful in distinguishing an S1 from an L5 radiculopathy. It is important to remember that H-reflexes are sensitive but not specific. Gastrocnemius–soleus H-reflex side-to-side latency differences of greater than 1.5 m/s are suggestive of S1 radiculopathy (as is unilateral absence of an H-reflex). F-wave latencies and amplitudes are so variable that their use in evaluating a patient for radiculopathy is not recommended.

Needle EMG is the most useful study in the electrodiagnostic evaluation to both localize a radiculopathy and predict its prognosis. The presence of spontaneous activity on needle EMG is the most objective evidence of acute denervation. Fibs and PSWs can be seen in the paraspinal muscles within 5 to 7 days of initial injury. This is followed by findings in the peripheral muscles within 3 to 6 weeks. In order to diagnose radiculopathy, the corresponding paraspinal muscle and two peripheral muscles innervated by different peripheral nerves, but the same nerve root, should have positive findings (see Tables 17-7 and 17-8). With axon loss, MUs will fire with increasing frequency (>20 Hz); this is also known as "decreased recruitment." With reinnervation, the abnormal spontaneous activity may disappear (in the paraspinals at 6 to 9 weeks followed by proximal muscles at 2 to 5 months and distal muscles at 3 to 7 months). MUAPs will become polyphasic with a long duration (>15 ms). After 6 months to 1 year, large-amplitude (>7 mV using a monopolar needle) MUAPs may be noted.

TABLE 17-7 Clinical Presentation Associated with Levels of Radiculopathy

Root level	Muscle group	Clinical signs
C5	Rhomboid (dorsal-scapular n.) Supraspinatus/infraspinatus (suprascapular n.) Deltoid/teres minor (axillary n.) Biceps/brachialis (musculocutaneous n.)	1. Positive neck distraction/ compression test 2. Decreased/absent biceps tendon reflex 3. Decreased/absent sensation to lateral arm (axillary n.) 4. Weakness of shoulder abduction
C6	Extensor carpi radialis longus/ brevis (radial n.) Pronator teres/flexor carpi radialis (median n.) Deltoid/teres minor (axillary n.)	1. Decreased/absent brachioradialis reflex 2. Decreased/absent sensation to lateral forearm 3. Weakness of wrist extension
C7	Triceps/extensor digitorum communis/extensor indicis/ extensor digiti minimi (radial n.) Flexor carpi radialis (median n.) FCU (ulnar n.)	1. Decreased/absent triceps reflex 2. Decreased/absent sensation to middle finger 3. Weakness of wrist flexion

(Continued)

TABLE 17-7 Clinical Presentation Associated with Levels of Radiculopathy (Continued)

Root level	Muscle group	Clinical signs
C8	FCU (ulnar n.) Flexor pollicis longus/flexor digitorum superficialis (median n.) Flexor digitorum profundus (median/ulnar n.) Extensor indicis/extensor pollicis brevis (radial n.) First dorsal interosseous (ulnar n.)	1. Decreased/absent sensation to ring/little finger and to distal half of the forearm's ulnar side 2. Weakness of finger flexion 3. Intrinsic weakness/atrophy
T1	APB (median n.) ADM/first dorsal interosseous (ulnar n.)	1. Decreased/absent sensation to medial side of the upper half of the forearm and arm (medial brachial cutaneous n.) 2. Weakness of finger abduction/adduction

TABLE 17-8 Clinical Presentation Associated with Levels of Radiculopathy

Root level	Myotomes	Clinical signs
L2, L3, L4	Iliacus/vastus medialis (femoral n.) L2,3 and adductor longus/gracilis (obturator n.) L2,3,4	1. Pain in the thigh 2. Weakness in hip flexion/adduction
L4	Vastus lateralis and rectus femoris Tibialis anterior (deep peroneal n.) Vastus medialis/lateralis (L2-4)	1. Decreased/absent patellar reflex 2. Knee extension weakness 3. Pain in the medial side of leg
L5	Gluteus medius/TFL (superior gluteal n., L4-S2) Flexor hallucis longus/flexor digitorum longus/lateral gastrocnemius/tibialis posterior (tibial n., L5-S2) Extensor hallucis longus/extensor digitorum longus (deep peroneal n., L5)	1. Pain and paresthesias in lateral aspect of the leg and dorsum of the foot 2. Ankle dorsiflexor weakness
S1[a]	Medial gastrocnemius/soleus/flexor hallucis brevis (tibial n., L5-S2) Peroneus longus/brevis (superficial peroneal n., L5-S1), TFL/gluteus maximus (sup/inf gluteal n., L4-S1, L5-S2) Extensor hallucis longus and extensor digitorum longus (deep peroneal n., L4, L5, S1)	1. Decreased/absent ankle reflex 2. Pain and paresthesias at the lateral border of the foot 3. Weakness of foot plantarflexion and toe extension

[a]H-reflex may help to confirm the diagnosis and distinguish S1 from L5 radiculopathy.

Motor Neuron Diseases

Motor neuron diseases may affect both the UMNs and lower motor neurons (LMNs). These disorders specifically affect the motor cortex, corticospinal tracts, and/or anterior horn cells. Clinical signs of LMN lesions include atrophy, flaccidity, hyporeflexia, and fasciculations. UMN signs include weakness, spasticity, hyperreflexia, and upgoing plantar reflex (positive Babinski sign). There are usually no sensory changes. With EMG testing, only the LMN aspect of the disorder can be assessed.

Electrodiagnostic Findings – SNAP has *normal* amplitude and conduction velocities. CMAP conduction velocities are *normal or mildly decreased.* The amplitude of the CMAP may be *decreased* due to axonal loss if significant atrophy is present. EMG findings (in at least three limbs or two limbs and bulbar muscles) include abnormal spontaneous potentials (fibs and PSW), fasciculations, and CRDs. Decreased recruitment with increased firing frequency may be noted. Large-amplitude, long-duration polyphasic potentials may be noted if reinnervation has occurred.
LMN: Poliomyelitis/postpolio syndrome (PPS) and SMA
UMN and LMN: Amyotrophic lateral sclerosis (ALS)
UMN: Primary lateral sclerosis (PLS)

ALS – Characterized by degeneration of anterior horn cell. UMN and LMN signs are usually present. Clinical presentation includes asymmetric atrophy, weakness and fasciculations, dysphagia, and dysarthria. Pseudobulbar signs may be noted. Bowel and bladder are typically spared. EMG findings include abnormal spontaneous potentials (fibs and PSWs). MUAPs demonstrate decreased recruitment with increased MUAP duration and amplitude.

PPS – Loss of anterior horn cell decades (typically 30 years) after polio. This disorder is hypothesized to be due to burnout of MU from increased metabolic demand or normal axon loss with aging. *Halstead-Ross criteria* include the onset of two or more of the following: fatigue, arthralgia, myalgia, and cold intolerance with history of previous stable polio diagnosis. Electrodiagnostically, this may resemble poliomyelitis, so clinical findings must be considered. NCSs show normal SNAPs and abnormal CMAP. EMG shows increased amplitude and duration of MUAPs with decreased recruitment.

EMG Findings in Myopathies

Electrodiagnostic testing is an important tool in the diagnosis of myopathies. EMG testing helps to make a diagnosis, determine the extent of a disease, prognosticate, and guide further studies, such as muscle biopsies. Generally, only one side of the body is tested on EMG, leaving the muscles on the other side preserved for muscle biopsy. It is important to rule out other diseases by performing at least one sensory and one motor nerve study in addition to the EMG study.

Typical Findings

NCS: Usually normal since myopathies typically affect proximal muscles initially (and in nerve studies, the active electrode is usually placed over a distal muscle). As the disease progresses, distal muscles may become involved and the motor NCS may be abnormal.

SNAP: normal (sensory fibers are not affected).

CMAP: amplitudes may be reduced due to muscle fiber atrophy; distal latency and CV are normal as the myelin is not affected.

EMG – MUs will usually show early recruitment, polyphasia (due to the variability in muscle fiber diameter), and small-amplitude (due to muscle fiber dropout) and short-duration potentials (see Fig. 17-8). Fib potentials and PSWs as well as myotonic discharges can be seen. In long-standing myopathies, there may be little activity at rest due to loss of muscle fiber. Increased insertional activity is also common in many myopathies.

Typically in myopathies, the proximal lower extremity muscles will show more positive EMG findings. It is important to sample a sufficient number of muscles to differentiate between a myopathy and a focal injury. Muscles should be sampled based on weakness as seen in the clinical examination. However, muscles that are extremely weak (<2/5 in manual testing) can be too deteriorated to provide a good signal.

In steroid myopathy, EMG testing would be normal, as it predominantly affects the type II muscle fibers (EMG tests primarily the type I fibers).[14–16]

NMJ Disorders

The NMJ is divided into the presynaptic terminal, the synaptic cleft, and a postsynaptic muscle end plate. Neuromuscular transmission involves (1) presynaptic terminal depolarization and ACh release, (2) ACh binding and ion channel opening, and (3) postsynaptic membrane depolarization and muscle AP generation. Disorders of the NMJ hinder the production, release, or uptake of ACh at the NMJ. The most well-known postsynaptic disorder is *myasthenia gravis (MG)*. Presynaptic abnormalities include *Lambert-Eaton myasthenic syndrome (LEMS)* and botulism. A *repetitive nerve*

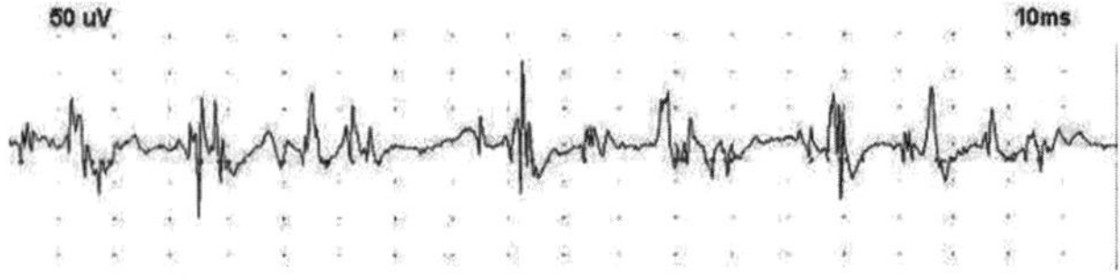

Figure 17-8 In this EMG of a patient with inclusion body myositis, many MUs are activated simultaneously at a low level of muscle contraction (early recruitment). Note the low amplitude and short duration of individual units.

stimulation (RNS) study and *SFEMG* are useful electrodiagnostic tests when trying to evaluate for NMJ disorders.

Routine sensory and motor conduction studies will usually be normal. Only in profound weakness, as in myasthenic crisis, will borderline or slightly decreased CMAP amplitudes be observed. Routine EMG examination may demonstrate unstable MUAPs, where moment-to-moment variations in amplitude and configuration may be seen.

RNS after routine NCS is performed by delivering trains of supramaximal stimuli to a peripheral nerve while recording CMAPs. This depletes stores of releasable ACh from diseased NMJs, producing a progressive amplitude decrement from the first to the fifth waveform in patients with disorders of the NMJ. When RNS is performed at low rates (2 to 5 Hz), a decrement of >10% is considered abnormal. Although the proximal muscles are usually more affected than the distal muscles, the proximal muscles are more difficult to test (the limb must be restrained as the entire limb is often stimulated with proximal stimulation) (Fig. 17-9).

Postactivation facilitation occurs when there is recovery of the CMAP amplitudes on repeat slow RNS following a 10-second isometric contraction or rapid RNS (20 to 50 Hz) studies. This is due to calcium

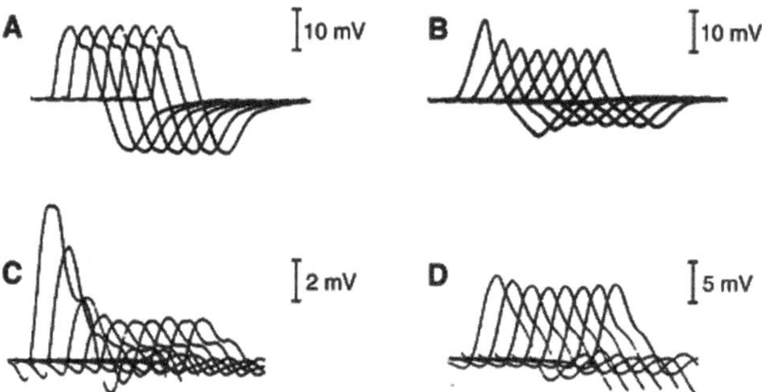

Figure 17-9 CMAPs recorded from the ADM of human subjects during repetitive stimulation of the ulnar nerve at three stimuli per second. **A.** A recording from a normal individual shows no change in the amplitude of the muscle electrical response during the stimulation interval. **B.** In a patient with *MG*, the same stimuli produce a 40% decrement in response amplitude over the first five stimuli, with a slow partial recovery during subsequent stimulations. Similar studies from a patient with severe MG before (**C**) and 2 minutes after (**D**) intravenous administration of 10 mg edrophonium, a short-acting acetylcholinesterase inhibitor. Note the change in amplitude scale between the two recordings and the reversal of the abnormal decrement by edrophonium.

facilitation. Although present to a lesser degree in MG and botulism, it is a hallmark finding in LEMS where increments as high as 500% may be observed.

If initial studies are unrevealing and suspicion for an NMJ disorder is high, consider testing more proximal muscles (e.g., spinal accessory and facial n.) and/or proceeding to SFEMG of at least one symptomatic muscle. SFEMG is the most sensitive test for NMJ disorders. Findings consistent with, but not specific for, NMJ disorders include increased *jitter*. Jitter refers to time variations between interpotential discharges of two different muscle fibers of the same MU. The most extreme abnormality of jitter is failed transmission, or *blocking*. In MG, jitter and blocking increase with increased firing rate. In LEMS and botulism, jitter and blocking decrease with increased firing rate (Fig. 17-10).

Prerequisites for performing a reliable RNS study include immobilization of the limb and recording electrode, supramaximal stimulation, optimization of limb temperature (≈30° C), and withholding of acetylcholinesterase inhibitors 12 to 24 hours prior to testing (if not medically contraindicated). Distal nerves that can be easily tested for RNS are the median and ulnar nerves, with recording electrodes at APB and ADM, respectively. If proximal studies are indicated, spinal accessory nerve with the recording electrode on the upper trapezius muscle is commonly utilized. In patients suspected of having ocular MG, facial RNS recording at orbicularis oris can be performed (Tables 17-9A–E).

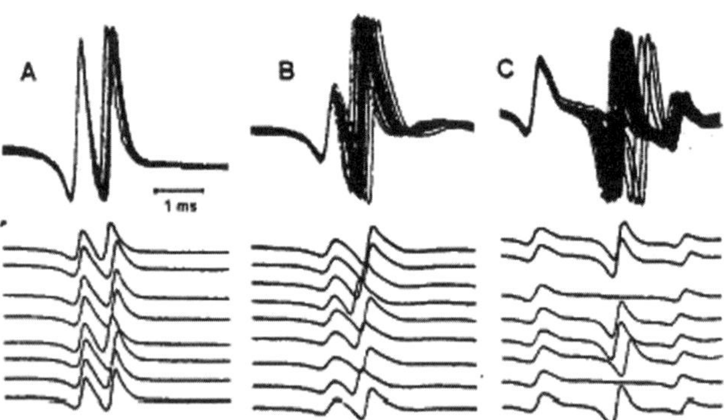

Figure 17-10 [Q46] SFEMG recordings. *Top*: superimposed view. *Bottom*: rastered view. **A.** Normal. **B.** Increased jitter. **C.** Increased jitter with blocking.

From Stalberg E. Clinical electromyography in myasthenia gravis. *J Neurol Neurosurg Psychiatry.* 1980;43:622-633, BMJ Publishing, with permission.

TABLE 17-9A Table of Normals

Upper Extremity – Motor[a]

Nerve	Active electrode	Stimulation site	Distance (cm) from active to first stimulation site	Onset latency (ms)	Amplitude (mV)[b]	Segment name	Velocity (m/s)
Median	APB	Wrist elbow	8	<4.2	>4.0 >4.0	Elbow–wrist	>50.0
Ulnar	Abductor digiti minimi	Wrist Below elbow (BE) Above elbow (AE)	8	<3.4	>4.0 >4.0 >4.0	BE–wrist AE–BE	>50.0 >50.0
Radial	Extensor indicis proprius	Forearm Erb's point	4	2.4 ± 0.5	14 ± 8.8	AE–EIP Erb's point–AE	61.6 ± 5.9 72 ± 6.3
Musculocutaneous	Distal to midpoint biceps brachii	Erb's point	23.5–41.5	4.5 ± 0.6	—	Erb's point–biceps brachii	—
Axillary	Middle deltoid	Erb's point	14.8–26.5	3.9 ± 0.5	—	Erb's point–deltoid	—

(Continued)

TABLE 17-9A Table of Normals (Continued)

Upper Extremity – Sensory[a]

Nerve	Active electrode	Stimulation site	Distance (cm)	Onset latency (ms)	Amplitude (μV)	Segment name	Velocity (m/s)
Median	Second digit	Mid-palm Wrist	7 7	<1.9 <3.5	>20.0 >20.0	Mid-palm–second digit Wrist–mid-palm	>45.0 >45.0
Ulnar	Fifth digit	Wrist BE AE	↑14	↑<3.1	↑ >18.0 >15.0 >14.0	↑ Wrist–fifth digit BE–wrist AE–BE	>44.0 >53.0 >54.0
Superficial radial	First dorsal web space	Forearm	14	1.8 ± 0.3 2.1 ± 0.3 2.4 ± 0.3	31 + 20 (13–60) 31 + 20 (13–60) 31 + 20 (13–60)	First web space–forearm	
Musculocutaneous	Forearm	Elbow	12	1.8 ± 0.1 (1.6–2.1)	24.0 ± 7.2 (12–50)	Forearm–elbow	65 ± 3.6

[a]Skin temperature should be maintained at 32° C.

[b]Side-to-side amplitude difference of >50% is significant or >20% amplitude drop distal to proximal is significant.

TABLE 17-9B Table of Normals: Lower Extremity – Motor[a]

Nerve	Active electrode	Stimulation site	Distance (cm)	Onset latency (ms)	Amplitude (mV)	Segment name	Velocity (m/s)[b]
Peroneal	EDB	Ankle Fib head Popliteal	↑8	↑<5.5	↑>2.5	Fibular head–ankle Popliteal–fibular head	>40.0 >40.0
Posttibial	Abductor hallucis	Ankle–knee	10	<6.0	>3.0	Knee–ankle	>40.0
Sciatic	ADM	Popliteal[b] Gluteal skin fold[c]	15.9–19.9 ± 2.4 32.9 ± 2.4	—	—	—	51.3±4.4

[a]Skin temperature should be maintained at 30° C.
[b]Popliteal fossa – surface electrodes.
[c]Gluteal skin fold – needle electrode.

TABLE 17-9C Table of Normals: Lower Extremity – Sensory[a]

Nerve	Active electrode	Stimulation site	Distance (cm)	Onset latency (ms)	Amplitude (μV)	Segment name	Velocity (m/s)
Sural	Lateral malleolus	Calf	14	<3.8	>10.0	Calf–lateral malleolus	>36.0
Lateral femoral cutaneous	1 cm medial to anterior superior iliac spine (ASIS)	Anterior thigh	12–16	2.6 ± 0.2	10–25	ASIS–anterior thigh	47.9 ± 3.7
Superficial peroneal	Anterior to lateral malleolus	Anterolateral calf	14	3.4 ± 0.4	18.3 ± 8.0	Lateral malleolus to calf	51.2 ± 5.7

[a]Skin temperature should be maintained at 30° C.

TABLE 17-9D Table of Normals: H-Reflex[a]

Site	Active	Latency (ms)	Stimulation site
Medial gastrocnemius–soleus muscle	Halfway from midpopliteal crease – proximal flare medial malleolus	28.0–35.0	Popliteal fossa (cathode proximal); use submaximal stimulation

[a]Skin temperature should be maintained at 30° C.

TABLE 17-9E Table of Normals: F Waves and F-Ratio Upper Extremities

Motor nerve	Pickup site	F-latency (ms)	F-wave velocity (ms)	F-ratio[a]
Median	APB	Wrist 29.1 ± 2.3	Wrist–spinal cord 59.2 ± 3.9	$0.7 < F < 1.3$
		Elbow 24.8 ± 2.0	Elbow–spinal cord 62.2 ± 2.2	
		Axilla 21.7 ± 2.8	Axilla–spinal cord 64.3 ± 6.4	
Ulnar	Abductor digiti quinti	Wrist 30.5 ± 3.0	Wrist–spinal cord 56.7 ± 2.9	$0.7 < F < 1.3$
		BE 26.0 ± 2.0	BE–spinal cord 58.2 ± 2.9	
		AE 23.5 ± 2.0	AE–spinal cord 61.1 ± 5.4	
		Axilla 11.2 ± 1.0	Axilla–spinal cord 63.1 ± 5.9	
Peroneal	EDB	Ankle 51.3 ± 4.7	Ankle–spinal cord 53.3 ± 3.8	$0.7 < F < 1.3$
		Knee 42.7 ± 4.0	Knee–spinal cord 56.3 ± 4.9	
Tibial	Abductor hallucis	Ankle 52.3 ± 4.3	Ankle–spinal cord 51.3 ± 2.9	$0.7 < F < 1.3$
		Knee 43.5 ± 3.4	Knee–spinal cord 54.4 ± 3.6	

AE, above elbow; BE, below elbow.
[a]F-ratio $F - M - 1$ as measured at elbow or knee 2 m.
Adapted from Weiss LD, Silver JK, Weiss J. *Easy EMG: A Guide to Performing Nerve Conduction Studies and Electromyography*. Edinburgh: Butterworth-Heinemann; 2004, with permission.

REFERENCES

1. Weiss L, Silver J, Weiss J. *Easy EMG*. Edinburgh: Elsevier; 2004:4-6, 13-14, 45.
2. Gooch CL, Weimer LH. The electrodiagnosis of neuropathy: basic principles and common pitfalls. *Neurol Clin*. 2007;25:1-28.
3. Weiss L, Weiss J, Pobre T, Kalman A. Nerve conduction studies. In: *Easy EMG*. Edinburgh: Elsevier; 2004:17-39: chap 4.

4. Canale S, Beaty J. Peripheral nerve injuries. In: *Campbell's Operative Orthopaedics.* 11th ed. St. Louis, MO: Mosby. chap 59.
5. Weiss L, Weiss J, Pobre T, Kalman A. Injury to peripheral nerves. In: Weiss L, Silver J, eds. *Easy EMG.* Edinburgh: Elsevier; 2004:81-84.
6. Preston DC, Shapiro B, eds. *Electromyography and Neuromuscular Disorders: Clinical-Electrophysiologic Correlations.* 2nd ed. Philadelphia, PA: Butterworth-Heinemann; 2005.
7. Preston DC, Shapiro BE. Blink reflex. In: *Electromyography and Neuromuscular Disorders.* 2nd ed. Philadelphia, PA: Elsevier; 2005:59-64.
8. Dumitru D, ed. *Electrodiagnostic Medicine.* 2nd ed. Philadelphia, PA: Hanley & Belfus; 2002.
9. Weiss L, Silver J, Weiss J. *Easy EMG.* Edinburgh: Elsevier; 2004.
10. Preston DC, Barbara ES. *Electromyography and Neuromuscular Disorders: Clinical-Electrophysiologic Correlations.* Philadelphia, PA: Butterworth-Heinemann; 2005:215-225.
11. Weiss LD, Silver JK, Weiss J. *Easy EMG: A Guide to Performing Nerve Conduction Studies and Electromyography.* Edinburgh: Butterworth-Heinemann; 2004:50-54.
12. Weiss L, Silver JK, Weiss J. Peripheral neuropathy. In: *Easy EMG.* Edinburgh: Butterworth Heinemann; 2004:161-166.
13. Braddom RL, Dillingham TR, et al. Electrodiagnostic medicine II: clinical evaluation and findings: generalized disorders: polyneuropathy. In: *Physical Medicine and Rehabilitation.* 3rd ed. Edinburgh: Saunders Elsevier; 2007:219-220.
14. Braddom RL. *Physical Medicine and Rehabilitation.* Edinburgh: Elsevier Saunders; 2007.
15. Cuccurullo SJ. *Physical Medicine and Rehabilitation.* New York, NY: Demos Medical Publishing; 2009.
16. EMedicine – Medical Reference. Motor unit recruitment in EMG: EMedicine neurology. Web. http://emedicine.medscape.com/article/1141359-overview. Accessed March 15, 2012.

RECOMMENDED READING

Ball RD. Electrodiagnostic evaluation of the peripheral nervous system (plexopathy). In: Delisa JA, Gans BM, eds. *Rehabilitation Medicine Principles and Practice.* Philadelphia, PA: Lippincott-Raven; 1998:358-359.

Braddom RL. *Physical Medicine & Rehabilitation.* 3rd ed. Philadelphia, PA: W.B. Saunders; 2007.

Cuccurullo SJ. *Physical Medicine and Rehabilitation Board Review.* 2nd ed. New York, NY: Demos Medical Publishing; 2010:365-366.

DeLisa JA. *Physical Medicine & Rehabilitation Principles and Practice.* 4th ed. Philadelphia, PA: Lippincott; 2005.

Gaudino W. Brachial plexopathies. In: Weiss L, Silver JK, Weiss J, eds. *Easy EMG.* Philadelphia, PA: Butterworth-Heinemann; 2004:171-180.

Gaudino W. Lumbosacral plexopathies. In: Weiss L, Silver JK, Weiss J, eds. *Easy EMG.* Philadelphia, PA: Butterworth-Heinemann; 2004:181-187.

Katirji B. *Electromyography in Clinical Practice: A Case Study Approach.* 2nd ed. Philadelphia, PA: Mosby; 2007.

Preston DC, Shapiro BE. Lumbosacral plexopathy. In: *Electromyography and Neuromuscular Disorder.* 2nd ed. Philadelphia, PA: Elsevier; 2005:471-489.

Weiss LD, Weiss J, Pobre T. *Oxford American Handbook of Physical Medicine and Rehabilitation.* New York, NY: Oxford University Press; 2010:187.

Weiss LD, Silver JK, Weiss J. *Easy EMG.* New York, NY: Butterworth-Heinemann; 2004: 23-24.

Chapter 18

ACUTE INFLAMMATORY DEMYELINATING POLYNEUROPATHY

Acute Inflammatory Demyelinating Polyradiculoneuropathy (AIDP, Guillain-Barré syndrome) – an acquired disease of autoimmune etiology characterized by ascending paresthesias and weakness that can progress to total body paralysis, autonomic disturbances, and respiratory failure. *Campylobacter jejuni*, mycoplasm, cytomegalovirus, Epstein-Barr virus, and *Haemophilus influenza* are pathogens commonly associated with AIDP. Global incidence is about 0.4 to 1.7/100,000; a mild flulike illness precedes ≈60% of cases by 1 to 4 weeks. More than 50% of patients will complain of pain that is initially described as muscular aching and may transition to neuropathic pain as disease progresses. Extraocular muscles and sphincter function are typically spared. Diagnosis is supported by areflexia, progressive weakness in all limbs, relative symmetry of involvement, CSF cytoalbuminologic dissociation (elevated protein, <10 mononuclear cells/mm^3), and electrodiagnostic findings.

Plasmapheresis or *IV Ig* (400 mg/kg/day × 5 days) given during the evolution of symptoms (within 2 weeks of onset) is effective and has proven to decrease the overall recovery time. Glucocorticoids are *not* effective. Early rehabilitation should emphasize *stretching* and *gradual strengthening*; aggressive therapies may cause overwork weakness. A *tilt table* may be useful in patients with autonomic instability. Prescription of appropriate assistive mobility devices and lower limb orthotics is often indicated.

Mortality is about 3% to 5%, usually due to respiratory or cardiovascular causes from autonomic dysfunction. Most patients recover completely or nearly completely. Recovery time can be weeks to months, or up to 6 to 18 months if axonal damage has occurred. About 10% have a pronounced residual disability, most often lower leg weakness and numbness of the feet; ≈5% to 10% may suffer one or more recurrences of acute polyneuropathy and some cases may evolve into a chronic, progressive inflammatory polyneuropathy.

Chronic Inflammatory Demyelinating Polyradiculoneuropathy (CIDP) – CIDP is pathologically similar to AIDP, but tends to have a slower onset of at least 2 months and may recur multiple times. Weakness is symmetrical with more distal than proximal muscle involvement. Treatment is the same as with AIDP, but CIDP patients with both sensory and motor involvement will respond to high-dose corticosteroids (usual regimen is 80 mg prednisone qd, tapered over months to the lowest effective dose). As with AIDP, diagnosis is supported by electrodiagnostics, CSF findings, nerve biopsy, and MRI abnormalities.

RECOMMENDED READING

Victor M. *Adams & Victor's Principles of Neurology*. 7th ed. New York, NY: McGraw Hill; 2001.

Cuccurullo SJ. *Physical Medicine & Rehabilitation Board Review*. 2nd ed. New York, NY: Demos Medical Publishing; 2004.

Chapter 19

MULTIPLE SCLEROSIS

Introduction and Epidemiology[1] – MS is a CNS inflammatory disease of unknown etiology (thought to be autoimmune) that is characterized by areas of demyelination that are disseminated in time and space. US prevalence is ≈400,000, ranging from 40 to 220/100,000 with ♀:♂ = 2:1 and Caucasian>Asian>African American. Mean onset is ≈30 years of age. Incidence and death rates are higher in the northern latitudes, although this differential appears to be decreasing. An important factor appears to be where one lives prior to 15 years of age.

Diagnosis and Clinical Features – *Definite MS* has been classically defined as ≥2 attacks, separated by ≥1 month, with clinical, imaging, or laboratory evidence (e.g., ↑ CSF protein with oligoclonal bands on electrophoresis and delayed visual evoked potential [VEP]/somatosensory evoked potential [SSEP] latencies) of ≥2 lesions.[2] Each attack lasts >24 hours. Ovoid plaques that are bright on T2 MRI are typically found in the periventricular white matter, cortical–subcortical junction, brainstem, and/or cerebellum. Corpus callosum lesions are relatively specific for MS. In 2005, revisions were made to the McDonald criteria for the diagnosis of MS (see Table 19-1).[3]

TABLE 19-1 2005 Revised McDonald Criteria for MS

Clinical (attacks)	Objective lesions	Additional requirements to make diagnosis
Two or more	Two or more	None; clinical evidence alone will suffice; additional evidence desirable but must be consistent with MS
Two or more	One	Dissemination in space by MRI *or* two or more MRI lesions consistent with MS plus positive CSF *or* await further clinical attack implicating another site
One	Two or more	Dissemination in time by MRI *or* second clinical attack
One	One	Dissemination in space by MRI *or* two or more MRI lesions consistent with MS plus positive CSF *and* dissemination in time by MRI or second clinical attack

(Continued)

TABLE 19-1 2005 Revised McDonald Criteria for MS (Continued)

Clinical (attacks)	Objective lesions	Additional requirements to make diagnosis
Zero (progression from onset)	One or more	Disease progression for 1 year (retrospective or prospective) *and* at least two of the following: • Positive brain MRI (nine T2 lesions or four or more T2 lesions with positive VEP) • Positive spinal cord MRI (two or more focal T2 lesions) • Positive CSF

McDonald WI, Compston A, Edan G, et al. Recommended diagnostic criteria for multiple sclerosis: guidelines from the International Panel on the Diagnosis of Multiple Sclerosis. *Ann Neurol.* 2001;50:121-127.
Polman CH, Reingold SC, Edan G, et al. Diagnostic criteria for multiple sclerosis: 2005 revisions to the McDonald criteria. *Ann Neurol.* 2005;58:840-846.

Common *presenting symptoms* include sensory changes, visual loss, motor changes, and diplopia. Common *clinical features* include paresthesias, weakness, spasticity, fatigue (may be worsened by heat, Uhthoff's phenomenon), bladder and sexual dysfunction, cognitive changes, depression, dysphagia, and neuropathic pain. Exacerbations are fewer during pregnancy but increased postpartum; fertility is unaffected. *Prognosis* is worse for males, older age of onset, high lesion burden on MRI at onset, initially polysymptomatic, predominantly cerebellar or motor symptoms, and rapidly progressive symptoms.

Clinical Categories and Treatment – *Relapsing–remitting* MS is characterized by acute attacks (<1 per month) followed by recovery (within weeks to months) with little or no residual neurologic deficit. Interferon β-1a (Avonex, Rebif), interferon β-1b (Betaseron), and glatiramer acetate (Copaxone) are effective therapies. Half will develop a *secondary progressive* course with or without relapses. Interferon β-1b may delay progression of disability in secondary progressive MS (i.e., wheelchair dependence). These two types comprise ≈85% of persons with MS.

Primary progressive MS (10% to 15%) is characterized by an insidious onset and gradual progression without acute relapses. It typically presents at around 40 years of age; males and females are equally affected. No proven pharmacotherapy assists treatment.

Progressive relapsing MS (<5%) is a progressive disease from the onset with superimposed acute relapses with or w/o some recovery.

IV steroids, which are a mainstay of acute treatment (e.g., methylprednisolone IV 500 mg qd × 5 days or 1 g qd × 3 days), shorten the exacerbation period, but do *not* change the ultimate extent of recovery. *Rehabilitation* management includes treatment of bowel/bladder spasticity and pain issues. Fatigue can be addressed with energy conservation techniques and/or pharmaceuticals (e.g., amantadine, *pemoline*, modafinil, and methylphenidate). Exercise, once considered contraindicated in MS, should be prescribed to help delay secondary disability.[4]

REFERENCES

1. Anderson DW. Revised estimate of MS prevalence in the U.S. *Ann Neurol.* 1992;31:331-336; Kurtzke JF. Epidemiology and etiology of multiple sclerosis. In: Brown T, Kraft GH, eds. *Physical Medicine and Rehabilitation Clinics of North America: Multiple Sclerosis: A Paradigm Shift.* Philadelphia, PA: Saunders; 2005;331-336.
2. Poser CM. New diagnostic criteria for MS. *Ann Neurol.* 1983;13:227-231.
3. Polman CH, Reingold SC, Edan G, et al. Diagnostic criteria for multiple sclerosis: 2005 revisions to the "McDonald Criteria". *Ann Neurol.* 2005;58:840-846.
4. Petajan JH. Impact of aerobic training on fitness and quality of life in MS. *Ann Neurol.* 1996;39:432-441.

Chapter 20

MOVEMENT DISORDERS

Definition – A group of CNS degenerative diseases associated with involuntary movements or abnormalities of skeletal muscle tone and posture. They can be broadly classified as hypokinetic (too little) or hyperkinetic (too much) movement disorders.

Pathophysiology of Parkinson's Disease (PD; Hypokinetic Movement Disorder) – The predominant area of involvement is basal ganglia, which are primarily inhibitory in function. Affects the dopamine-producing cells (substantia nigra and locus ceruleus) of basal ganglia, resulting in degeneration of nigrostriatal pathway and thereby causing decreased dopamine in the corpus striatum. This results in loss of inhibitory input to the cholinergic system, allowing excessive excitatory output.

Etiology – Unknown. The most common movement disorder is Parkinson's disease, affecting 1% of the population over 50 years of age. Incidence is 20/100,000 per year. Male:female ratio is 3:2. Associated with pesticide and herbicide use; 5% to 10% is hereditary (five genes identified so far).

Clinical Presentation

- The most common initial symptom is resting tremor (pill-rolling tremor) in the hands
- Characterized by a triad of resting tremor, bradykinesia, and muscle rigidity
- Features of advanced disease include masked facies, festinating gait (shuffling), and postural instability due to loss of postural reflexes, resulting in fall to side or backward
- Freezing phenomenon (transient inability to perform or restart certain tasks)
- Depression
- Dementia (40%)

Treatment – Medical or surgical.

The goal of medical treatment is to increase dopamine action and decrease cholinergic effect. A guiding principle is to start treatment when symptoms interfere with performing ADLs.

1. L-Dopa: Precursor of dopamine. Given with carbidopa (a dopa decarboxylase inhibitor), which prevents systemic metabolism of L-dopa (example: Sinemet).
2. Dopaminergic agonists:
   a. Ergot derivatives – bromocriptine (stimulates D2 receptors) and pergolide (stimulates D1 and D2 receptors).
   b. Nonergot derivatives – ropinirole (Requip) and pramipexole (Mirapex).

3. Amantadine – an antiviral that potentiates release of endogenous dopamine and has mild anticholinergic activity.
4. Anticholinergics – effective in relieving tremor. Includes trihexiphenidyl (Artane), benztropine (Cogentin), procyclidine, and orphenadrine.
5. Inhibitors of dopamine metabolism – inhibits monoamine oxidase (MAO)-B that is predominant in the striatum.
   a. Selegiline – decreases oxidative damage in substantia nigra and slows disease progression.
   b. Tolcapone – catechol-*O*-methyltransferase inhibitor, inhibits metabolism of dopamine in the liver, GI tract, and other organs.

Surgical treatment is indicated in patients with advanced disease in whom medical treatment is ineffective or poorly tolerated. Mostly effective in relief of tremor. Complications include brain hemorrhage, infection, and device failure.

1. Destructive surgery – thalamotomy or pallidotomy.
2. Deep brain stimulator – electrode placed into ventral intermediate nucleus of the thalamus.

Causes for Disability

1. Social isolation
2. Manual dexterity (inability to perform ADLs such as dressing, cutting food, writing, and fine motor skills)
3. Stooped posture, resulting in loss of balance and increased risk of falls
4. Slowness of gait, resulting in retropulsion (staggering backward) or propulsion (stumble forward)
5. Speech impairment
6. Dysphagia, resulting in silent aspiration
7. Drooling due to decreased frequency of spontaneous swallowing

Rationale for Rehabilitation – Functionally based, i.e., objectively assessed using unified PD rating scale (UPDRS), which includes assessment of walking speed, distance, backward and forward stepping, ability to navigate obstacles, fine motor tasks, equilibrium, and simultaneous and sequential tasks.

Rehabilitation Strategies

Physical therapy

- Posture training (hip extension, pelvic tilt, and standing)
- Postural reflexes
- ROM (passive/active and relaxation techniques)
- Ambulation – use of walker with wheels. Sometimes may use weighted walker to prevent retropulsion
- Conditioning (quadriceps and hip extensor strengthening)
- Frenkel's exercises for coordination of foot placement
- Wobble board or balance feedback trainers to improve body alignment and postural reflexes

Occupational therapy

- Adaptive equipments such as plate guards, cups/utensils with large handles, and swivel forks and spoons
- Replace buttons on clothing with Velcro/zipper closures

Other strategies

- Swallow evaluation
- Diaphragmatic breathing exercises to improve dysarthria

Hyperkinetic Movement Disorders

Include tremors, tics, Tourette's syndrome, dystonia (generalized and focal), dyskinesia, chorea, hemiballismus, myoclonus, and asterixis.

Tremor – Rhythmic oscillation of a body part. Occurs in 6% of the population. Treatment includes propranolol, primidone, benzodiazepines (BZDs; alprazolam), anticonvulsants (gabapentin and topiramate), and Botox.

Tics – Sustained nonrhythmic muscle contractions that are rapid and stereotyped and often occurring in the same extremity or body part during stress.

Tourette's Syndrome – Involuntary use of obscenities (coprolalia) and obscene gestures (copropraxia). Treated using neuroleptics (pimozide and haloperidol).

Dystonia – Slow sustained contractions of muscles that frequently cause twisting movements or abnormal postures.

- Idiopathic
- Focal (torticollis, blepharospasm, oromandibular dystonia, and writer's cramp)
- Generalized (Wilson's disease and lipid storage disorders)
- Neurodegenerative diseases such as PD and Huntington's disease
- Acquired with perinatal brain injury, CO poisoning, and encephalitis

Treatment includes anticholinergics, baclofen, carbamazepine, clonazepam, and Botox for focal dystonias.

Tardive Dyskinesia – Involuntary choreiform movements of face and tongue such as chewing, sucking, licking, puckering, and smacking due to hypersensitivity of dopamine receptors due to long-term blockade.

- Associated with long-term neuroleptic medication use (20%)
- Decreased since the advent of atypical neuroleptics such as clozapine, risperidone, and olanzapine
- Treatment includes BZDs

Ataxia – Usually associated with cerebellar disease

- Causes include stroke, MS, acute/chronic alcohol toxicity, and hereditary (slowly progressive) Friedreich's ataxia
- Treatment includes compensatory techniques, gait training, and assistive devices

Athetosis – Slow, writhing, and repetitive movements affecting face and upper extremities.

Chorea – Nonstereotyped, unpredictable, jerky movements involving oral structures.

Hemiballismus – Extremely violent flinging of unilateral arm and leg secondary to infarct or bleeding in subthalamic nuclei.

Myoclonus – Sudden jerky irregular contraction of muscle.

- Can be physiological (sleep jerks and hiccups)
- Essential (increasing with activity)
- Epileptic
- Symptomatic (part of underlying encephalopathy or stroke)
- Spinal myoclonus (group of muscles innervated by spinal segments). Occurs in spinal cord disorders such as tumor, trauma, or MS
- Treatment includes clonazepam, valproate, and Keppra

Chapter 21

SPINAL CORD INJURY

Epidemiology of Traumatic SCI

There are ≈12,000 new patients who survive SCI in the United States each year.[1] Since 2005, the mean age at time of injury is 40.2 years.[1] ♂:♀ = 4:1. Incomplete tetraplegia is the most common category, followed by complete paraplegia (22.9%), incomplete paraplegia (21.5%), and complete tetraplegia (16.9%).[1]

Since 2005, the most common etiologies are vehicular crashes (41.3%), followed by falls (27.3%), acts of violence (15.0), unknown (8.5%), and sports (7.9%).[1] The proportion of injuries from falls has increased and that from sports has decreased.[2]

Selected Tracts

The majority of descending *corticospinal motor fibers* cross at the medulla to become the lateral corticospinal tract (CST). A small number of CST fibers do not decussate at the medulla and descend via the anterior CST before crossing at the level of the anterior white commissure. Although often depicted in many representations of the spinal cord (see Fig. 21-1, right), the existence of a somatotopic organization of the lateral CST has been challenged.[3]

The ascending *dorsal white columns* cross in the medulla, via the medial lemniscus, then go on to the thalamus. These fibers carry joint position, vibration, and light touch (LT) sensation. The *spinothalamic tracts*, which carry pain, temperature, and nondiscriminative tactile sensations, cross to the contralateral side shortly after entry to the cord in the ventral white commissure of the spinal cord.

Classification of SCI: International Standards for the Neurologic Classification of SCI

1. Perform a supine sensory examination of the 28 dermatomes at the key sensory points for pin prick (PP) and LT, including rectal sensation. The sensory level is the most caudal level with intact (grade 2) sensation for both PP and LT.

   Rectal sensory examination includes evaluation of deep rectal sensation as determined by the patient's ability to feel the examiner's finger during digital rectal examination.
2. Perform a supine motor examination of 10 key muscle groups and voluntary anal contraction. The motor level for each side is the most caudal level with grade ≥3, where all muscles rostral to it are grade 5.

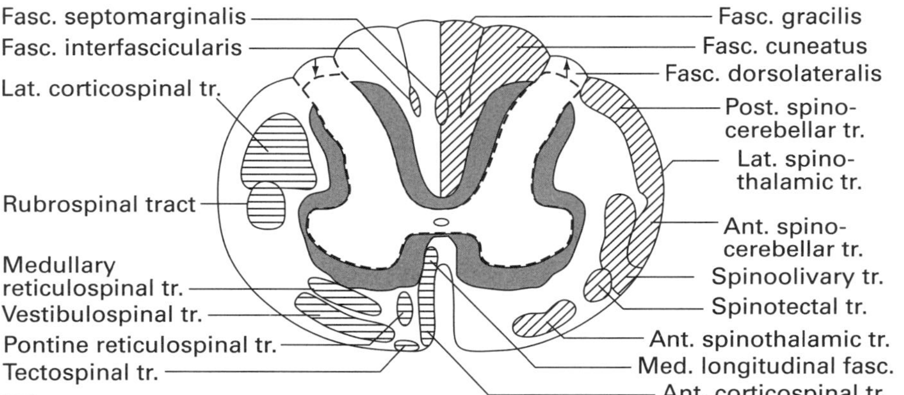

Figure 21-1 Ascending and descending pathways of the spinal cord. Two different types of *hatched areas* are used to differentiate ascending from descending pathways. The fasciculus proprius system (*shaded areas*) and dorsolateral fasciculus contain both ascending and descending nerve fibers (ligature present).

Adapted from Adams M, ed. *Adams & Victor's Principles of Neurology.* 7th ed. McGraw-Hill, 2001.

3. Determine the single neurologic level, which is the most caudal level at which both sensory and motor modalities are intact bilaterally, as defined earlier.
4. Classify injury as complete or incomplete. Complete injuries have no motor or sensory function, including deep anal sensation, preserved in sacral segments S4-5. Somatosensory evoked potentials (SSEPs) may be useful in differentiating complete versus incomplete SCI in patients who are uncooperative or unconscious.
5. Categorize by American Spinal Injury Association (ASIA) Impairment Scale (AIS) A to E.

   Determine the zone of partial preservation (ZPP) if ASIA A. ZPP is defined as preserved segments below the neurologic level of injury (NLOI) and used in complete injuries.

Important ASIA Key Sensory Points

C2	Occipital protuberance	T1	Medial epicondyle elbow	L3	Medial anterior knee
C3	Supraclavicular fossa	T2	Apex of the axilla	L4	Medial malleolus
C4	Top of the AC joint	T4	Medial to nipple	L5	Web space between first and second toes
C5	Lateral antecubital fossa	T10	Lateral to umbilicus	S1	Lateral heel
C6	Dorsal proximal thumb	T12	Inguinal ligament	S2	Lateral popliteal fossa
C7	Dorsal proximal middle finger	L1	Between T12 and L2	S3	Ischial tuberosity
C8	Dorsal proximal fifth finger	L2	Medial anterior thigh	S4-5	Anal mucocutaneous junction

ASIA Key Muscles

C5	Elbow flexors	T1	Small finger abductors	L5	Extensor hallucis longus
C6	Wrist extensors	L2	Hip flexors	S1	Ankle plantar flexors
C7	Elbow extensors	L3	Knee extensors		
C8	Flexor digitorum profundus of third digit	L4	Ankle dorsiflexors		

Sensory levels are scored as 0 (absent), 1 (impaired, including hyperesthesia), 2 (normal), or not testable (NT). When scoring PP, inability to distinguish PP from LT is scored 0/2. Muscles are graded from 0 (total paralysis) to 5 (normal active movement with full ROM against full resistance), or NT.

ASIA Impairment Scale, Revised (2000)

A Complete – No sensory or motor function is preserved in the lowest sacral segments S4-5. The ZPP (only used in ASIA A) refers to the most caudal segment below the level of injury with partial sensory or motor function.

B Incomplete – Sensory but no motor function is preserved below the neurologic level and must include sacral segments S4-5.

C Incomplete – Motor function is preserved more than three levels below the neurologic level, and more than half of the key muscles below the neurologic level have a muscle grade <3.

D Incomplete – Motor function is preserved more than three levels below the neurologic level, and at least half of the key muscles below the neurologic level have a muscle grade ≥3.

E Normal – LT, PP, and motor function of the key muscles are normal.[4]

Note: For an individual to receive a grade of ASIA C or D, there must be sensory or motor S4-5 sparing. In addition, the individual must have either (1) voluntary anal sphincter contraction or (2) sparing of motor function more than three levels below the motor level.

SCI Clinical Syndromes

Central Cord – This incomplete syndrome is typically seen in older persons with cervical spondylosis who experience neck hyperextension injury, resulting in greater upper limb rather than lower limb impairment. Bowel, bladder, and sexual dysfunction are variable. The postulated mechanism of injury involves cord compression both anteriorly and posteriorly, with inward bulging of the ligamentum flavum during hyperextension in a stenotic spinal canal.[5] *Penrod*[6] retrospectively studied 51 patients with central cord syndrome and noted better overall recovery of ambulation, self-care, and bowel/bladder function in patients <50 years of age than their older counterparts at time of discharge from rehabilitation.

Brown-Séquard – Hemisection of the cord produces ipsilateral weakness and proprioceptive loss and contralateral loss of PP and temperature sense. The prognosis for ambulation is best among the incomplete SCI syndromes.

Anterior Cord – There is variable loss of motor and PP sensation, with relative preservation of proprioception and LT. Prognosis for motor recovery is generally considered poor. Typically, the anterior cord syndrome results from a vascular lesion in the territory of the anterior spinal artery, but it may also be seen resulting from retropulsed disks/vertebral fragments. Intraoperative SSEPs, which primarily monitor the posterior column pathways, may miss the development of an anterior cord syndrome.

Cauda Equina – Cauda equina injuries may be due to neural canal compression or fractures of the sacrum or spine at L2 or below. While the damage occurs within the spinal cord, the syndrome can be described as "multiple lumbosacral radiculopathies," since the cauda is comprised of lumbosacral nerve roots. Sequelae depend on the roots involved but usually involve impairment of bowel, bladder, and sexual function. Areflexia, saddle anesthesia, and lower limb weakness are also characteristic. Radicular neuropathic pain is common and can be severe. Recovery is possible because the nerve roots can recover. Consultation for possible early surgery is indicated.

Conus Medullaris – A pure conus medullaris lesion (e.g., intramedullary tumor) results in saddle anesthesia and bladder, sphincter, and sexual dysfunction due to cord injury at the S2-4 segments. Anal cutaneous and bulbocavernosus (S2-4) and ankle deep tendon reflexes (S1,S2) may be either absent or preserved depending upon whether the lesion is "high" in the conus. Prognosis for recovery is poor. Conus lesions due to trauma (e.g., L1 vertebral body fracture) are typically accompanied by injury of some of the lumbosacral nerve roots, resulting in a variable degree of lower limb dysfunction.

Basis for Acute Interventions

High-dose steroids have been reported to be neuroprotective in acute SCI by inhibiting lipid peroxidation and scavenging free radicals. The use of IV methylprednisolone (MP) in acute nonpenetrating traumatic SCI is supported by the *National Acute Spinal Cord Injury Studies* (NASCIS).[7,8] The results of the NASCIS trials, however, have been challenged by some authors and organizations.[9,10]

In the *NASCIS 2* trial, segmental and long-tract neurologic function modestly improved at 6 weeks, 6 months, and 1 year post-SCI in patients receiving MP within 8 hours of SCI as compared with placebo or naloxone. MP was given as a 30 mg/kg bolus over 1 hour, then as a 5.4 mg/kg/h drip for an additional 23 hours. The *NASCIS 3* trial further refined the MP protocol such that when steroid treatment is initiated within 3 hours of SCI, MP is administered for 24 hours; if initiated at 3 to 8 hours post-SCI, MP is administered for an additional 24 hours, for a total of 48 hours.

GM-1 *ganglioside* (Sygen) has never been approved for the treatment of SCI. A study demonstrated neuroprotective and neuroregenerative effects in vitro. The *Sygen Multicenter Acute SCI Study*[11] showed a more rapid time course of neurologic recovery in the Sygen + IV MP versus the IV MP group. However, the outcomes in both groups were found to be similar at 26 weeks.

The optimal timing for *surgery* after SCI is unknown. Retrospective data suggest a role for urgent decompression in the setting of bilateral facet dislocation or incomplete SCI with progressive neurologic deterioration.[12]

Prognosis and Recovery in Traumatic SCI

Complete SCI – Only 2% to 3% of patients who are AIS A at 1 week post-SCI improve to AIS D by 1 year.[13] In persons with *complete tetraplegia*, >95% of key muscles in the ZPP with grade 1 or 2 at 1 month post-SCI will reach grade 3 at 1 year[13]; ≈25% of the most cephalad grade 0 muscles at

1 month recover to grade 3 at 1 year,[13] those having pin sensation being the most likely to recover motor function. Most upper limb recovery occurs during the first 6 months, with the greatest rate of change during the first 3 months. Motor level is superior to the neurologic or sensory level in correlating with function. In patients who are *complete paraplegics* at 1 week post-SCI, NLOI has been found to remain unchanged at 1 year in 73%, improve 1 level in 18%, and improve ≥2 levels in 9%.[13] Waters[14] reported that only 5% of complete paraplegics eventually achieve community ambulation.

Incomplete SCI – *Incomplete tetraplegics* often recover multiple levels below the initial level. Waters[15] reported that 46% of incomplete tetraplegics recover sufficient motor function to ambulate at 1 year; 80% of *incomplete paraplegics* regain hip flexors and knee extensors (KEs; grade ≥3) by 1 year.[13]

In a review of 27 patients who were initially sensory incomplete, Crozier[16] reported that partial (or greater) preservation of PP sensation below the zone of injury was predictive of eventual functional ambulation.

Miscellaneous – The 72-hour post-SCI neurologic examination may predict recovery more reliably than an examination performed on the day of injury. Absence of the *bulbocavernosus reflex* beyond the first few days can signify a lower motor neuron lesion and have implications on bowel, bladder, and sexual function. On *MRI*, presence of hemorrhage and length of edema are independent negative predictors of motor function at 1 year.[13] Strength ≥3/5 in the b/l HFs and one KE correlates with community ambulation.[17]

Expected Functional Levels

(I, independent; A, assist; D, dependent; predicted outcomes are based on patients of typical age for traumatic SCI – older patients have overall poorer expected outcome)

C1-3 – ventilator dependent (or may have phrenic nerve pacing); D for secretion management. I with power WC mobility and pressure relief with equipment; otherwise essentially D for all care (but I for directing care).

C4 – may be able to breathe w/o a ventilator. May use a mobile arm support for limited ADLs if there is some elbow flexion and deltoid strength. May be able to use a sip–puff or head-control WC.

C5 – may require A to clear secretions. May be I for feeding after setup and with adaptive equipment, e.g., a long opponens orthosis with utensil slots and mobile arm support. Requires A for most upper body ADLs. Most patients will be *unable* to do self–clean intermittent catheterization. I with power WC; some users may be I with manual WC on noncarpeted, level, indoor surfaces. Some may drive specially adapted vans.

C6 – May use a tenodesis orthosis and short opponens orthosis with utensil slots. I with feeding except for cutting food. I for most upper body ADLs after setup and with modifications (e.g., Velcro straps on clothing);

A to D for most lower body ADLs, including bowel care. Some males may be I with self–intermittent catheterization (IC) after setup; females are usually D. Some patients may be I for transfers using a sliding board and heel loops, but many will require A. May be I with manual WC, but power WCs are often used, especially for longer distances and outdoors. May drive an adapted van.

C7 – Essentially I for most ADLs, often using a short opponens splint and universal cuff. May require A for some lower body ADLs. Women may have difficulty with IC. Bowel care may be I with adaptive equipment, but suppository insertion may still be difficult. I for mobility at a manual WC level, except for uneven transfers. Patients may be I with a nonvan automobile with hand controls if the patient can transfer and load/unload the WC.

C8 – Completely I with ADLs and mobility using manual WC and adapted car.

Paraplegia – Trunk stability improves with lower lesions. *Upper and mid-thoracics* may stand and ambulate with b/l KAFOs and Lofstrand crutches (i.e., swing-through or swing-to gait), but the intent is usually exercise, not functional mobility. Using orthoses and gait-assistive devices, *lower thoracics* and *L1* SCI patients can do household ambulation and may be I community ambulators. *L2-S5* SCI patients may be community ambulators with or w/o orthoses (i.e., KAFOs or AFOs) and/or gait-assistive devices. (AFOs generally compensate for the ankle weakness, while canes and crutches primarily compensate for hip abduction and extension weakness.)

Selected Issues in SCI

Autonomic Dysreflexia (AD) – can occur in 48% to 85% of patients with SCI at T6 or above.[18] Since resting SBPs can be 90 to 110 mm Hg in this population, SBPs of 20 to 40 mm Hg > baseline may signify AD.[18] A noxious stimulus below the level of injury causes reflex sympathetic vasoconstriction (BP ↑). Due to the SCI, higher CNS centers cannot directly modulate the sympathetic response. The body attempts to lower BP by carotid and aortic baroreceptor/vagal-mediated bradycardia, but this is usually ineffective (Fig. 21-2).

The primary treatment of AD entails removing the source of noxious stimulus. This is most commonly bladder dysfunction, and the second most common cause is bowel distention. Other causes include pressure ulcers, undiagnosed fractures, abdominal emergencies, ingrown toenails, and body positioning. Table 21-1 gives a complete chart of the causes of AD.

Long-Term Routine Urinary Tract Surveillance after SCI – *Upper tract* follow-up can include *renal scan with GFR* or *renal scan with 24-hour Cr clearance* yearly to follow renal function. *Renal and bladder ultrasound* can be done annually to detect hydronephrosis and stones. *Lower tract* evaluation can include *urodynamics* once the bladder starts exhibiting uninhibited contractions (or at around 3 to 6 months postinjury) and then as determined by the clinician (often done annually). Routine

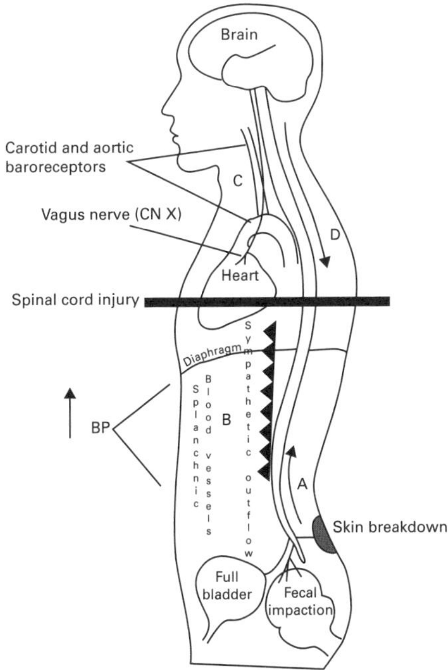

Figure 21-2 **A.** A strong sensory input (not necessarily noxious) is carried into the spinal cord through intact peripheral nerves. The most common origins are bladder and bowel. **B.** This strong sensory input travels up the spinal cord and evokes a massive reflex sympathetic surge from the thoracolumbar sympathetic nerves. This sympathetic surge causes widespread vasoconstriction, most significantly in the subdiaphragmatic (or splanchnic) vasculature. Thus, peripheral arterial hypertentaion occurs. **C.** The brain detects this hypertensive crisis through intact baroreceptors in the neck delivered to the brain through cranial nerves IX and X (vagus). **D.** The brain attempts two maneuvers to halt the progression of this hypertensive crisis. First, the brain attempts to shut down the sympathetic surge by sending descending inhibitory impulses. Unfortunately, these inhibitory impulses do not reach most syspathetic outflow levels because of the spinal cord injury at T6 or above. Therefore, inhibitory impluses are blocked in the injured spinal cord. The second maneuver orchestrated by the brain, in an attempt to bring down peripheral blood pressure, is heart rate slowing through an intact vagus (parasympathetic) nerve. This may result in a compensatory bradycardia but is inadequate, and hypertension continues. In summary, the sympatheitc nerves prevail below the level of neurologic injury, and the parasympathetic nerves prevail above the level of injury. Once the inciting stimulus is removed, the relex hypertension resolves.

Adapted from American Spinal Injury Association. *Standards for Neurological and Functional Classification of SCI*. 3rd ed. Chicago, IL: ASIA; 1990.

TABLE 21-1 Stimuli and Conditions Associated with the Development of Autonomic Dysreflexia

Gastrointestinal system
Bowel distention
Anal fissures
Esophageal reflux
Enemas
Gastric dilatation
Gastric ulcer
Cholecystitis or cholelithiasis
Urogenital system
Penile stimulation and intercourse
Urethral and bladder distention
Vaginal dilatation
Urinary tract infections
Epididymitis
Renal calculus
Testicular torsion
Skin
Cutaneous stimulation
Sunburns
Pressure sores
Extremities
Deep venous thromboses
Ingrown toenails
Functional electrical stimulation
Spasticity
Bone fractures
Range-of-motion exercises
Position changes
Procedures and conditions
Urodynamics and cystoscopy
Surgical procedures
Radiologic procedures
Pulmonary emboli
Electroejaculation
Labor
Miscellaneous
Medications
Emergence in cold water
Self-induced autonomic dysreflexia (intentional boosting)
Sentinel event of another serious medical complication

Adapted from Teasell RW, Arnold JM, Krassioukov A. Cardiovascular consequences of loss of supraspinal control of the sympathetic nervous system after spinal cord injury. *Arch Phys Med Rehab.* 2000;81(4):506-516, with permission.

cystoscopy to potentially diagnose neoplasm at an earlier rather than a later stage should be performed annually as patients approach 10 years of chronic indwelling (urethral or suprapubic) catheter use or sooner (after 5 years) if there are additional risk factors (heavy smoker, age > 40 years, and history of many UTIs).

Posttraumatic Syringomyelia – seen in ≈3% to 8% of posttraumatic SCI patients as manifested by neurologic decline or up to 20% on autopsy. It can develop as early as 2 months post-SCI.[19] Pain is often worsened by coughing or straining, but not by lying supine. Ascending sensory loss, progressive weakness (including bulbar muscles), ↑ sweating, orthostasis, and Horner's syndrome may also be seen. Diagnosis is by MRI. Treatment is usually observational and symptomatic. Surgical interventions are available for large, progressive lesions.

Sexual Function and Fertility – *Females*: 44% to 55% of women with SCI can achieve orgasm.[20] Menses typically returns within 6 months post-SCI, and reproductive function is preserved. Incidence of prematurity and small-for-date infants is high, but there is no increase in spontaneous abortions. Spinal anesthesia is recommended during delivery for patients with SCI at T6 or above to avoid AD.

Males: With *complete* upper motor neuron SCI, reflexogenic erections can usually be achieved, although ejaculation is rare. With *incomplete* SCI, reflexogenic erections are usually attainable; ejaculation is less rare than for those with complete SCI; and some patients can achieve psychogenic erections. Complete or incomplete injuries *below T11* may result in erections of poor quality and duration. Infertility is common after SCI, due to factors including retrograde ejaculation and poor sperm quantity and motility. *Vibratory* ejaculation in which the ventral penile shaft is stimulated requires that the postinjury period is >6 months and L2-S1 is intact. *Electroejaculation* (seminal vesicle and prostatic stimulation through the rectum) is another option.

Tendon Transfer Surgery in Tetraplegia – Triceps function can be restored in the C5,6 SCI patient with a posterior deltoid-to-triceps or a biceps-to-triceps transfer. Lateral key grip can be restored in a C6 SCI patient via the modified *Moberg procedure*, which involves attachment of the brachioradialis (C5,6) to the flexor pollicis longus (C8,T1) and stabilization of the thumb carpometacarpal and IP joints.

REFERENCES

1. NSCISC National Spinal Cord Injury Statistical Center. The University of Alabama at Birmingham. https://www.nscisc.uab.edu. Accessed March 15, 2012.
2. Devivo M. Epidemiology of traumatic SCI. In: Kirshblum S, ed. *Spinal Cord Medicine*. Philadelphia, PA: Lippincott Williams & Wilkins; 2002:69.
3. Levi AD. Clinical syndromes associated with disproportionate weakness of the upper versus the lower extremities after cervical spinal cord injury. *Neurosurgery*. 1996;38:179-183.
4. American Spinal Injury Association. *International Standards for Neurological Classification of SCI, Revised 2000, Reprinted 2003*. Chicago, IL: ASIA; 2003.

5. Kirshblum S. Neurologic assessment and classification of traumatic SCI. In: Kirshblum S, ed. *Spinal Cord Medicine.* Philadelphia, PA: Lippincott Williams & Wilkins; 2002:88.
6. Penrod LE. Age effect on prognosis for functional recovery in acute, traumatic central cord syndrome. *Arch Phys Med Rehabil.* 1990;71:963-968.
7. Bracken MB. NASCIS 2. *N Engl J Med.* 1990;322:1405-1411.
8. Bracken MB. NASCIS 3. *JAMA.* 1997;277:1597-1604.
9. Nesathurai S. Steroids and SCI: revisiting NASCIS 2 and 3. *J Trauma.* 1998;45:1088-1093.
10. Hurlbert RJ. Methylprednisolone for acute SCI: an inappropriate standard of care. *J Neurosurg.* 2000;93(1 suppl):1-7.
11. Geisler F. Sygen multicenter study. *Spine.* 2001;26(suppl):87-98.
12. Fehlings MG. The role and timing of decompression in acute SCI. *Spine.* 2001;26(suppl):101-109.
13. Ditunno JF. Predicting outcome in traumatic SCI. In: Kirshblum S, ed. *Spinal Cord Medicine.* Philadelphia, PA: Lippincott Williams & Wilkins; 2002:87.
14. Waters RL. Donald Munro lecture: functional and neurologic recovery following acute SCI. *J Spinal Cord Med.* 1998;21:195-199.
15. Waters RL. Motor and sensory recovery following incomplete tetraplegia. *Arch Phys Med Rehabil.* 1994;75:306-311.
16. Crozier KS. SCI: prognosis for ambulation based on sensory examination in pts who are initially motor complete. *Arch Phys Med Rehabil.* 1991;72:119-121.
17. Hussey RW. SCI: requirements for ambulation. *Arch Phys Med Rehabil.* 1973;54:544-547.
18. Campagnolo D. Autonomic and CV complications of SCI. In: Kirshblum S, ed. *Spinal Cord Medicine.* Philadelphia, PA: Lippincott Williams & Wilkins; 2002:123-132.
19. Little JW. Neuromusculoskeletal complications of SCI. In: Kirshblum S, ed. *Spinal Cord Medicine.* Philadelphia, PA: Lippincott Williams & Wilkins; 2002:241-239.
20. Sipski ML. Sexual arousal and orgasm in women: the effects of SCI. *Ann Neurol.* 2001;49:35-44.

Chapter 22

TRAUMATIC BRAIN INJURY

Introduction and Epidemiology

TBI is a serious public health problem in the United States.

Each year, an estimated 1.7 million people sustain a TBI.[1] Of them

- 52,000 die,
- 275,000 are hospitalized, and
- 1.365 million, nearly 80%, are treated and released from an emergency department.

TBI is responsible for a third (30.5%) of all injury-related deaths in the United States.[1]

TBI is more common in children aged 0 to 4 years, adolescents aged 15 to 19 years, and adults aged 65 years and older. Adults aged 75 years and older have the highest rates of TBI-related hospitalization and death. TBI rates are higher for males than for females.

The leading causes of TBI are

- falls (35.2%);
- motor vehicle – traffic (17.3%);
- struck by/against events (16.5%); and
- assaults (10%).[1]

Blasts are a leading cause of TBI for military personnel in war zones.[2]

Direct medical costs and indirect costs such as lost productivity because of TBI totaled an estimated $60 billion in the United States in 2000.[3]

Primary injury occurs at the time of impact and results from the shear forces of the impact (Fig. 22-1).

Secondary injury follows primary injury and is the effect of cerebral and extracerebral insults. It occurs at both a macroscopic level and a cellular level.

The mechanisms of secondary injury are classified under four categories[4] (Table 22-1):

1. Ischemia, excitotoxicity, energy failure, and cell death
2. Cerebral swelling
3. Axonal injury
4. Inflammation and regeneration

Theories of Recovery: At least three different theories have been proposed to explain the recovery that follows a brain injury and include a reversal of diaschisis, compensation, and adaptive plasticity. Diaschisis is a temporary reduction in function of structures interconnected with an injured brain. Functional recovery is likely to be related to a gradual reduction in diaschisis.

Compensation is the use of alternative strategies as an individual attempts to supplement lost function.

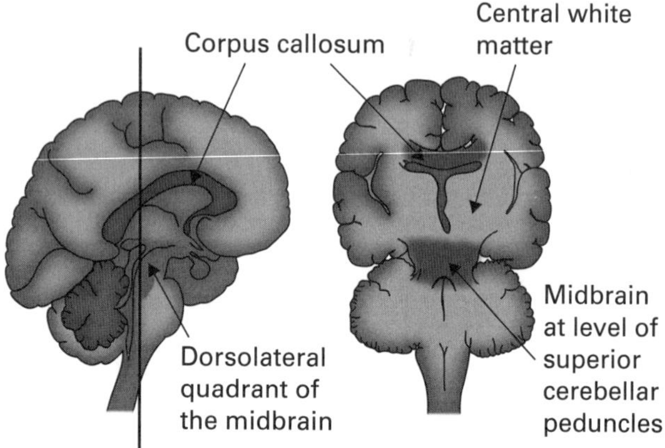

Figure 22-1 Brain regions particularly involved in diffuse axonal injury include the corpus callosum and parasagittal white matter as well as the dorsolateral quadrants of the midbrain.

Adapted from Auergach SH. Neuroanatomical correlates of attention and memory disorders in traumatic brain injury: an application of behavioral subtypes. *J Head Trauma Rehabil.* 1986;1:1-12.

A third theory is that functional recovery is largely dependent upon neuroplasticity of intact remaining brain structure. Underlying mechanisms include unmasking of existing connections, long-term potentiation, long-term depression, axonal sprouting, dendritic sprouting, synaptogenesis, and angiogenesis (Table 22-2).[5]

Glasgow Outcome Scale: The Glasgow Outcome Scale (GOS) is a five-level score:

Dead
Vegetative state
Severely disabled
Moderately disabled
Good recovery

Posttraumatic Amnesia (PTA): the duration during which patients neither encode nor retain any new information and experience and can be assessed by Galveston Orientation Amnesia Test (GOAT). The end of PTA is marked by a score of >75 on GOAT on two consecutive days (Table 22-3).

In the future, a combination of clinical, laboratory (serum biomarkers and genetic markers), evoked potentials, and radiological techniques (functional MRI and MR spectroscopy) may need to be used for prognostication (Table 22-4).

TABLE 22-1 Comparison of Clinical Features Associated with Coma, Vegetative State, Minimally Conscious State, and Locked-In Syndrome

Condition	Consciousness	Sleep/wake	Motor function	Auditory function	Visual function	Communication	Emotion
Coma	None	Absent	Reflex and postural responses only	None	None	None	None
Vegetative state	None	Present	Postures or withdraws to noxious stimuli Occasional nonpurposeful movement	Startle Briefly orients to sound	Startle Brief visual fixation	None	None Reflexive crying or smiling
Minimally conscious state	Partial	Present	Localizes noxious stimuli Reaches for objects Holds or touches objects in a manner that accommodates size and shape Automatic movements (e.g., scratching)	Localizes sound location Inconsistent command following	Sustained visual fixation Sustained visual pursuit	Contingent vocalization Inconsistent but intelligible verbalization or gesture	Contingent smiling or crying

Adapted from Disorders of Consciousness: Giacino JT, Ashwal S, Childs N, et al. The minimally conscious state: definition and diagnostic criteria. *J Neurol.* 2002;58:349-353, Special Article.

TABLE 22-2 Glasgow Coma Scale

		Score
Eye opening	Spontaneously	4
	To speech	3
	To pain	2
	None	1
Verbal response	Orientated	5
	Confused	4
	Inappropriate	3
	Incomprehensible	2
	None	1
Motor response	Obeys commands	6
	Localizes to pain	5
	Withdraws from pain	4
	Flexion to pain	3
	Extension to pain	2
	None	1
Maximum score		15

Adapted from Teasdale G. Assessment of coma and impaired consciousness. *Lancet* 1974;2:81-84.

TABLE 22-3 Summary of Evidence-Based Guidelines for Prognostication after Severe TBI

Severe disability according to GOS is unlikely when
- time to follow command is less than 2 weeks
- duration of PTA is less than 2 months

Good recovery according to GOS is unlikely when
- time to follow commands is longer than 1 month
- duration of PTA is greater than 3 months
- age is more than 65 years

Adapted from Kothari S. Prognosis after severe TBI: a practical evidence based approach. In: Zasler ND, Katz DI, Zafonte RD, eds. *Brain Injury Medicine Principles and Practice.* New York, NY: Demos Medical Publishing; 2007.

TABLE 22-4 Rancho Los Amigos Cognitive Functioning Scale

Rancho level	Clinical correlate
I	No response
II	Generalized response
III	Localized response
IV	Confused, agitated response
V	Confused, inappropriate, nonagitated response
VI	Confused, appropriate response
VII	Automatic, appropriate response
VIII	Purposeful and appropriate response

This is a descriptive scale used for communication between members of the rehabilitation team.
Adapted from Rehabilitation of the Head Injured Adult: Comprehensive Physical Management. *Professional Staff Association, Ranchos Los Amigos Hospital*; 1979.

Acute Treatment

The "ABCs," airway maintenance, breathing, and circulation, are addressed first. The spine is immobilized due to a risk of associated cervical spine injury.

Intracranial Pressure (ICP) Monitoring in Severe TBI: ICP monitoring is appropriate in

- Patients with Glasgow Coma Scale scores postresuscitation ≤8.
- Head CT showing contusions, hemorrhages, edema, or compressed basilar cisterns.
- ICP monitoring may also be appropriate in patients with postresuscitation scores ≤8 with a normal head CT and two of the following: age >40 years, motor posturing, or a systolic pressure of <90 mm Hg.[6]

ICP is monitored by external ventricular drain that can both monitor and drain CSF if necessary. Increased ICPs can be managed by elevating the head end of the bed, preventing hyperthermia, and using diuretics like mannitol. Additional modalities may include use of hyperventilation, barbiturates, and decompressive hemicraniectomy. Steroids have not been shown to reduce ICP and are not recommended for use in TBI.

Use of hypothermia has not shown to reduce all-cause mortality. Brain Trauma Foundation recommendations (Guidelines for the management of severe TBI, 3rd edition, 2007) do not show any level 1 or level 2 evidence for use of hypothermia. However, patients treated with hypothermia were more likely to have a neurological favorable outcome of GOS 4 or 5.

Issues Unique to TBI

Sleep Disturbances – Sleep disturbances occur commonly in patients who have suffered a TBI and may occur during all stages of recovery. Establishing an adequate sleep–wake cycle plays a vital role. Nonpharmacological and pharmacological techniques may need to be utilized. Medications for sleep initiation and for sleep maintenance may need to be considered.

Pharmacotherapy of Arousal and Alertness – Dopaminergic agents (amantadine and bromocriptine) and adrenergic agents like methylphenidate are considered in issues related to impaired arousal and alertness.

Agitation – Posttraumatic agitation is defined as a delirium present during the period of PTA, manifested by behavioral excesses such as aggression, akathisia, disinhibition, emotional lability, destructiveness, or combativeness.[7] The Agitated Behavior Scale is commonly used to quantify agitation in the rehabilitation setting. Medical reasons are always considered first (infections, pain, hypoxia, and metabolic abnormalities). Treatment includes nonpharmacological interventions (quiet room, dim light, limited visitors, Vail bed, and ambulation). Atypical antipsychotics are considered an option in managing TBI-related agitation. Cochrane database review reported that the best evidence for medication management in the treatment of TBI-related agitation exists for inderal (2003).

Endocrine Dysfunction after TBI – Approximately 30% to 50% of patients who survive a TBI demonstrate endocrine abnormalities. Syndrome of Inappropriate Antidiuretic Hormone is the common TBI endocrinopathy causing hyponatremia and is associated with euvolemia, low BUN, and urine osmolality greater than serum osmolality. The treatment in most cases is fluid restriction and in rare cases hypertonic saline. A less common cause of hyponatremia is cerebral salt wasting where patients are dehydrated. Hence, treatment includes replacement of fluids and salt. Diabetes insipidus is rare and usual onset is 5 to 10 days after trauma. Features include polyuria, low urine osmolality, high serum osmolality, and normal to high sodium. Treatment includes hormonal replacement. Anterior hypopituitarism may present weeks to months after moderate to severe TBI and may have an insidious onset with malaise, hypothermia, bradycardia, hypotension, hyponatremia, or stagnation of rehabilitation progress. Workup includes serum hormonal assays and treatment includes hormonal replacement.

Dysautonomia – manifests as tachycardia, increased BP, tachypnea, fever, and sweating. Treatment options include NSAIDs, β-blockers, and symptomatic treatment.

Posttraumatic Epilepsy (PTE) – a disorder characterized by recurrent late seizure episodes in patients with TBI, not attributable to any other etiology. Posttraumatic seizures (PTS) refer to a single or recurrent seizure episode after TBI. PTS have further been classified as early (<1 week after TBI) and late (>1 week after TBI).[8] The incidence of early seizures is approximately 5% among nonpenetrating TBI patients and is higher in younger children and that of late seizures is 4% to 7% in nonpenetrating TBI. PTS are observed in 35% to 65% of patients with penetrating TBI. Studies do not recommend the use of prophylactic anticonvulsants for the prevention of late PTS. Routine seizure prophylaxis beyond 1 week after TBI is not recommended. Prophylactic phenytoin has been shown to reduce the risk of early seizures after severe TBI, but no benefit has been found between 8th day and 2 years post-TBI. Prophylactic use of phenytoin or valproate is not recommended to prevent late PTS, and treatment duration is not clearly established.[9]

Carbamazepine and valproic acid are the preferred agents for treatment of PTE, and treatment duration is not clearly established.

Role of Technology in Rehabilitation of TBI Patients – Use of virtual reality (for driving simulation and to simulate real-life scenarios), as these sessions have been shown to facilitate neuroplasticity and promote motor recovery. Neuroprosthetics to improve ambulation and robotic trainers to maximize therapy intensity and make mass practice more convenient.

No evidence exists to recommend the use of hyperbaric oxygen therapy in the treatment of TBI.

REFERENCES

1. Faul M, Xu L, Wald MM, Coronado VG. *Traumatic Brain Injury in the United States: Emergency Department Visits, Hospitalizations, and Deaths.* Atlanta, GA: Centers for Disease Control and Prevention, National Center for Injury Prevention and Control; 2010.
2. Champion HR, Holcomb JB, Young LA. Injuries from explosions. *J Trauma.* 2009;66(5):1468-1476.
3. Finkelstein E, Corso P, Miller T, et al. *The Incidence and Economic Burden of Injuries in the United States.* New York, NY: Oxford University Press; 2006.
4. Kochanek P, Clark R, Jenkins L. TBI: Pathobiology. In: Zasler ND, Katz DI, Zafonte RD, eds. *Brain Injury Medicine: Principles and Practice.* New York, NY: Demos Medical Publishing; 2007:81-96.
5. Nudo R, Dancause N. Neuroscientific basis for occupational and physical therapy interventions. In: Zasler ND, Katz DI, Zafonte RD, eds. *Brain Injury Medicine: Principles and Practice.* New York, NY: Demos Medical Publishing; 2007:913-928.
6. Narayan RK, Kishore PR, Becker DP, et al. Intracranial pressure: to monitor or not to monitor. A review of our experience with severe head injury. *J Neurosurg.* 1982;56:650-659.
7. Sandel ME, Mysiw WJ. The agitated brain injured patient, part 1: definitions, differential diagnosis and assessment. *Arch Phys Med Rehabil.* 1996;77:617-623.
8. Brain Injury Special Interest group of the AAPMR. Practice parameter: antiepileptic drug treatment of post traumatic seizures. *Arch Phys Med Rehabil.* 1998;79:594-597.
9. Temkin NR. A randomized double blind study of phenytoin for the prevention of post traumatic seizures. *N Engl J Med.* 1990;323:497-502.

Chapter 23

STROKE

EPIDEMIOLOGY AND RISK FACTORS

A stroke is defined by the WHO as the rapid development of clinical signs of cerebral dysfunction, with signs lasting at least 24 hours or leading to death with no apparent cause other than that of vascular origin.[1]

About 795,000 Americans suffer a new or recurrent stroke. This means that, on average, a stroke occurs every 40 seconds. Stroke kills more than 137,000 people a year, which is about 1 of every 18 deaths. It is the No. 3 cause of death behind diseases of the heart and cancer. On average, every 4 minutes, someone dies of stroke. About 40% of stroke deaths occur in males and 60% in females. The 2006 US stroke death rates per 100,000 population for specific groups were 41.7 for white males, 41.1 for white females, 67.7 for black males, and 57.0 for black females.

The two major types of stroke are *ischemic* (≈83%) and *hemorrhagic* (17%).[2] On further categorizing, 32% are embolic, 31% large vessel thrombotic, 20% small vessel thrombotic, 10% intracerebral hemorrhagic, and 7% subarachnoid hemorrhagic.[2] The Framingham Heart Study data revealed 30-day survival rates to be 73% to 81% following cerebral infarction and 36% after intracerebral hemorrhage,[3] although survival figures vary widely in the literature and have generally been improving with time.

Males, African Americans, and the elderly are at increased risk for developing stroke. Modifiable risk factors include HTN, DM, hypercholesterolemia, hyperhomocysteinemia, hypercoagulable states, heart disease, carotid arteriosclerosis, substance abuse, obesity, and a sedentary lifestyle.

SELECTED ISCHEMIC STROKE SYNDROMES

MCA – Deficits can include c/l hemiplegia/hypesthesia (face and arm worse than leg), c/l homonymous hemianopia, and i/l gaze preference.

With *dominant* hemisphere involvement, receptive aphasia (inferior division of MCA to Wernicke's area) and/or expressive aphasia (superior division of MCA to Broca's area) can occur, but classically patients can learn from demonstration and mistakes. *Gerstmann's syndrome* (parietal lobe) consists of asomatognosia (right–left confusion), dyscalculia, finger agnosia, and dysgraphia.

With *nondominant* hemisphere involvement, spatial dyspraxia and c/l hemineglect may be seen; insight/judgment are often affected (likely to need supervision); ADL recovery is often said to be slower.

Acrodermatitis Chronica Atrophican (ACA) – Deficits can include c/l hemiplegia/hypesthesia (leg worse than arm; face and hand spared), alien arm/hand syndrome, urinary incontinence, gait apraxia, abulia (inability to make decisions), perseveration, amnesia, paratonic rigidity (*Gegenhalten*, or variable resistance to passive ROM), and transcortical motor aphasia (with a dominant hemisphere ACA lesion).

Posterior Cerebral Artery (PCA) – Deficits can include c/l homonymous hemianopia, c/l hemianesthesia, c/l hemiplegia, c/l hemiataxia, and vertical gaze palsy. *Dominant*-sided lesions can lead to amnesia, color anomia, dyslexia w/o agraphia, and simultagnosia (defunct perceptual analysis). *Nondominant*-sided lesions can lead to prosopagnosia (cannot recognize familiar faces).

The *central poststroke pain (Dejerine-Roussy or thalamic pain) syndrome* can occur with involvement of the thalamogeniculate branch. *Weber's syndrome* (penetrating branches to the midbrain) consists of i/l CN III palsy and c/l limb weakness). A b/l PCA stroke can cause *Anton syndrome* (cortical blindness, with denial) or *Bálint's* syndrome, which consists of optic ataxia, loss of voluntary but not reflex eye movements, and an inability to understand visual objects (asimultagnosia).

Brain Stem – The *lateral medullary (Wallenberg) syndrome* (posterior inferior cerebellar artery) consists of vertigo, nystagmus, dysphagia, dysarthria, dysphonia, i/l Horner's syndrome, i/l facial pain or numbness, i/l limb ataxia, and c/l pain and temporary sensory loss. The "locked-in" *syndrome* (basilar artery) is due to b/l pontine infarcts affecting the corticospinal and bulbar tracts, but sparing the reticular activating system. Patients are awake and sensate, but paralyzed and unable to speak. Voluntary blinking and vertical gaze may be intact. The *Anton syndrome* (basilar artery) is characterized by cortical blindness with denial. The *Millard-Gubler syndrome* is a unilateral lesion of the ventrocaudal pons that may involve the basis pontis and the fascicles of cranial nerves VI and VII. Symptoms include contralateral hemiplegia, ipsilateral lateral rectus palsy, and ipsilateral peripheral facial paresis. When the penetrating branches of the PCA to the midbrain get affected, it could result in *Weber syndrome*. Symptoms are ipsilateral characterized by the presence of an oculomotor nerve palsy and contralateral hemiparesis or hemiplegia.

Lacunar – The more common syndromes include *pure motor hemiplegia* (posterior limb internal capsule [IC]), *pure sensory stroke* (thalamus or parietal white matter), the *dysarthria-clumsy hand syndrome* (basis pontis), and the *hemiparesis-hemiataxia syndrome* (pons, midbrain, IC, or parietal white matter). "Pseudobulbar palsy" is caused by anterior IC and corticobulbar pathway lacunes (loss of volitional bulbar motor control [e.g., dysarthria, dysphagia, dysphonia, and face weakness], but involuntary motor control of the same muscles is intact, e.g., can yawn or cough). Emotional lability may be seen.

Ischemic Stroke Pharmacotherapy and Intervention

Guidelines for Acute Stroke Pharmacotherapy

IV tissue plasminogen activator (tPA) is indicated for acute ischemic stroke within 3 hours of symptom onset. Contraindications for the use of tPA are as follows:

1. Minor stroke symptoms/tPA
2. Head CT positive for blood
3. BP > 185/100 despite medical treatment
4. Coagulopathy
   a. PT > 15 seconds or INR > 1.7
   b. Heparin within 48 hours prior with elevated PTT
   c. Patient on warfarin
5. Platelets > 100 k
6. Blood sugar <50 or >400
7. Stroke/severe brain injury in past 3 months
8. History of IVH, arteriovenous malformation, or aneurysm
9. History of GI or GU bleed in past 30 days
10. Major surgery in past 14 days
11. Seizure at onset of stroke
12. Acute myocardial infarct

Early anticoagulation is likely to be beneficial in acute cardioembolic and large-artery ischemic strokes, in patients with severe CHF, and for progressing stroke when the suspected mechanism is ongoing thromboembolism.[4] Clinical trials, in general, do *not* show clear benefits for *SC heparin, low-molecular-weight heparin, or heparinoids* in the treatment of acute ischemic stroke,[4] but they are recommended for DVT/pulmonary embolism (PE) prophylaxis in the absence of contraindications.

Low-dose *ASA* (160 to 325 mg) is recommended within 48 hours for patients with acute ischemic strokes not receiving thrombolytics or anticoagulation.[4] ASA can be safely used with low-dose SC heparin for DVT prophylaxis.

In general, elevated BPs in the acute period should *not* be aggressively managed unless mean arterial BP (which is (SBP + 2DBP)/3) > 130 or SBP > 220 mm Hg.[5]

Recommendations for Secondary Prevention

Ongoing lifestyle and medical risk factor modifications, such as those identified in the *Framingham Heart Studies* (a series of >1,000 papers originally identifying smoking, HTN, and hypercholesterolemia among others as risk factors for cardiovascular diseases), are warranted.

For *noncardioembolic* cerebral ischemic events (strokes or transient ischemic attacks [TIAs]), one of the three following long-term prophylactic *options* is recommended[4]:

a. ASA 50 to 325 mg qd;
b. ASA 25 mg bid + extended-release dipyridamole 200 mg bid (*Aggrenox*);
c. Clopidogrel (*Plavix*) 75 mg qd (acceptable for ASA-allergic patients).

The *CAPRIE* (Clopidogrel versus Aspirin in Patients at Risk of Ischemic Events)[6] trial demonstrated that clopidogrel is slightly better than ASA (5.33% vs. 5.83% overall incident rate) in reducing ischemic events (e.g., MI and stroke) in a study of 19,185 patients with known atherosclerotic disease (8.7% risk reduction vs. ASA, $p = 0.045$).

For *cardioembolic* cerebral ischemic events, oral anticoagulation with a target INR of 2.5 (range 2.0 to 3.0) is recommended.[4] INRs > 3.0 are associated with a higher risk of brain hemorrhage that outweighs the potential benefits.[4]

The *NASCET* (North American Symptomatic Carotid Endarterectomy Trial)[7] study demonstrated a 6 to 10× reduction in the long-term risk of stroke following carotid endarterectomy (CEA) versus medical management alone for patients with recent stroke or TIA with extracranial internal carotid artery stenosis of 70% to 99%. The benefit, however, was largely dependent on the skill of the surgeon. CEA for stenosis <70% was not supported. ASA, 81 to 325 mg qd, is recommended before and after the CEA.[4] Guidelines for incidentally discovered asymptomatic carotid stenosis are less clear.

Patent foramen ovale (PFO) is relatively common in the general population, but its prevalence is higher in patients with cryptogenic stroke (i.e., stroke with no identifiable cause). Importantly, paradoxical embolism through a PFO should be strongly considered in young patients with cryptogenic stroke. There is no consensus on the optimal management strategy, but treatment options include antiplatelet agents, warfarin sodium, percutaneous device closure, and surgical closure.

Postacute Medical Complications

The major *causes of death* poststroke are the stroke itself (i.e., progressive cerebral edema and herniation), pneumonia, cardiac disease, and PE. Complications noted during the *postacute stroke rehabilitation period* include pneumonia and pulmonary aspiration (51% to 78%), falls (22% to 73%), urinary incontinence (37% to 79%), DVT (up to 45%), musculoskeletal pain, and central poststroke pain.[8]

Urinary incontinence typically improves but may still be present in 15% to 20% after 6 months.[8] Treatment can include timed-voiding, fluid intake regulation, and treatment of UTIs.

Glenohumeral subluxation, seen in 30% to 50% of patients, may play a role in poststroke shoulder pain.[4] Arm trough or lapboard use while sitting, stretching of the shoulder depressors/internal rotators, and avoiding pulling on the affected arm during transfers can be key aspects of management during the early rehabilitation phase. If spasticity becomes severe, a subscapularis phenol/botulinum toxin injection can sometimes be helpful.[9]

Factors that predict transfer to acute medical facilities are elevated admission WBC count, low admission hemoglobin level, greater neurologic deficit, and history of cardiac arrhythmia.[3]

Motor Recovery Following Stroke

Twitchell[10] gave the first systematic clinical description of motor recovery following stroke. In particular, tone and "stereotypic" movements, characterized by a tight coupling of movement at adjacent joints (later termed "synergy" by Brunnstrom), were noted to develop before isolated voluntary motor control was reestablished. In addition, it was noted that motor control returned proximally before distally and LEx function recovered earlier and more completely than UEx function. Poor prognostic indicators included severe proximal spasticity, proprioceptive facilitation response not present by 9 days, onset of movement at >2 to 4 weeks, absence of voluntary hand movement at 4 to 6 weeks, or a prolonged flaccid period. Full recovery, when it occurred, was usually complete within 12 weeks (Fig. 23-1).

Brunnstrom[11] later formalized the stages of motor recovery:

1. Flaccid limb
2. Some spasticity with weak flexor and extensor synergies
3. Prominent spasticity; voluntary motion occurs within synergy patterns

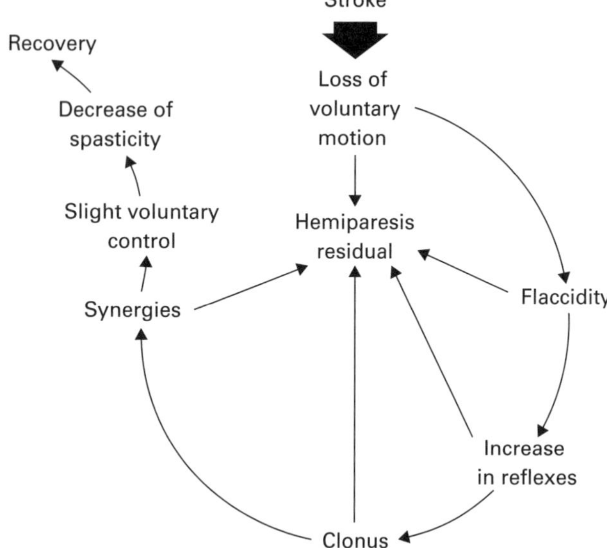

Figure 23-1 Stroke recovery pattern, per Cailliet.

Figure courtesy of Cailliet R. *The Shoulder in Hemiplegia*. Philadelphia, PA: FA Davis; 1980.

4. Some selective activation of muscles outside of synergy patterns. Spasticity reduced
5. Most limb movement independent from limb synergy; spasticity further reduced but still present with rapid movements
6. Near-normal coordination with isolated movements
7. Restoration to normal

NEUROPHYSIOLOGICAL THERAPIES

1. **Neurodevelopmental approach/Bobath approach**
   - The most commonly used approach ("hands-on" approach, touch and pressure applied by therapist). The goal is to normalize tone, inhibit primitive patterns of movement, and facilitate selective automatic, voluntary reactions and subsequent normal patterns.
   - Suppress abnormal muscle patterns, which is contradictory to Brunnstrom's approach. Proximal key points include shoulders and pelvis; distal key points include upper and lower extremities (typically the hands and feet).
   - Focuses on the relationship between sensory input and motor output.
2. **Proprioceptive neuromuscular facilitation (PNF)**
   - Developed by Kabat in the 1940s for the treatment of paralysis. Knott and Voss applied PNF to all types of therapeutic exercises and began presenting the technique in workshops in 1952.
   - It is often a combination of passive stretching and isometric contractions.
   - Uses spiral and diagonal components of movement with the goal of facilitating movement patterns that will have more functional relevance than the traditional technique of strengthening individual group muscles.
   - Resistance is used during spiral and diagonal movement patterns with the goal of facilitating irradiation of impulses to other parts of the body associated with the primary movement.
3. **Brunnstrom approach**
   - Uses primitive synergistic patterns in training in an attempt to improve motor control through central facilitation.
   - Synergies and primitive refluxes are considered normal processes of recovery.
   - Enhances specific synergies through the use of cutaneous proprioceptive stimuli and central facilitation using Twitchell's recovery.
4. **Rood approach/sensorimotor approach**
   - Uses sensorimotor stimulation to modify muscle tone and voluntary motor activity.
   - Inhibitory or facilitatory input through the use of quick stretching, icing, fast brushing, slow stroking, tendon tapping, and vibration and joint compression to promote contraction of proximal muscles.

5. **Constraint-induced movement therapy**
   - Constraint-induced movement therapy (CI or CIMT) is a technique pioneered by UAB behavioral neuroscientist Edward Taub.[19]
   - Requires the patient to be able to extend their wrist and fingers.
   - The focus of CI lies in forcing the patient to use the affected limb by restraining the unaffected one. The affected limb is then used intensively for either 3 or 6 hours a day for at least 2 weeks.

Functional Outcome Following Stroke

A common observation is that physical performance, functional ability, and quality of life are considerably better after rehabilitation and during long-term care than immediately after the stroke. Outcomes after a stroke can be assessed via medical morbidity, mortality, level of impairment, length of hospital stay, cost of care, functional limitations, placement at the time of discharge and follow-up, amount of handicap or social functioning, quality of life, and life satisfaction. The *Framingham Heart Study* not only showed that 78% of 148 stroke survivors were independent in mobility skills, 68% were independent in the performance of self-care activities, and 84% were living in home environments, but also saw reductions in vocational function, socialization outside the home, and pursuit of interests and hobbies.[12]

More recently, the *Auckland Stroke Outcomes Study* showed that of 418 five-year stroke survivors, two-thirds had good functional outcome in terms of neurologic impairment and disability (defined as modified Rankin score <3), 22.5% had cognitive impairment indicative of dementia, 20% had experienced a recurrent stroke, almost 15% were institutionalized, and 29.6% had symptoms suggesting depression.[13] *Admission functional ability* is the strongest and most consistent predictor of discharge,[14] and significant predictors of functional status at the time of discharge were admission functional status score and onset admission interval.[15] Paolucci et al.[16] provided further evidence of better functional prognosis in stroke survivors with hemorrhagic stroke versus ischemic stroke. The *Copenhagen Stroke Study* showed that those with severe strokes are characterized by younger age, the presence of a spouse at home, early neurological recovery, and decreasing body temperature.[17] *A Very Early Rehabilitation Trial (AVERT)*, a phase II randomized controlled trial made up of 71 patients with an average age of 74 years, concluded that earlier and more intensive mobilization after stroke may fast-track return to unassisted walking and improve functional recovery.[18] In general, about 75% to 85% of stroke patients are discharged home after formal acute rehabilitation care.[12]

Overall, the prognosis for a stroke survivor is good. Approximately 80% of stroke survivors walk within a year following stroke, 85% recover normal swallowing, 40% are able to return to work, and 90% are able to return home. *The Copenhagen Stroke Studies*[20,21] are an extensive, ongoing series of papers with descriptions of stroke rehabilitation outcomes. One recurrent theme is that short-term and long-term morbidity/mortality and rehabilitation outcome are positively affected by special stroke units (vs. general medical or neurologic units).[20] Generally, length of hospital stay is also significantly reduced. Another theme is that initial stroke recovery is generally the most important factor in both neurologic and functional recovery. The best neurologic recovery is seen by 11 weeks for 95% of patients; most ADL recovery (by Barthel Index) is by 12.5 weeks with daily PT/OT, but recovery could take 2 years or more.[21] Although the prognosis in patients with mild or moderate stroke is usually excellent, periodic rehabilitation interventions may be necessary to maintain function.

REFERENCES

1. Stewart DG. Stroke rehabilitation: epidemiologic aspects and acute management. *Arch Phys Med Rehabil.* 1999;80:S4-S7.
2. Cuccurullo. *Physical Medicine and Rehabilitation Board Review.* 2nd ed. New York, NY: Demos Medical Publishing; 2010:6.
3. Kelly-Hayes M. Factors influencing survival and need for institutionalization following stroke. *Arch Phys Med Rehabil.* 1988;69:415-418.
4. Albers GW. Antithrombotic and thrombolytic therapy for ischemic stroke. Sixth American College of Chest Physicians Consensus Conference on Antithrombotic Therapy. *Chest.* 2001;119(1 suppl):300S-320S.
5. Special Writing Group of the AHA Stroke Council. Guidelines for the management of pts with acute ischemic stroke. *American Heart Association* Pub. No. 71-0054, 1994.
6. CAPRIE Steering Committee. A randomised, blinded, trial of clopidogrel versus aspirin in patients at risk of ischaemic events (CAPRIE). *Lancet.* 1996;348:1329-1339.
7. North American Symptomatic Carotid Endarterectomy Trial Collaborators. Beneficial effect of carotid endarterectomy in symptomatic patients with high-grade carotid stenosis. *N Engl J Med.* 1991;325:445-453.
8. Stein J. *Stroke Recovery and Rehabilitation.* New York, NY: Demos Medical Publishing, 2009.
9. Brandstater ME. Stroke rehabilitation. In: DeLisa J, ed. *Rehabilitation Medicine: Principles and Practice.* 3rd ed. Philadelphia, PA: Lippincott-Raven; 1998:1006:1655-1676.
10. Twitchell TE. The restoration of motor function following hemiplegia in man. *Brain.* 1951;74:443-480.
11. Brunnstrom S. *Movement Therapy in Hemiplegia: A Neurological Approach.* Philadelphia, PA: Harper & Row; 1970.
12. Harvery RL, Roth EJ, Yu D. Rehabilitation in stroke syndromes. In: Braddom RL, ed. *Physical Medicine and Rehabilitation.* 3rd ed. St. Louis, MO: Saunders Elsevier; 2003: chap. 51.
13. Feigin VL, Barker-Collo S, Parag V, et al. ASTRO study group. Auckland stroke outcomes study. Part 1: gender, stroke types, ethnicity, and functional outcomes 5 years poststroke. *Neurology.* 2010;75(18):1597-1607.
14. Jongbloed L. Prediction of function after stroke: a critical review. *Stroke.* 1986;17;765-775.
15. Yavuzer G, Kucukdeveci A, Arasil T, Elhan A. Rehabilitation of stroke patients: clinical profile and function outcome. *Am J Phys Med Rehabil.* 2001;80:250-255.
16. Paolucci S, Antonucci G, Grasso MG. Functional outcome of ischemic and hemorrhagic stroke patients after inpatient rehabilitation: a matched comparison. *Stroke.* 2003;34:2861-2865.
17. Jorgensen HS, Reith J, Nakayama H. What determines good recovery in patients with the most severe strokes? The Copenhagen Stroke Study. *Stroke.* 1999;30(10):2008-2012.
18. Cumming TB, Thrift AG, Collier JM, et al. Very early mobilization after stroke fast-tracks return to walking: further results from the phase II AVERT randomized controlled trial. *Stroke.* 2011;42(1):153-158. Epub Dec 9, 2010.

19. Dromerick AW. Does the application of CIMT during acute rehabilitation reduce arm impairment after ischemic stroke? *Stroke.* 2000;31:2984-2988.
20. Jorgensen HS. The effect of a stroke unit: reductions in mortality, discharge rate to nursing homes, length of hospital stay, and cost. *Stroke.* 1995;26:1178-1182.
21. Jorgensen HS. Outcome and time course of recovery in stroke. *Arch Phys Med Rehabil.* 1995;76:406-412.

RECOMMENDED READING

Roth EJ. Stroke. In: O'Young BJ, ed. *Physical Medicine & Rehabilitation Secrets.* 2nd ed. Philadelphia, PA: Hanley & Belfus; 2002.

Cuccurullo SA. Physical medicine and rehabilitation board review. http://www.ncbi.nlm.nih.gov/books/bv.fcgi?highlight=techniques,brunnstrom&rid=physmedrehab.section.726#758. Accessed May 3, 2007.

Chapter 24

NEUROGENIC BLADDER

Neurophysiology – Bladder distention activates detrusor stretch (δ) receptors, which in turn activate the *sacral micturition center* at S2-4. During bladder filling, the intact cerebral cortex inhibits the sacral micturition center and reflex bladder contraction. Also, *sympathetic efferents* (arising from ≈T10-L2, hypogastric nerve) stimulate fundal β-receptors (relaxation) and trigonal/bladder neck α-receptors (contraction), the overall effect of which is storage. (Mnemonic: sympathetic is for storage; *p*arasympathetic is for *p*eeing.)

The first sensation of bladder filling is typically at ≈100 mL. Fullness may be appreciated at ≈300 to 400 mL. Voluntary continence is maintained via *somatic efferents* (Onuf's nucleus, S2-4, pudendal nerve), which innervate the external urethral sphincter.

With voiding, urethral sphincter pressure drops and the detrusor contracts (stimulated by *parasympathetic fibers* from the sacral micturition center, traveling in the pelvic nerves). This synergic interaction between sphincter and detrusor is coordinated by the *pontine micturition center* (Fig. 24-1).

Neurogenic Bladder – A *suprapontine* (i.e., TBI and stroke) lesion can cause detrusor hyperreflexia, w/o detrusor–sphincter dyssynergia (DSD). Symptoms can include frequency and incontinence ("failure to store"). *Treatment* options may include timed voids (i.e., offer bedpan q2h), urinary collection devices (i.e., condom catheter), or anticholinergics (e.g., oxybutynin).

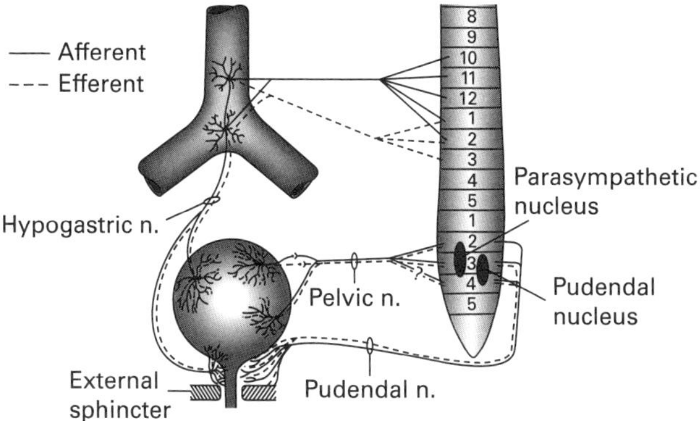

Figure 24-1 Innervation of the bladder.

A *suprasacral* SCI can cause DSD, which is characterized by the lack of sphincter relaxation during bladder contraction. This may manifest as urinary retention ("failure to empty") and eventually result in vesicoureteral reflux due to high bladder contraction pressures. *Treatment* options include clean intermittent catheterization (CIC) (e.g., volumes <400 to 500) and oral or intravesical anticholinergics (e.g., capsaicin and resiniferatoxin), α-adrenergic blockers, indwelling catheterization, stent placement, sphincterotomy, sphincter botulinum injection, or neurostimulation.

A *sacral or peripheral nerve lesion* can cause detrusor areflexia, which may manifest as retention or overflow incontinence. *Treatment* options may include Valsalva maneuver, suprapubic pressure (Crede) or percussion, cholinergic agonists (e.g., bethanechol), CIC, or indwelling catheter.

Chapter 25

SPEECH AND SWALLOWING

APHASIA

Defined as impairment of speaking, listening, reading, and/or writing secondary to brain insult. Broca's, Wernicke's, and global aphasias are the most common. Many cases do *not* fit all the features of the classic syndrome descriptions. It is important to assess patients for agnosia, a complex sensory and recognition disorder that can often be misdiagnosed as aphasia. The *cortical aphasias* (listed below) usually involve the dominant hemisphere and will have anomia. *Anomic aphasia* (temporal–parietal area and angular gyrus) is characterized by poor naming skills. *Subcortical aphasias* can involve the internal capsule and putamen and are characterized by sparse output and impaired articulation.

Cortical aphasias:

1. Global (MCA stem and multilobar)
2. Transcortical mixed (anterior cerebral artery [ACA]/posterior cerebral artery watershed area)
3. Broca's (sup. div. of MCA, Brodmann's area 44 and 45 in prefrontal gyrus)
4. Wernicke's (inf. div. of MCA, Brodmann's area 21 and 42 in the posterior, superior temporal gyrus)
5. Transcortical motor (ACA, prefrontal lobe near Broca's area). Patients also demonstrate echolalia
6. Conduction (MCA and arcuate fasciculus): 10% of cortical aphasias
7. Anomic (damage to left temporal/parietal lobe[s]) (Fig. 25-1)

Treatment of aphasia is individualized to take advantage of residual/recovering function and compensate for deficits, which can vary considerably, even for patients with the same aphasia syndrome. *Melodic intonation therapy* (thought to utilize "musical" areas in the nondominant hemisphere) may be helpful for patients with expressive aphasia. It has been shown that intensive therapy, on average of 98 hours postinsult, provides positive outcomes.[1] Family members should be trained to encourage participation of the aphasic patient in conversation and to allow plenty of time for the patient to regain expression.

APRAXIA AND DYSARTHRIA

Apraxia of speech is an impairment in the production of syllables and words due to abnormalities in the motor planning of speech; in the *absence* of weakness, verbal comprehension is intact. Difficulty with polysyllabic words and inconsistency of the phonemic error are typical, e.g., "*bopishmarter,* I mean *doppingor* (supermarket)." Treatment consists of intensive speech drills. *Melodic intonation therapy* (utilizing nondominant

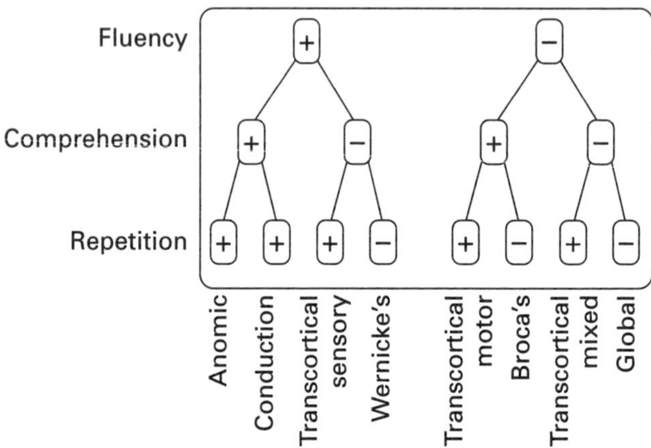

Figure 25-1 Flow chart to assess aphasia types. This flow (ligatures present) chart characterizes fluency (ligatures) of speech output, auditory comprehension, and repetition ability for brief bedside screening of patients with aphasia. The plus symbol (+) indicates that the specific function is intact or at least fairly good. The minus symbol (–) indicates the specific function is relatively impaired. Note that a plus symbol does not necessarily indicate that the function is normal, and a minus symbol does not necessarily indicate that a function is completely defective.

From Canter GJ. *Syndromes of apahasia in relation to cerebral connectionism*, South Bend, IN; 1979, Short course presented to the Indiana Speech and Hearing Association, with permission.

hemispheric musical areas) may be helpful for patients with concomitant expressive, but not receptive, aphasia.

Flaccid dysarthria can be the result of weakness of the muscles of articulation (i.e., brain stem or cranial n. pathology). It is characterized by a breathy, hypernasal, weak voice with imprecise consonant formation and monopitch. *Ataxic dysarthria* is due to cerebellar disease and is characterized by a slow, slurred, and monopitch harsh voice with distorted vowels and irregular articulation. *Spastic dysarthria* is due to a UMN lesion and is characterized by a voice that is strained, hypernasal, and low in pitch and loudness. Speech is slow and characterized by poor prosody. Spastic dysarthria is also associated with dysphagia.

The essentials of a typical *dysarthria treatment* plan include medical, prosthetic, and behavioral interventions. The focus of treatment is to (1) strengthen/coordinate orolingual musculature; (2) slow down the rate of speech; (3) enunciate clearly or "overarticulate"; and (4) become aware of and practice speech at an appropriate loudness.

Dysphagia Treatment

Along with modification of food and liquid, the treatment of dysphagia includes both compensatory swallowing maneuvers and swallowing exercises to strengthen and increase control of swallowing mechanisms. Other modalities used in the treatment of dysphagia include electrical stimulation, preprandial self-dilation of upper esophageal sphincter (UES) with balloon catheter, preprandial thermal tactile stimulation, surgical UES dilation, and pharyngeal bypass mechanisms when safe oral intake is not possible.

Suboptimal Cognitive Status – Feedings should be supervised. For *impulsivity*, present foods one at a time. For *poor judgment*, use small-bowled utensils, covered cups with small openings, and intermittently pinch straws closed to control drinking rate. For *poor attention*, a quiet, distraction-free environment should be utilized.

Oral Phase Dysphagia – For *facial weakness*, modify food texture and place food at the back of mouth or on the stronger side (i.e., tilt the head toward the stronger side). EMG biofeedback or sucking/blowing exercises may be helpful. For *poor lingual control*, tongue active ROM and strengthening can be prescribed (precise articulation should be encouraged). Neck extension may also be used to increase oral transit time.

Pharyngeal Phase Dysphagia – This is the most common type and is often accompanied by a wet, gurgly voice with coughing. (Note that an absent gag reflex does not necessarily connote an unsafe swallow; conversely, those with intact gags may aspirate.) Techniques for a *delayed swallow reflex* include chin tuck, rotation of the head to the weaker side, supraglottic swallow, and thickened liquids. The *chin tuck* maneuver widens the vallecula (allowing the bolus to rest there while the reflex is triggered), reduces the airway opening, and reduces the space between tongue base and posterior pharyngeal wall (increasing pharyngeal pressure). In the *supraglottic swallow*, the patient holds a deep breath with a concomitant Valsalva, swallows, clears the throat, then swallows again, before resuming breathing. Chin tuck and supraglottic swallow are also useful for *reduced laryngeal closure*.

The Mendelsohn maneuver can address *incomplete relaxation or premature closing of the cricopharyngeus*. The patient improves pharyngeal clearance by "holding" a swallow midway for 3 to 5 seconds (allowing more complete cricopharyngeal relaxation) before completing the swallow. The Shaker exercise works on the same deficits. The patient lying supine lifts head, looks at feet for 1 minute three times with a 1-minute rest interval, followed by 30 consecutive rapid head raises.

REFERENCE

1. Braddom RL. *Physical Medicine & Rehabilitation*. 4th ed. Philadelphia, PA: Elsevier; 2011.

Chapter 26

SPASTICITY

Spasticity is a disorder characterized by a velocity-dependent increased resistance to passive stretch, associated with exaggerated tendon jerks, resulting from hyperexcitability of the stretch reflex. Spasticity is part of the *UMN syndrome*, which includes the *positive* symptoms of spasticity and uninhibited flexor reflexes in the lower limbs and the *negative* symptoms of weakness and poor dexterity. Commonly used clinical scales are listed in Table 26-1.

TREATMENT

Indications for treating spasticity include pain, decreased function, poor hygiene, skin breakdown, poor cosmesis, and poor positioning. Potential factors that may be exacerbating spasticity (e.g., pressure ulcers, UTIs, bowel impaction, ingrown toenails, and SSRIs) should be addressed. Care should be taken before treating any spasticity that may be utilized functionally (e.g., hypertonia in the lower limbs assisting transfers or gait). One algorithm for treating spasticity may be as per Fig. 26-1.

TABLE 26-1 Commonly Used Clinical Scales

Modified Ashworth Scale[a,b] score[c]		**Spasm**	**frequency**
0	No increase in tone	0	No spasms
1	Slightly increased tone, with a catch/ release or minimal resistance at terminal ROM	1	Spasms induced by stimulation
1+	Slightly increased tone, with a catch, followed by minimal resistance throughout the remainder (less than half) of the ROM	2	Infrequent spontaneous spasms (<1/h)
2	Increased tone through most of the ROM, but affected part easily moved	3	Spontaneous spasms (>1/h)
3	Considerably increased tone; passive movement difficult	4	Spontaneous spasms (>10/h)
4	Affected part rigid in flexion or extension		

[a]Adapted from Bohannon RW. Interrater reliability on a modified Ashworth scale of muscle spasticity. *Phys Ther.* 1987;67:206-207.
[b]Adapted from Penn RD. Intrathecal baclofen for severe spasticity. *Ann N Y Acad Sci.* 1988;531:15-66.
[c]By subject self-report.

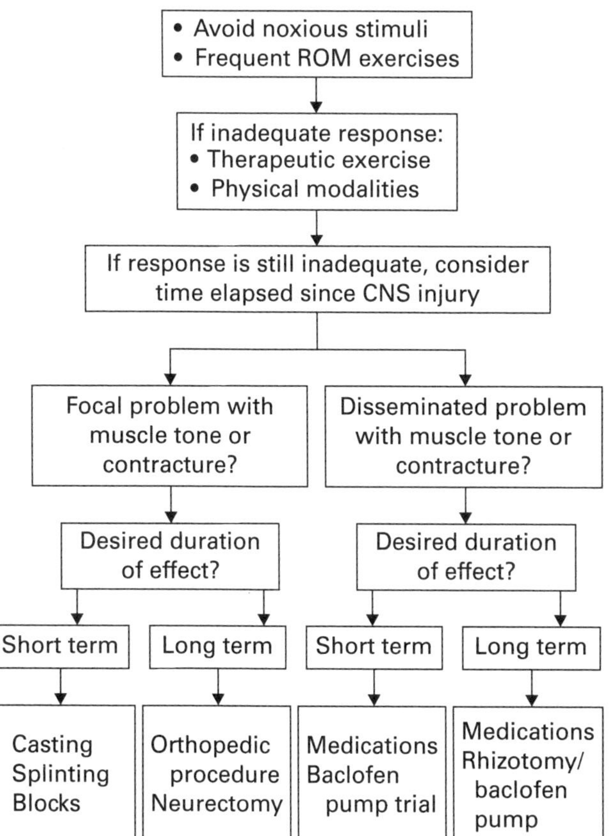

Figure 26-1 Algorithm for treating spasticity.

Courtesy of Katz R. Spasticity. In: O'Young BJ, ed. *Physical Medicine & Rehabilitation Secrets*. 2nd ed. Philadelphia, PA: Hanley & Belfus; 2002:144.

Physical Modalities

A *stretching program* should be the cornerstone for most spasticity treatment programs. *Splints, casting,* or *bracing* can help preserve ROM by "resetting the muscle spindles." Contractures can be reduced by serially casting a joint (i.e., increasing the stretch stepwise for 1 to 2 days at a time), although this technique is not always well-tolerated and may lead to skin breakdown. *Cryotherapy* (>15 minutes) may be helpful transiently by reducing the hyperexcitability of the muscle stretch reflex and reducing nerve conduction velocities. *Functional electrical stimulation* (>15 minutes) can improve function and reduce tone for hours after the stimulation (thought to be due to neurotransmitter modulation at the spinal cord level). Hippotherapy, which involves rhythmic movements, is found useful in spasticity reduction in lower limbs. Other modalities include application of tendon pressure, cold, warmth, vibration, massage, low-power laser, and acupuncture.[1]

Pharmaceutical Options

Oral Medications – These may be indicated for *nonfocal* spasticity. Efficacy is often limited by side effects. FDA-approved medications include baclofen, diazepam, dantrolene (*clonidine*), and tizanidine. Recently, off-label use of *gabapentin* has shown promising results in the treatment of spasticity in a small group of MS patients undergoing a crossover study.[2]

Botulinum Toxin-A (BTX-A) – BTX irreversibly blocks NMJ transmission by inhibiting presynaptic ACh release. BTX-A (Fig. 26-2; Botox and Allergan) is FDA-approved for blepharospasm, strabismus, and cervical dystonia and most recently for severe glabellar (between the eyebrows) frown lines. It is also widely used for spasticity and myofascial pain with favorable results. Onset of effect is typically 24 to 72 hours. Peak effect is at 2 to 6 weeks. Clinical efficacy is typically up to 3 to 4 months. Recovery is due to axonal sprouting.

The theoretical parenteral LD_{50} for a 75-kg adult is 3,000 U; the recommended maximum dose is 10 U/kg IM (up to 400 U) per visit. At least 3 months of interval between sessions is recommended to decrease the potential for antibody formation. BTX-A is contraindicated in pregnancy, lactation, NMJ disease, and concomitant aminoglycoside use and with human albumin USP allergy. BTX-A should be stored at –5° to –20° C and should be reconstituted with 0.9% preservative-free saline only. It is available for use for up to 4 hours if refrigerated (2° to 8° C).

Advantages of BTX-A over phenol include ready diffusion into the injected area (up to 3 to 4 cm), making injections technically easier, and the absence of dysesthesias (since it is selective for the NMJ; see Table 26-2 for suggested BTX-A dosing).

BTX-B (Myobloc) – BTX-B was FDA-approved in 2000 for cervical dystonia. Clinically, it is used for similar indications as BTX-A, although the units are markedly different (initially, 2,500 to 5,000 U of BTX-B divided among the affected muscles). BTX-B may be effective in patients who have developed resistance to BTX-A due to repeated use. It may be stored at room temperature for up to 9 months, or 21 months if refrigerated (2° to 8° C). It does not need to be reconstituted, but may be diluted with normal saline, in which case it must be used within 4 hours.

Phenol (carboxylic acid) – Phenol destroys nerves in a dose-dependent manner, with onset within 1 hour and a duration that can last years (duration varies widely in the literature). Target nerves are localized with

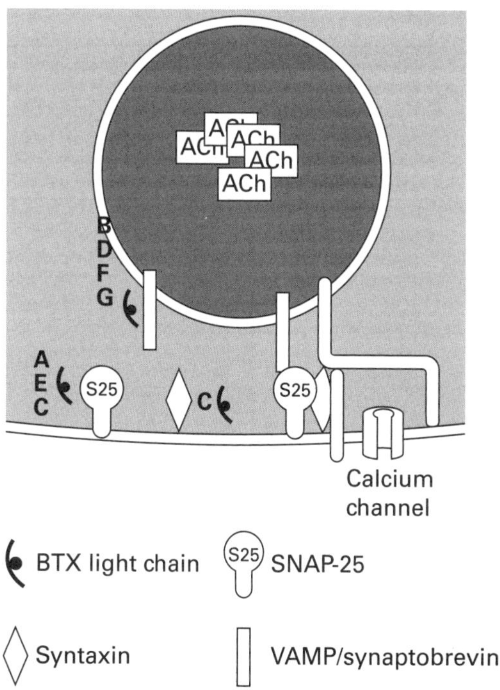

Figure 26-2 There are seven distinct BTX subtypes. The BTX heavy chain binds to the presynaptic end plate and the receptor–BTX complex is internalized by endocytosis. The light chain of BTX-A lyses SNAP-25, a protein needed for fusion of ACh vesicles with the presynaptic membrane.

Adapted from Cutter NC. Gabapentin effect on spasticity in MS: a placebo-controlled, randomized trial. *Arch Phys Med Rehabil.* 2000;81:164-169; Brin MF, ed. *Muscle & Nerve. Spasticity: Etiology, Evaluation, Management, and the Role of BTX-A.* Vol. 6 (Suppl). New York, NY: John Wiley & Sons; 1997:S151.

a nerve stimulator and destroyed by direct perineural injection (with subsequent Wallerian degeneration). Alternatively, the motor-point area (located by nerve stimulator) can be injected (e.g., 1 to 10 mL of 3% to 5% solution IM; max: 10 mL of 5%). Recovery with either option occurs by nerve fiber regeneration.

Phenol injections can be combined with BTX injections during a single session, which may be especially useful when there are BTX dosage concerns (i.e., phenol for large, proximal muscles and BTX for smaller, distal muscles). Advantages over BTX include low cost, lack of

TABLE 26-2 Suggested BTX-A Dosing (in Units)

Clinical pattern	Potential muscles involved	Avg starting dose	Range, per visit	Injection sites, #
Adducted/ internally rotated shoulder	Pectoralis complex	100	75–100	4
	Latissimus dorsi	100	50–150	4
	Teres major	50	27–75	1
	Subscapularis	50	25–75	1
Flexed elbow	Brachioradialis	50	75	1
	Biceps	100	50–200	4
	Brachialis	50	25–75	2
Pronated forearm	Pronator quadratus	25	10–50	1
	Pronator teres	40	25–75	1
Flexed wrist	Flexor carpi radialis	50	25–100	2
	Flexor carpi ulnaris	40	10–50	2
Thumb-in-palm	Flexor pollicis longus	15	5–25	1
	Adductor pollicis	10	5–25	1
	Opponens pollicis	10	5–25	1
Clenched fist	Flexor digitorum superficialis	50	25–75	4
	Flexor digitorum profundus	15	25–100	2
Intrinsic plus hand	Lumbricals interossei	15	10–50/hand	3
Flexed hip	Iliacus	100	50–150	2
	Psoas	100	50–200	2
	Rectus femoris	100	75–200	3
Flexed knee	Medial hamstrings	100	50–150	3
	Gastrocnemius	150	50–150	4
	Lateral hamstrings	100	100–200	3
Adducted thighs	Adductor brev/long/ magnus	200/leg	75–300	6/leg
Extended knee	Quadriceps femoris	100	50–200	4
Equinovarus foot	Gastrocnemius medial/ lateral	100	50–200	4
	Soleus	75	50–100	2
	Tibialis posterior	50	50–200	2
	Tibialis anterior	75	50–150	3
	Flexor digitorum long/ brevis	75	50–100	4
	Flexor hallucis longus	50	25–75	2

Striatal toe	Extensor hallucis longus	50	20–100	2
Neck	Sternocleidomastoid[a] Scalenus complex Trapezius Levator scapulae	40 30 60 80	15–75 15–50 50–150 25–100	2 3 3 3

[a]The dose should be reduced by half if both SCMs are being injected.
Dosing guidelines: The recommended maximum dose per visit is 10 U/kg, not to exceed 400 U. The maximum dose per injection site is 50 U. The maximum volume per site is typically 0.5 mL. Reinjection should occur no more frequently than q3 mos. Consider lowering the dosing if patients' Ashworth scores are in the low range, if patients' weight or **muscle bulk** is low, or if the likely duration of treatment is chronic.

Adapted from Brin MF. Dosing, administration, and a treatment algorithm for use of BTX-A for adult-onset spasticity. *Muscle Nerve.* 1997;6(suppl);S214.

antibody formation, and longer duration of effect. Disadvantages versus BTX include the greater technical skill involved and potential for dysesthesias, although the latter can be reduced by limiting injections to relatively accessible motor branches of nerves (e.g., pectoral, musculocutaneous, obturator, inferior gluteal, and branches to hamstrings, gastroc–soleus, and tibialis anterior) and avoiding mixed nerve injections (main tibial or median nerve). A trial with a local anesthetic (e.g., marcaine, 0.25% to 0.5%) prior to phenol neurolysis can be helpful in predicting the potential effects.

Intrathecal Baclofen (ITB) – ITB is indicated for severe spasticity (Ashworth grade ≥ 3) 2° to SCI (FDA-approved in 1992) and severe spasticity of cerebral origin (FDA-approved in 1996). It is also used with fair to good success off-label for severe muscle spasms in chronic back pain and radicular pain. Patients should have a history of poor response to conservative treatments and be older than 4 years or have adequate body weight (>40 1bs). A trial of epidural baclofen or a subarachnoid catheter with external pump is often given before implantation of an internal pump. A screening trial of epidural baclofen might be as follows: 50 mg epidural bolus on day 1; if not efficacious, 75 mg on day 2; if prior doses not successful, 100 mg on day 3. A drop in spasticity of ≈2 Ashworth grades during the trial may roughly predict efficacy of the implanted pump.

The pump is typically placed in the LLQ to be away from the appendix. The pump is typically refilled every 4 to 12 weeks depending on the dosage being administered and the size of the pump. The patient must be committed to being compliant with seeing the physician for refills of the medication. The battery lasts about 5 years (the pump must be removed to replace the battery). Advantages of ITB include reduced CNS side effects (e.g., sedations) versus oral medications. Potential problems with the implanted system include infection, catheter kinking or dislodgment, and headaches 2° to CSF leak out of the catheter site. The average infusion rate for a lumbar pump is 600 μg/day. Increased spasticity should be worked up and treated before adjusting the ITB dose.

Surgical Options

Numerous procedures exist, including tendon transfer, tendon/muscle lengthening, and neurosurgical (brain/spinal cord) lesioning (Fig. 26-3). The *split anterior tibial tendon transfer (SPLATT)* (right) procedure can be an effective treatment for the spastic equinovarus foot. The lateral portion of the split distal anterior tibialis tendon is reattached to the third cuneiform and cuboid bones. *Achilles tendon lengthening* usually accompanies the SPLATT.

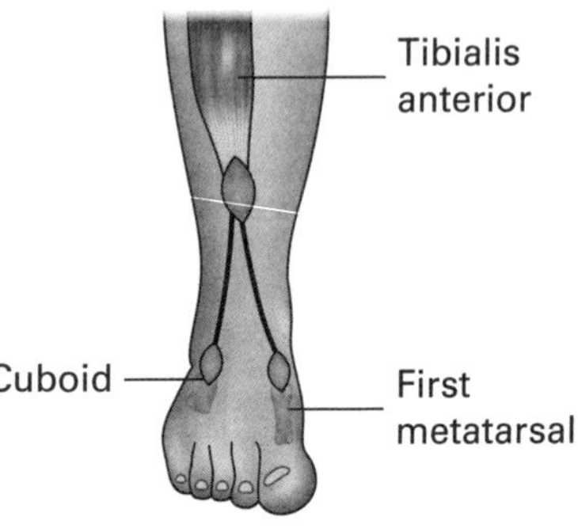

Figure 26-3 Tendons in lower leg.
Adapted from Keenan MA. *Manual of Orthopaedic Surgery for Spasticity.* Philadelphia, PA: Raven Press; 1993.

Selective dorsal rhizotomy may be of some benefit in CP. The procedure involves laminectomy and exposure of the cauda equina. The dorsal rootlets are stimulated individually, and rootlets that produce abnormal EMG responses in limb musculature (believed to be contributing to spasticity) are then severed. Anterior rootlet lesions are undesirable as denervation atrophy may follow, with resultant skin breakdown. Favorable selection criteria for rhizotomy include spastic CP (without athetosis), age between 3 and 8 years, HO prematurity, good truncal balance, and a supportive family.

References

1. Gracies JM. Physical modalities other than stretch in spastic hypertonia. *Phys Med Rehabil Clin North Am.* 2001;12:747-768.
2. Cutter NC. Gabapentin effect on spasticity in MS: a placebo-controlled, randomized trial. *Arch Phys Med Rehabil.* 2000;81:164-169.

Chapter 27

HETEROTOPIC OSSIFICATION

INTRODUCTION

Heterotopic ossification (HO) is the formation of bone at an abnormal anatomical site, usually in soft tissue, due to the metaplasia of mesenchymal cells into osteoblasts. There are two forms: acquired form, which is precipitated by a musculoskeletal trauma such as fracture, thermal injury, or THA, and neurogenic form, examples of which are SCI, stroke, and TBI. HO is typically seen near large joints and below levels of neurologic injury. Symptoms are nonspecific, such as edema, pain, and loss of joint mobility (in late stages). The differential diagnosis can include DVT, septic arthritis, cellulitis, thrombophlebitis, osteomyelitis, hematoma, osteosarcoma, hemarthrosis, or CRPS. If HO is suspected, a plain x-ray or three-phase bone scan may be obtained. The bone scan may be positive at least 1 week before x-ray is positive; phases 1 and 2 of the bone scan are highly sensitive.

Reports of incidence in the literature vary, depending on the methodology used and whether clinically silent HO is included. In *burns*, common sites include elbow (posterior > anterior) > shoulder (adult) or hip (children). HO location may not coincide with the area of the burn. In *SCI*, HO is seen at the hip (anterior > posterior) > knee > shoulder > elbow > feet. With *TBI*, UEx equals LEx; shoulder ≃ elbow ≃ hip. Hip HO is commonly seen following *THA*. HO may occur at the distal end of *amputated limbs*.

Complications – Some complications of HO include peripheral nerve entrapment, pressure ulcers, and functional impairment if joint ankylosis develops.

Treatment – *Resting* the acutely involved joint for ≤2 weeks is acceptable to ↓ inflammation and microscopic hemorrhages.[1] *Ice* may also be helpful. While still an area of controversy, gentle *ROM exercises*, such as painless passive ROM or active ROM, are recommended to maintain joint mobility.[2] More aggressive ROM may be initiated after the first 2 weeks, but must be curtailed if erythema or swelling increases.[1] Immobilization in a functional position is prudent if ankylosis is inevitable.

Medical options include NSAIDs (e.g., *indomethacin*, 25 mg po tid × ≥6 weeks) or *etidronate* (e.g., 20 mg/kg po qd × 2 weeks, then 10 mg/kg po qd × 10 weeks; other regimens exist). Etidronate is thought to reduce further HO formation by reducing osteoblastic/clastic activity and calcium phosphate precipitation.[1] It does *not*, however, treat HO that has already formed.

Radiation therapy has been used with success to prevent and/or treat HO in post-THA patients, although it is rarely used.[2]

Surgical resection may be indicated to address significant functional limitations. An ideal surgical candidate would have three factors: no joint pain or swelling, a normal alkaline phosphatase level (which tends to normalize with maturity), and a three-phase bone scan indicating mature HO. It is important to ensure that the HO has reached maturity before resection, because resection of immature HO leads to recurrence rates of nearly 100%. Gentle, early (within 48 hours) postoperative ROM is recommended.[1]

REFERENCES

1. Subbarao J. HO. In: O'Young BJ, Young MA, Steins SA, eds. *Physical Medicine & Rehabilitation Secrets.* 2nd ed. Philadelphia, PA: Hanley & Belfus; 2002:456-459.
2. Shehab D, Elgazzar A, Collier D. Heterotopic ossification. *J Nucl Med.* 2002;43: 346-353.

Chapter 28

DEEP VENOUS THROMBOSIS

Selected Prophylaxis Options

Low-Dose Unfractionated Heparin (LDUH) – LDUH binds with antithrombin III to inhibit factor IIa (thrombin) and factor Xa (intrinsic clotting pathway).

Low-Molecular-Weight Heparin (LMWH) – Mechanism of action is similar to LDUH, but the reduced binding with plasma proteins results in a longer and more predictable half-life. It is contraindicated in heparin-induced thrombocytopenia (HIT).[1] *Enoxaparin* (Lovenox), 30 mg SC bid or 40 mg qd, is FDA-approved for s/p THA; 30 mg bid is approved for s/p TKA. *Dalteparin* (Fragmin), 5,000 U SC qd, is FDA-approved for s/p THA.

Vitamin K antagonist (VKA or Warfarin[1]) – It inhibits the vitamin K–mediated production of *pro*coagulant factors X, IX, VII, and II (extrinsic pathway) and *anti*coagulant proteins C and S. There is an initial paradoxical procoagulant effect since proteins C and S are depleted first (thus, initiating therapy with "loading" doses >5 mg qd is not usually recommended).

For INRs 5 to 9 w/o significant bleeding, give 1 to 2.5 mg po vitamin K or follow INRs w/o vitamin K. For INRs > 9 w/o significant bleeding, give 3 to 5 mg po vitamin K and monitor INRs (repeat vitamin K if necessary). For elevated INRs with serious bleeding, give 10 mg vitamin K by slow IV infusion (repeat q12h if necessary) and supplement with plasma or prothrombin complex concentrate.

Fondaparinux, 2.5 mg SC qd (Arixtra) – This is a heparin derivative that selectively inhibits factor Xa and is FDA-approved for s/p hip fracture surgery (HFS), THA, and TKA.

Others – *Hirudins* (e.g., lepirudin, 15 mg SC bid) are direct thrombin inhibitors indicated in the setting of HIT. *Heparinoids* (e.g., danaparoid, no longer available for nonmedical reasons) have a similar mechanism of action as that of UH, but do *not* contain heparin and are also used in the setting of HIT. *ASA* inhibits platelet aggregation, but is *not* recommended by the American College of Chest Physicians (ACCP) for DVT prophylaxis because other measures are more efficacious.[1] *Inferior vena cava filters* are used for pulmonary embolism (*not* DVT) prophylaxis.

DVT Prophylaxis in Selected Conditions

Orthopedic surgery[1]: THA or TKA – LMWH, fondaparinux, or VKA (INR 2 to 3).

HFS – Fondaparinux, LMWH, VKA, or LDUH.

Duration – THA/HFS 10 to 35 days, TKA at least 10 days. Optimal use of intermittent pneumatic compression or graduated compression stockings may provide additional efficacy.

Medical/Neuro Patients[1] – LMWH, LDUH, or fondaparinux is recommended for patients with general medical issues (e.g., cancer and bed rest) or following *ischemic stroke* with impaired mobility. The ideal time to start anticoagulation after hemorrhagic stroke has not been determined.

SCI[2] – Mechanical and anticoagulation treatment should be initiated as early as possible, provided there is no active bleeding or coagulopathy. Compression hose and boots should be applied for 2 weeks (r/o DVT first if thromboprophylaxis has been delayed >72 hours).

For American Spinal Injury Association (*ASIA*) *A, B* – UH adjusted to high-normal aPTT (activated PTT) or LMWH for ≥8 weeks. For *ASIA A, B with other risk factor(s)* (e.g., LEx fracture, cancer, previous thrombosis, heart failure, obesity, and age >70 years) – UH adjusted to high-normal aPTT or LMWH for 12 weeks or discontinue from rehabilitation. *ASIA C* – UH 5,000 U q12h or LMWH for up to 8 weeks. *ASIA D* – UH 5,000 U q12h or LMWH while in hospital. The ACCP recommends against the use of inferior vena cava filters as thromboprophylaxis following acute SCI.[1]

DVT Treatment

In the absence of contraindications, initial treatment is typically *IV heparin*. *Warfarin* is usually started within 24 hours of DVT diagnosis, once the heparin is therapeutic. A 5-mg initial dose of warfarin is preferred over a 10-mg dose due to early paradoxical hypercoagulability. Heparin is discontinued when the INR has been ≥2 for two consecutive days. Warfarin is typically instituted for 3 to 6 months.

LMWH (e.g., enoxaparin, 1 mg/kg SC bid, or dalteparin, 200 U/kg SC qd) + warfarin is an alternative for the outpatient treatment of uncomplicated DVT; LMWH can be discontinued after 5 days and when INR > 2.[3] *Thrombolytics* may have a role in patients with extensive proximal DVT and low bleed risk. The treatment of isolated calf DVT remains controversial.

REFERENCES

1. Geerts WH, Berggvist D, Pineo, et al. Prevention of venous thromboembolism. American College of Chest Physicians Evidence-Based Clinical Practice Guidelines (8th edition). *Chest.* 2008;133:381S-453S.
2. Consortium for Spinal Cord Medicine. *Clinical Practice Guideline: Thromboembolism.* 2nd ed. Washington, DC: Paralyzed Veterans of America; 1999.
3. Levine M. A comparison of home LMWH vs. hospital UH for proximal DVT. *N Engl J Med.* 1996;334:677-681.

Chapter 29

PRESSURE ULCERS

The National Pressure Ulcer Advisory Panel (NPUAP) defines a *pressure ulcer* as a "localized injury to the skin and/or underlying tissue, usually over a bony prominence as a result of pressure or pressure combined with shear and/or friction."

Kosiak[1] showed that 70 mm Hg of pressure applied continuously over 2 hours produced moderate histologic changes in rat muscle. Dinsdale[2] showed that shear can significantly reduce the amount of pressure necessary to disrupt blood flow.

Secondary factors include

- Immobility
- Diminished sensation or mental status
- Advanced age
- Incontinence (leading to skin maceration)
- Elevated tissue temperatures
- Circulatory deficiencies
- Anemia
- Nutritional deficits

Bony prominences are particularly at risk; muscle is more sensitive to breakdown from pressure than skin. Ulcers are commonly staged according to NPUAP guidelines as follows:

Stage I – Intact epidermis with nonblanchable erythema not resolved within 30 minutes. Warmth, edema, induration, or discoloration may be indicators of stage I ulcers in patients with darker skin.

Stage II – Partial-thickness epidermal or dermal skin loss. These may appear as blisters with erythema.

Stage III – Full-thickness skin loss and subcutaneous involvement, but not through the underlying fascia.

Stage IV – Full-thickness skin loss with involvement of muscle, tendon, bone, or joint.

An ulcer with slough or necrotic tissue is deemed *unstageable.* Figure 29-1 depicts the stages of ulcers.

Pressure ulcer *prevention* should include appropriate seating/bed equipment, proper positioning, and education about pressure relief (i.e., weight shifting every 15 to 20 min for ≥30 seconds while sitting; turning in bed q2h).

Treatment of pressure ulcers includes addressing the etiologic factors, treatment of infections, debridement of necrotic tissue (sharp, mechanical, enzymatic, or autolytic), regular wound cleansing, and use of appropriate wound dressings. A trial of topical antibiotics (e.g., silver sulfadiazine) may be helpful in wounds not healing with optimal debridement and cleansing. Wound cultures are *not* generally thought to be helpful because most wounds are colonized with bacteria. Systemic antibiotics should be reserved

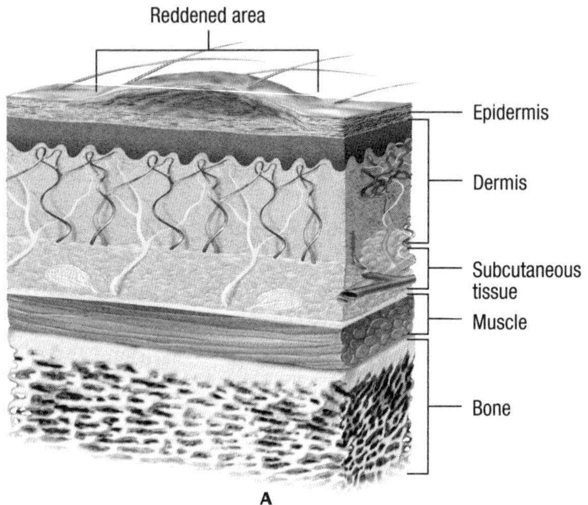
Stage I
Reddened area
Epidermis
Dermis
Subcutaneous tissue
Muscle
Bone

A

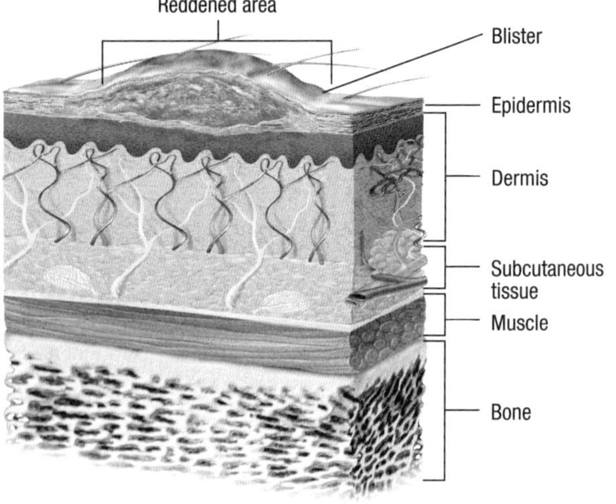
Stage II
Reddened area
Blister
Epidermis
Dermis
Subcutaneous tissue
Muscle
Bone

B

Stage III

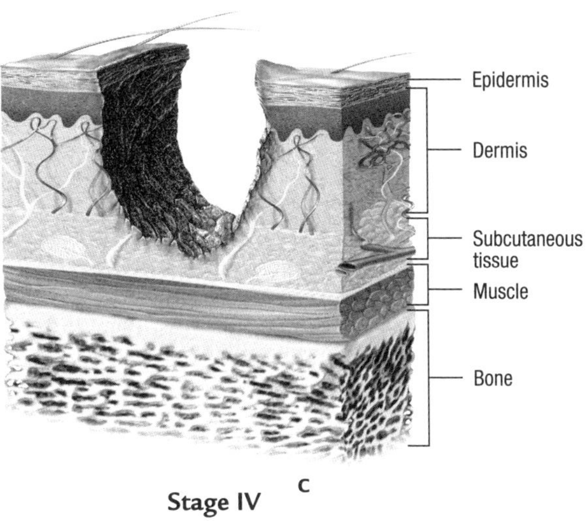

C

Stage IV

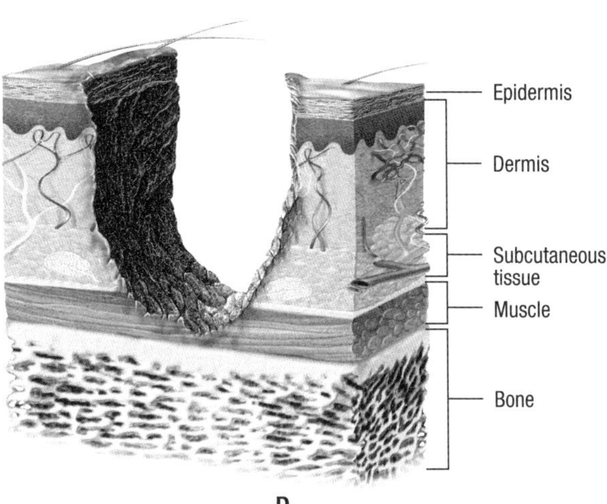

D

Figure 29-1 Stages of a pressure ulcer: **A.** Stage I; **B.** Stage II; **C.** Stage III; and **D.** Stage IV.

From the Anatomical Chart Company, Lippincott Williams & Wilkins, with permission.

for cases with evidence of osteomyelitis, cellulitis, or systemic infection. Modalities such as UV light, laser radiation, US, hyperbaric O_2, and electrical stimulation may be helpful in accelerating wound repair, although only *E-stim* has sufficient supportive evidence to receive endorsement by the AHCPR (now the AHRQ).[3] Surgical flaps may expedite the healing of noninfected deep ulcers by filling the void with well-vascularized healthy tissue (they do not provide a "cushion").

REFERENCES

1. Kosiak M. Etiology of decubitus ulcers. *Arch Phys Med Rehabil.* 1961;42:19-29.
2. Dinsdale SN. Decubitus ulcers: role of pressure and friction in causation. *Arch Phys Med Rehabil.* 1974;55:147-154.
3. *Clinical Practice Guideline No. 3.* AHCPR publication No. 92-0047, 1994.

Chapter 30

PHARMACEUTICALS

Selected Common "Rehab Drugs"

Note – The following doses are for adults. Contraindications always include hypersensitivity to the drug itself. "Warn/Prec" are some warnings that should be made and conditions where the medication may impose additional risk of adverse reaction. "Most common" side effects may be marked with an asterisk. The information presented here is abridged; please refer to the PDR or product inserts for more information, including pediatric dosing guidelines. (*Drugs are listed in alphabetical order.*)

Acetaminophen – oxycodone hydrochloride (Percocet, Endo; Roxicet, Roxane) – [tabs 325/2.5, 325/5, 325/7.5, 325/10, 500/7.5, 650/10 mg]

Indic/dosage: pain, moderate to moderate-severe: acetaminophen 325 to 650 mg/oxycodone 2.5 to 10 mg orally q6h prn; max 4,000 mg acetaminophen/day

Action: acetaminophen is a nonopiate and nonsalicylate analgesic and antipyretic drug; oxycodone hydrochloride, a semisynthetic pure opioid agonist, has actions similar in quality with those of morphine and acts predominantly on the CNS and organs composed of smooth muscle

Contra: bronchial asthma, known or suspected paralytic ileus, and respiratory depression

Warn/prec: chronic administration may result in psychic and physical dependence and tolerance, concomitant use of other CNS depressants (including alcohol), elderly or debilitated patients, and in pregnancy C (acetaminophen) and B (oxycodone)

Adverse reactions: constipation, nausea/vomiting, dizziness, light-headedness, and somnolence

Alendronate (Fosamax, Merck) – [tabs 5, 10, 35, 40, 70 mg]

Indic/dosage: osteoporosis prevention: 5 mg qd or 35 mg qwk; osteoporosis treatment: 10 mg qd or 70 mg qwk; Paget's disease: 40 mg qd × 6 months; all tablets should be taken ≥30 minutes before first food or beverage of the day, with a full glass of water; avoid lying down for at least 30 minutes

Action: bisphosphonates act to inhibit normal and abnormal bone resorption; as a result, an asymptomatic reduction in serum Ca and PO_4 is noted

Contra: hypocalcemia, severe renal dysfunction, and dysphagia

Warn/prec: upper GI disease and pregnancy C

Adverse reactions: esophagitis, GI distress, headache, myalgias, arthralgias, back pain, dysphagia, abdominal distension, chest pain, peripheral edema, flulike symptoms, and esophageal ulcer

Amantadine (Symmetrel, Endo) – [caps 100 mg, syrup 50 mg/5 mL]

Indic/dosage: Parkinson's disease/syndrome: 100 mg bid, can increase to 400 mg/day after one to several weeks, start at 100 mg qd for those on other anti-Parkinson's medications or medically ill patients; treatment or prophylaxis for influenza A: 200 mg initially, then 100 mg qd; off-label for poor arousal or inattention in TBI: 100 mg bid; off-label for postpolio syndrome pain, fatigue in MS as well as TBI, and hyperthermia of central origin in TBI

Action: blocks ion channels (nicotinic ACh, M2 ionic channel in influenza A); also believed to release dopamine from intact dopaminergic terminals

Warn/prec: seizure disorder, CHF, renal disease, and pregnancy C; withdrawal from amantadine should be gradual

Adverse reactions: (usually well-tolerated) dizziness, nausea, nervousness, ataxia, insomnia, dry mouth, GI hypomotility, urinary retention, changes in mood, confusion, hallucinations, CHF, edema, orthostatic hypotension, and livedo reticularis (particularly women)

Amitriptyline (Elavil, Merck) – [tabs 10, 25, 50, 75, 100, 150 mg]

Indic/dosage: depression: 50 to 150 mg qhs (for elderly 10 mg tid and 20 mg qhs may be sufficient; reduce dose for hepatic impairment); off-label for neuropathic pain (start at lower doses than for depression)

Action: tertiary amine tricyclic, norepinephrine (NE)/serotonin reuptake inhibitor; also has anti-α1-adrenergic and potent antimuscarinic properties; may potentiate analgesic effect of opioids

Contra: acute post-MI and concomitant monoamine oxidase inhibitor (MAOI) use

Warn/prec: cardiovascular (CV) disorders (can cause HTN), hyperthyroidism, schizophrenia/paranoia, pregnancy D, and discharge before elective surgery; withdraw gradually after long-term use to avoid insomnia and abdominal discomfort

Adverse reactions: dry mouth, blurred vision, constipation, urinary retention, CV effects (tachycardia and prolongation of AV conduction), weight gain, somnolence, seizures, photosensitivity, GI distress, leukopenia, gynecomastia, testicular swelling, sexual dysfunction, and menstrual irregularity

Monitoring: baseline and periodic leukocyte and differential counts, LFTs, and ECG. Patients with CV issues require surveillance

Baclofen (Lioresal, Novartis) – [tabs 10, 20 mg, intrathecal (IT)]

Indic/dosage: spasticity: titrate to a maximum dose of 20 mg qid as follows: 5 mg tid × 3 days, then 10 mg tid × 3 days, then 15 mg tid × 3 days, then 20 mg tid × 3 days, increase as needed; consider IT if oral in effective but titration limited by side effects; no indication of oral form for spasticity due to stroke, Parkinson's disease, or CP

Action: analog of γ-aminobutyric acid (GABA) thought to bind to GABA-B receptors, inhibiting Ca influx into presynaptic terminals and suppressing spinal cord excitatory neurotransmitters

Warn/prec: impaired renal function, risk of seizure if withdrawn too quickly (therefore, should taper off over ≈1 week), and pregnancy C

Adverse reactions: *Oral baclofen*: drowsiness, dizziness, headache, nausea/vomiting, lassitude, GI upset, urinary frequency, CNS depression, confusion, slurred speech, nasal congestion, seizures, blurred vision, weakness, hypotonia, HTN, CV collapse, respiratory failure, rash, pruritus, and increased LFTs; *IT baclofen*: fatigue and drowsiness

Overdosage: IV physostigmine 1 to 2 mg. Also see p. 213 for details on IT baclofen

Bisacodyl (Dulcolax, Boehringer Ingelheim) – [oral tab 5 mg, rectal suppository 10 mg]

Indic/dosage: constipation: 5 to 15 mg po qd up to 30 mg/day- or 10 mg suppository rectally qd

Action: stimulates enteric nerves to cause colonic mass movements, a contact laxative; increases fluid and NaCl secretion and increases peristalsis

Contra: appendicitis, intestinal obstruction, and gastroenteritis

Warn/prec: abdominal pain, nausea, vomiting, rectal bleeding, inflammatory bowel disease, use for more than 7 days is not recommended, and pregnancy A

Adverse reactions: abdominal colic, abdominal discomfort, diarrhea, and proctitis

Capsaicin (Zostrix, Medicis) – [cream 0.025%, 0.075%, both OTC]

Indic/dosage: FDA-approved for postherpetic neuralgia; commonly used for OA and neuropathic pain: apply a thin film to affected areas tid to qid; may require ongoing use for effect; experimental intravesical instillation inhibits contractions in neurogenic bladders

Action: evidence suggests that capsaicin depletes the pain neurotransmitter substance P from unmyelinated peripheral neurons

Warn/prec: wash hands after application, avoid contact with eyes, and avoid heating pads in treated areas

Adverse reactions: local burning sensation, which typically improves with repeated use, but may not be tolerated by some

Carbamazepine (Tegretol, Novartis) – [tabs 100, 200 mg, oral suspension 100 mg/5 mL]

Indic/dosage: epilepsy: start at 200 mg bid; trigeminal neuralgia: start at 100 mg qd; off-label for neuropathic pain: start at 100 mg bid; maximum dose for all indications is 1,200 mg/day, usually divided in tid doses, increase doses each week by ≤200 mg/day

Action: unknown, but related to the tricyclic antidepressants (TCAs); may be a result of Na channel blockade in rapidly firing neurons and reduced excitatory synaptic transmission in the trigeminal nucleus

Contra: TCA hypersensitivity, history of bone marrow depression, and concomitant use of MAOIs (or within 14 days of discharge)

Warn/prec: impaired liver/renal function, hyponatremia, pregnancy C, and numerous drug interactions

Adverse reactions: initially dizziness, ataxia, drowsiness, nausea/vomiting, but usually subside spontaneously within a week, bone marrow suppression, hepato/nephrotoxicity, nystagmus, rash, Stevens-Johnson syndrome (SJS), and arrhythmias

Monitoring: pretreatment CBC, BUN, LFTs, and Fe, with periodic follow-up (frequency guidelines not established)

Celecoxib (Celebrex, Pfizer/Searle/Pharmacia) – [caps 100, 200 mg]

Indic/dosage: OA: 200 mg qd or 100 mg bid; rheumatoid arthritis (RA): 100 to 200 mg bid; acute pain/dysmenorrhea: 400 mg initially, followed by 200 mg if needed on first day, then 200 mg bid prn

Action: COX-2 selective NSAIDs

Contra: hypersensitivity to sulfonamides, ASA, and NSAIDs

Warn/prec: HTN, CHF, history of GI bleed, and renal insufficiency; monitor INRs closely with concomitant warfarin treatment, pregnancy C, and nasal polyps

Adverse reactions: edema, GI distress/bleed, thrombocytopenia, nephro/hepatotoxicity, bronchospasm, and agranulocytosis. *Note*: In the CLASS study,[1] annual incidence of upper GI ulcer complications (bleeding, perforation, and obstruction) for celecoxib 200 mg bid versus NSAIDs (ibuprofen 800 mg tid or diclofenac 75 mg bid) was 0.76% versus 1.45%; when combined with symptomatic ulcers, annual incidence was 2.08% versus 3.54% ($p = 0.02$)

Clonidine (Catapres, Boehringer Ingelheim) – [tabs 0.1, 0.2, 0.3 mg, transdermal therapeutic system (TTS) qwk patch 0.1/24, 0.2/24, 0.3 mg/24 h]

Indic/dosage: HTN: start orally at 0.1 to 0.3 mg bid or TTS 0.1 mg/24 h qwk, maximum dose is 2.4 mg/day orally or TTS 0.3 mg/24 h qwk; off-label for spasticity: dosing similar to HTN; IT clonidine used investigationally for spasticity and neuropathic pain

Action: central α-adrenergic agonist that ↓ sympathetic discharge

Warn/prec: CV disease, impaired liver/renal function, withdraw gradually to avoid rebound HTN, and pregnancy C

Adverse reactions: dry mouth/eyes, headache, dizziness, nausea, constipation, sedation, weakness, fatigue, orthostatic hypotension, edema, anorexia, erectile dysfunction, joint pain, and leg cramps

Cyclobenzaprine (Flexeril, Merck) – [tab 10 mg]

Indic/dosage: muscle spasm due to acute painful musculoskeletal conditions: 10 mg tid, maximum 60 mg/day, not to exceed 2 to 3 weeks

Action: structurally related to the TCAs; thought to act on the brain stem to reduce skeletal muscle hyperactivity, but not effective for spasticity of central origin

Contra: TCA hypersensitivity, concomitant MAOIs (or within 14 days of discharge), and recovery from acute MI, CHF, arrhythmias, conduction disturbances, and hyperthyroidism

Warn/prec: glaucoma, prostatic hypertrophy, and pregnancy B

Adverse reactions: drowsiness, dizziness, dry mouth, weakness, taste changes, fatigue, paresthesias, nausea, insomnia, blurred vision, seizures, hepatitis, and tachycardia

Dantrolene (Dantrium, Procter & Gamble) – [caps 25, 50, 100 mg, injection]

Indic/dosage: spasticity: start at 25 mg qd, increase by 25 mg q4-7d to a maximum of 400 mg/day divided into bid–qid (considered the oral agent of choice in TBI due to peripheral action and less CNS side effects); off-label for malignant hyperthermia: 2 mg/kg IV push until symptoms subside or cumulative dose of 10 mg/kg reached; also off-label for heat stroke and cocaine overdose rigidity

Action: reduces excitation–contraction coupling via reduction of sarcoplasmic reticulum Ca release

Contra: active liver disease and lactation

Warn/prec: risk of hepatic dysfunction higher in women or if >35 years, cardiomyopathy or pulmonary disease present, and pregnancy C

Adverse reactions: weakness, malaise, sedation, dizziness, nausea, diarrhea, acnelike rash, pruritus, headache, insomnia, photosensitivity, fatal/nonfatal hepatotoxicity (most commonly 3 to 12 months after initiation of treatment, most cases resolve with discharge), and seizures

Monitoring: baseline/periodic LFTs

Diazepam (Valium, Roche) – [tabs 2, 5, 10 mg, oral solution 5 mg/5 mL, 5 g/1 mL, injection]

Indic/dosage: skeletal muscle spasticity due to local reflex spasm, UMN spasticity, athetosis, and stiff-man syndrome: 2 to 10 mg po/IM tid–qid (geriatric patient, 1 to 2.5 mg qd–bid); anxiety dosing similar to spasticity; EtOH withdrawal: initially 2 to 5 mg IV, repeat q3-4h prn; status epilepticus: 0.2 to 0.5 mg/kg/dose IV q15-30min to a maximum of 30 mg

Action: proposed mechanism for antispasticity effect is a postsynaptic facilitation of spinal cord GABA w/o a direct GABA-mimetic effect

Contra: CNS depression and acute angle glaucoma

Warn/prec: class IV, impaired liver/renal function, depression may worsen with use, and pregnancy D

Adverse reactions: sedation, "hangover," dizziness, ataxia, diplopia, hypotension, confusion, constipation, urinary retention/incontinence, anterograde amnesia, dependency, withdrawal syndrome, bone marrow suppression, rash, fever, hepatotoxicity, blood dyscrasias, and injection site reaction (local pain and thrombophlebitis); apnea/cardiac arrest (rare, typically only after IV administration or in elderly or medically ill patients)

Docusate sodium (Colace, Purdue Products LP) – [tabs 50, 100 mg]

Indic/dosage: constipation: 50 to 200 mg po qd or in divided doses 2 to 4× daily; 50 to 100 mg rectally as an enema

Action: actively draws water into stool, thus softening stool and achieving ease in bowel movement

Contra: concomitant use of mineral oil, intestinal obstruction, acute abdominal pain, and nausea/vomiting

Warn/prec: sudden change in bowel habits > 2 weeks duration, use > 1 week, rectal bleeding, and pregnancy A

Adverse reactions: abnormal taste in mouth, diarrhea, nausea, cramping, and hepatotoxicity (rare)

Etanercept (Enbrel, Amgen) – [subcutaneous (SC) powder for solution 25 mg, SC: 50 mg/mL]

Indic/dosage: ankylosing spondylitis, psoriatic arthritis, RA (moderate to severe): in each case, 50 mg SC qwk given as one 50 mg injection or two 25 mg injections in one day or one 25 mg injection given twice weekly, 72 to 96 hours apart

Action: dimeric soluble form of the p75 TNF receptor that specifically binds TNF-α and TNF-β, binding of etanercept to TNF renders it biologically inactive; also modulates biologic responses that are induced or regulated by TNF, including expression of adhesion molecules responsible for leukocyte migration, serum levels of cytokines, and serum levels of matrix metalloproteinase

Contra: sepsis

Warn/prec: infection, chronic or recurring, TB, alcoholic hepatitis, demyelinating disorders, pancytopenia, aplastic anemia, malignancies, concomitant use of abatacept, anakinra, cyclophosphamide, or live vaccines is not recommended, and pregnancy C

Adverse reactions: injection site reaction, headache, and abdominal pain

Etidronate (Didronel, Procter & Gamble) – [tabs 200, 400 mg]

Indic/dosage: Paget's disease: 5 to 10 mg/kg qd, not to exceed 6 months, or 11 to 20 mg/kg qd, not to exceed 3 months; HO following SCI: 20 mg/kg qd × 2 weeks, then 10 mg/kg qd × 10 weeks; HO following total hip replacement: 20 mg/kg qd × 1 month preoperative, 20 mg/kg qd × 3 months postoperative

Action: as with other bisphosphonates, it inhibits hydroxyapatite crystal growth by preventing precipitation of soluble amorphous $CaPO_4$; also slows osteoblastic and osteoclastic activities

Contra: renal impairment

Warn/prec: CHF, enterocolitis, long bone fracture, and pregnancy C

Adverse reactions: nausea/vomiting, GI distress, osteomalacia/inhibition of bone mineralization, fractures, bone pain, seizures, angioedema, and stomatitis

Gabapentin (Neurontin, Parke-Davis) – [caps 100, 300, 400 mg, tabs 600, 800 mg, solution 50 mg/mL]

Indic/dosage: partial seizures with or w/o 2° generalization: 300 mg qhs on day 1, 300 mg bid on day 2, 300 mg tid on day 3, continue to titrate as tolerated to effect, up to 3,600 mg/day; off-label for neuropathic pain: similar dosing; off-label second-line treatment for spasticity (see p. 210)

Action: unknown; a GABA analog w/o activity at GABA receptors; hypothesized to alter the concentration or metabolism of cerebral amino acids

Warn/prec: impaired renal function and pregnancy C; discharge gradually over 1 week (no known drug interactions)

Adverse reactions: initially somnolence, dizziness, ataxia, but these usually resolve within 2 weeks of starting the drug, fatigue, nystagmus, tremor, diplopia, nausea, nervousness, dysarthria, weight gain, leukopenia, thrombocytopenia, dyspepsia, depression, periorbital edema, and myalgias.

Infliximab (Remicade, Centocor Ortho Biotech, Inc.) – [IV powder for solution 100 mg]

Indic/dosage: ankylosing spondylitis: 5 mg/kg IV over at least 2 hours given at weeks 0, 2, and 6, then q6wk thereafter; psoriatic arthritis: 5 mg/kg IV over at least 2 hours given at weeks 0, 2, and 6, then every 8 weeks; may be given with or without methotrexate; RA (moderate to severe), in combination with methotrexate: 3 mg/kg IV over at least 2 hours given at weeks 0, 2, and 6, then every 8 weeks in combination with methotrexate; may increase dose up to 10 mg/kg IV or give 3 mg/kg IV every 4 weeks in patients with an incomplete response

Action: chimeric human-murine immunoglobulin (IgG1κ) monoclonal antibody that binds specifically to TNF-α, a proinflammatory cytokine; neutralizes the biological activity of TNF-α (induction of proinflammatory cytokines, enhancement of leukocyte migration, and stimulation of neutrophil and eosinophil functions)

Contra: CHF

Warn/prec: serious infections, TB, CHF, COPD, CNS/peripheral demyelinating disorders, concomitant use of anakinra or live vaccines is not recommended, and pregnancy C

Adverse reactions: headache, nausea, rash, and fatigue

Lactulose (Enulose, Barre-National) – [oral solution, oral syrup, solution: all 10 g/15 mL]

Indic/dosage: constipation: 15 to 30 mL po qd for 24 to 48 hours; may be increased to 60 mL/day if needed

Action: synthetic disaccharide; bacteria in the colon degrade lactulose into lactic acid, acetic acid, and formic acid, resulting in an increase in osmotic pressure and acidification of intestinal contents which in turn softens the stool by promoting stool water content

Contra: galactosemia

Warn/prec: diabetes and pregnancy B

Adverse reactions: bloating, diarrhea, epigastric pain, flatulence, and nausea/vomiting

Leflunomide (Arava, Sanofi Aventis) – [oral tab: 10, 20 mg]

Indic/dosage: RA: loading dose, 100 mg po qd for 3 days; for maintenance in RA, 20 mg po qd; may reduce dose to 10 mg daily if higher doses not tolerated

Action: immunomodulatory agent, inhibits dihydroorotate dehydrogenase; antiinflammatory effects have been demonstrated in in vivo and in vitro experimental models; antiproliferative activity

Contra: pregnancy or potential for pregnancy

Warn/prec: liver injury, bone marrow dysplasia, pancytopenia, agranulocytosis, thrombocytopenia, immunodeficiency, infections, and pregnancy X

Adverse reactions: diarrhea, alopecia, rash, HTN, increased liver enzymes, and SJS

Lidocaine patch (Lidoderm, Endo Pharmaceuticals) – [patch 5% (10 × 14 cm)]

Indic/dosage: FDA-approved in 1999 to treat postherpetic neuralgia: apply ≤3 patches on intact skin over the most symptomatic area qd (12 hours on/12 hours off); off-label for other types of neuropathic pain

Action: diffusion of lidocaine into the local epidermis/dermis is thought to block conduction of impulses (inhibits Ca-mediated Na and K ion fluxes) and stabilize neuronal membranes; provides direct local analgesia w/o complete anesthetic block

Warn/prec: do not reuse patches; avoid showers/swimming with patch on; when used appropriately, mean peak serum levels due to systemic absorption may reach about one-tenth the therapeutic level used for antiarrhythmia (these patches are safe); caution in patients with hepatic failure or on antiarrhythmics; and pregnancy B

Adverse reactions: initially, local erythema, edema, and/or paresthesias, usually mild and resolves within minutes to 1 hour

Magnesium citrate (Citroma, Swan) – [oral solution 1.75 g/30 mL]

Indic/dosage: constipation: 150 to 300 mL (1.745 g/30 mL solution) po once, may repeat prn

Action: attracts water through the tissues via osmosis, once in the intestine can attract enough water into the intestine to induce defecation; additional water helps to create more feces, which naturally stimulates bowel motility

Contra: heart block, severe renal disease, and rectal bleeding

Warn/prec: rectal blood, saline cathartics without adequate fluid replacement can produce dehydration, and pregnancy A

Adverse reactions: diarrhea, dizziness, and hypermagnesemia

Metaxalone (Skelaxin, Pfizer, Inc.) – [tab 400 mg]

Indic/dosage: relief of discomfort associated with acute, painful musculoskeletal conditions: 800 mg tid–qid

Action: not established, but may be due to general CNS depression; no direct action on contractile mechanism of striated muscle, motor end plate, or nerve fiber

Contra: history of anemias and significantly impaired renal/hepatic function

Warn/prec: liver impairment and pregnancy (unknown)

Adverse reactions: drowsiness, paradoxic CNS excitation, nervousness, nausea/vomiting, irritability, dizziness, rash, leukopenia, hemolytic anemia, and jaundice

Methylphenidate (Ritalin, Novartis) – [tabs 5, 10, 20 mg]

Indic/dosage: ADHD; narcolepsy; off-label for depression (as a stimulant) in elderly, cancer, and poststroke patients: 10 to 15 mg/day up to 40 to 60 mg/day in 2 to 3 divided doses, typically 30 to 45 minutes before meals

Action: a mild CNS stimulant with action similar to amphetamines (believed to facilitate NE and dopamine release)

Contra: glaucoma, Tourette syndrome, severe anxiety, and agitation

Warn/prec: class II, HTN, seizure disorder, CV disease, numerous drug interactions, and pregnancy C

Adverse reactions: nervousness, insomnia, anorexia, headache, dizziness, dyskinesia, rash, HTN, tachycardia, palpitations, GI distress, dependency, leukopenia, exfoliative dermatitis, erythema multiforme, motor tics, elevated LFTs, ventricular arrhythmias, and thrombocytopenia

Midodrine (ProAmatine, Shire Pharmaceuticals) – [tabs 2.5, 5, 10 mg]

Indic/dosage: 10 mg, 3× daily at approximately 4-hour intervals for the treatment of symptomatic orthostatic hypotension. Dosing should primarily take place during the daytime hours when the patient is upright. Renal dosing: initiate treatment using 2.5 mg doses

Action: long-acting, selective α-adrenergic agonist

Contra: acute renal disease/urinary retention, pheochromocytoma, severe organic heart disease or CHF, supine HTN, and persistent and excessive thyrotoxicosis

Warn/prec: OTC drugs that cause elevations in BP, concomitant use with other therapeutic agents that may cause vasoconstriction, concurrent use with digitalis glycosides, β-blockers, or other agents that directly or indirectly reduce heart rate, DM, hepatic insufficiency, patients receiving fludrocortisone for vision disorders (risk of elevated intraocular pressure), and urinary retention

Adverse reactions: bradyarrhythmia, HTN, orthostatic hypotension exacerbation, urinary urgency, urinary retention, urinary frequency, sleep disturbances, headache, dizziness, restlessness, heartburn, and nausea; pregnancy C

Modafinil (Provigil, Caphalon, Inc.) – [tabs 100, 200 mg]

Indic/dosage: FDA-approved in 1998 for excessive daytime sleepiness (EDS) due to narcolepsy: 200 mg qd, 100 mg in liver impairment; off-label for fatigue due to MS and to improve alertness post-TBI; being studied in Alzheimer's disease, age-related memory decline, and EDS due to sleep and neurologic disorders

Action: thought to act on the anterior hypothalamus and other CNS centers; increases glutaminergic while reducing GABAergic transmission

Contra: cardiac disease

Warn/prec: class IV, impaired liver/renal function, and pregnancy C

Adverse reactions: headache, nausea, infection (2° to decreased immune function due to sleep reduction), nervousness, anxiety, insomnia, rhinitis, diarrhea, dry mouth, anorexia, dizziness, and depression

Monitoring: consider periodic LFTs

Oxybutynin (Ditropan, Janssen) – [tab 5 mg, oral suspension 5 mg/5 mL]

Indic/dosage: bladder instability: 5 mg bid–tid, maximum 5 mg qid

Action: muscarinic blocker with a direct antispasmodic effect on smooth muscle

Contra: myasthenia gravis, GI obstruction, ileus, ulcerative colitis, megacolon, obstructive uropathy, and glaucoma

Warn/prec: impaired liver/renal function and pregnancy B

Adverse reactions: dry mouth, nausea, blurred vision, tachycardia, flushing, decreased sweating, dry eyes, constipation, urinary retention, dizziness, drowsiness, insomnia, hallucinations, restlessness, cycloplegia, and erectile dysfunction

Oxycontin (OxyContin, Purdue Pharma LP; Roxicodone, Xanodyne Pharmaceuticals, Inc.) – [oral caps 5 mg; oral solution 5 mg/5 mL, 20 mg/mL; oral tabs 5, 10, 15, 20, 30 mg]

Indic/dosage: pain (moderate to severe; immediate-release capsules): initial, 5 mg po q6h prn; adjust based on pain severity and patient response; pain (moderate to severe; controlled-release tablets): opioid-naive patients, 10 mg po q12h; titrate up to 40 mg po q12h prn based on patient's response; maximum daily dose, 80 mg; maximum single dose, 40 mg; single dose greater than 40 mg or a total daily dose greater than 80 mg is reserved for opioid-tolerant patients only

Action: opioid analgesic with actions similar to morphine, a pure agonist opioid; exact mechanism is unknown, specific CNS opioid receptors for endogenous compounds with opioidlike activity that have been identified throughout the CNS may play a role in the analgesic effects of this drug

Contra: bronchial asthma, paralytic ileus, known or suspected, and respiratory depression

Warn/prec: abuse potential, crushing, cutting, breaking, chewing, or dissolving controlled-release tablets prior to ingestion leads to rapid release and absorption of a potentially fatal dose of oxycodone; concomitant use of other CNS depressants (including alcohol), and elderly or debilitated patients

Adverse reactions: constipation, nausea/vomiting, dizziness, light-headedness, somnolence, and pruritus

Phenytoin (Dilantin, Pfizer, Inc.) – [caps 30, 50, 100 mg; chewable tab 50 mg; oral suspension 125 mg/5 mL; injection]

Indic/dosage: seizure prophylaxis: 4-6 mg/kg/d IV BID-TID. Start by loading 10-20 mg/kg IV divided in 3 doses, 2-4 h apart. max is 400/ dose.

Action: centrally acting modifier of Na, Ca, and K ion transport that results in membrane "stability"; blocks Na channels in a use-dependent manner

Contra: sinus bradycardia, SA block, second/third-degree AV block, and Adams-Stokes syndrome

Warn/prec: hypotension, CV disease, DM, impaired liver/renal function, arrhythmias, thyroid disease, pregnancy D, porphyria, and elderly

Adverse reactions: anorexia, dyspepsia, nausea, ataxia, nystagmus, diplopia, lethargy, insomnia, constipation, tremor, slurred speech, headache, rash, blood dyscrasias, megaloblastic anemia, severe dermatologic reactions, hepatotoxicity, severe CV abnormalities, purple glove syndrome, toxic delirium, lymphoma, SLE, gingival hyperplasia, coarse facies, and osteomalacia

Monitoring: trough level should be drawn after 1 week of regular use to determine steady-state level; draw level 2 to 4 hours after IV loading dose; no strict guidelines for drawing levels after oral loading

Prednisone (Organon) – [tabs 1, 2.5, 5, 10, 20, 50 mg; oral solution 5 mg/5 mL]

Indic/dosage: inflammatory disorders: 5 to 60 mg qd

Action: adrenocorticosteroid with glucocorticoid and mineralocorticoid activities

Contra: systemic fungal infection

Warn/prec: seizure disorder, osteoporosis, CHF, DM, HTN, TB, impaired liver function, and pregnancy C

Adverse reactions: edema, mood swings, psychosis, adrenal insufficiency, immunosuppression, peptic ulcer, CHF, insomnia, anxiety, hypokalemia, osteoporosis, appetite change, headache, dizziness, HTN, hyperglycemia, acne, cushingoid features, skin atrophy, ecchymosis, impaired wound healing, and menstrual irregularities

Pregabalin (Lyrica, Pfizer) – [caps 25, 50, 75, 100, 150, 200, 225, 300 mg]

Indic/dosage: diabetic peripheral neuropathy: initial, 50 mg po tid, may be increased to 100 mg po tid within 1 week; fibromyalgia: initial, 75 mg po bid, may be increased to 150 mg po bid within 1 week, no evidence of additional benefit with doses above 450 mg/day; postherpetic neuralgia: initial, 75 mg po bid or 50 mg po tid, may be increased to 300 mg/day within 1 week based on efficacy and tolerability

Action: GABA analog that strongly binds to $\alpha 2\delta$ site (a subunit of voltage-gated calcium channels) in CNS tissues and reduces calcium-dependent release of several neurotransmitters, possibly by modulation of calcium channel function; however, exact mechanism of action is unknown

Contra: hypersensitivity to pregabalin or any other component of the product

Warn/prec: abrupt discontinuation, risk of adverse events, and increased seizure frequency; angioedema, CHF, increased risk of suicidality, and pregnancy C

Adverse reactions: peripheral edema, weight gain, dizziness, headache, somnolence, and blurred vision

Psyllium (Metamucil, Proctor and Gamble) – [seed husks 3 g; seed 5 to 10 g; liquid extract 2 to 4 mL]

Indic/dosage: constipation: seed husks: 3 g, up to tid; seed: 5 to 10 g, up to tid; liquid extract: 2 to 4 mL up to tid

Action: absorbs water from the GI tract, increasing stool bulk

Contra: intestinal obstruction and fecal impaction

Warn/prec: adequate fluid intake is required, inadequate water may cause psyllium to swell and block the throat or intestines, GI obstruction, and pregnancy C

Adverse reactions: abdominal cramps, bronchospasm, diarrhea, and esophageal/GI obstruction

Sennosides (Senokot, Purdue Pharma, LP) – [tablet, granules, syrup, tea, suppository]

Indic/dosage: constipation: tablets, oral: 0.5 to 2 g of the crude drug or 20 to 40 mg sennosides with water qhs; granules, oral: 5 mL (326 mg, 1 teaspoon) up to a maximum of 10 mL bid; extra strength tablets, oral: 1 tablet (364 mg) qhs, up to a maximum of 2 tablets bid; syrup, oral: 10 to 15 mL (436 to 654 mg), up to a maximum of 30 mL daily; suppository, rectal: 1 suppository (652 mg) qhs, repeat in 2 hours if necessary

Action: hydroxyanthracene glycosides are not absorbed but converted by microflora of the large intestine into active aglycones; exert a laxative effect on the colon resulting in stimulation of colonic motility and accelerated colonic transit, reducing opportunity for fluid absorption and enhancing the laxative effect

Contra: bowel obstruction, acute inflammation (Crohn's disease and appendicitis), and pregnancy C

Warn/prec: abdominal pain, nausea/vomiting, and rectal bleeding

Adverse reactions: abdominal pain, nausea, cramps, electrolyte abnormalities, and diarrhea

Sildenafil (Viagra, Pfizer, Inc.) – [tabs 25, 50, 100 mg]

Indic/dosage: erectile dysfunction: start at 50 mg about 1 hour prior to sexual activity, increase up to 100 mg or decrease to 25 mg prn; 25 mg recommended for age >65 years

Action: selective PDE-5 inhibitor that increases cGMP levels and promotes smooth muscle relaxation in the corpus cavernosum

Contra: regular or intermittent nitrate use (may result in death due to severe hypotension); MI/stroke within 6 months

Warn/prec: liver/renal disease, hypotension, penile deformities, seek medical attention for erections >4 hours, no nitrates for cardiac events or autonomic dysreflexia for 24 hours after sildenafil ingestion

Adverse reactions: headache, flushing, dyspepsia, nasal congestion, visual problems (blurred vision, blue tinge, and photophobia), priapism, UTI, diarrhea, dizziness, hypotension, tachycardia, MI, TIAs, and stroke

Tamsulosin (Flomax, Boehringer Ingelheim Pharmaceuticals, Inc.) – [oral caps 4 mg]

Indic/dosage: benign prostatic hyperplasia: initial, 0.4 mg orally once daily; if no response after 2 to 4 weeks may increase dose to 0.8 mg orally once daily

Action: α1A adrenoceptor antagonist, selectively blocks sympathetic nervous stimulation of the receptor, resulting in relaxation of the smooth muscles of the prostate, prostatic urethra, and bladder neck

Contra: hypersensitivity to tamsulosin or to any component of the product

Warn/prec: orthostasis (postural hypotension, dizziness, and vertigo), concomitant use with strong CYP3A4 inhibitors or other α-adrenergic blocking agents should be avoided, and pregnancy B

Adverse reactions: dizziness, headache, rhinitis, abnormal ejaculation, infectious disease, retinal detachment, and priapism

Tizanidine (Zanaflex, Acorda) – [tab 2, 4 mg]

Indic/dosage: spasticity: no set dosing; sample regimen: start at 2 mg qhs, then q3d increase to 2 mg qam/2 mg qhs→2 mg qam/4 mg qhs→ until 4 mg tid is achieved; maximum dose is 36 mg/day

Action: central α2-adrenergic agonist that reduces spasticity by increasing presynaptic inhibition of motoneurons; reportedly ≈10% of the BP effects of clonidine; peak effects at 1 to 2 hours after administration

Warn/prec: impaired renal/hepatic function and pregnancy C

Adverse reactions: somnolence, weakness, hypotension, dry mouth, dizziness, hepatotoxicity, severe bradycardia, hallucinations, asthenia, UTI, constipation, urinary frequency, flulike symptoms, pharyngitis, rhinitis, and increased spasms

Tolterodine (Detrol, Pfizer, Inc.) – [tabs 1, 2 mg; LA tabs 2, 4 mg]

Indic/dosage: bladder instability: 2 mg bid, 1 mg bid in hepatic dysfunction (with Detrol LA, 2 or 4 mg qd)

Action: muscarinic blocker that exerts a direct antispasmodic effect on smooth muscle

Contra: narrow-angle glaucoma and gastric or urinary retention

Warn/prec: impaired liver/renal function and pregnancy C

Adverse reactions: dry mouth, blurred vision, dry eyes, urinary retention, UTI, somnolence, headache, dizziness, GI distress, upper respiratory infection, flulike symptoms, arthralgia, and pruritus

Topiramate (Topamax, Janssen) – [tabs 25, 100, 200 mg; caps 15, 25 mg]

Indic/dosage: FDA-approved in 1997 as an adjunct treatment for partial-onset seizures and mood stabilizer: start at 25 mg bid and increase daily dose to 50 mg/week until therapeutic (typically 200 to 400 mg/day); Ortho-McNeil pursuing indication for diabetic neuropathy (initial J&J studies not promising); off-label use for neuropathic pain: no established dosing regimen, may start at 25 mg qhs with weekly increases of 25 mg/day; clinical trial to study possible slowing of ALS progression in progress

Action: Na channel blocker, but analgesic mechanisms unclear

Warn/prec: pregnancy C

Adverse reactions: somnolence, dizziness, vision problems, unsteadiness, nausea, paresthesias, psychomotor slowing, nervousness, speech/memory problems, tremor, and confusion

Tramadol (Ultram, Janssen) – [tab 50 mg]

Indic/dosage: FDA-approved in 1993 for moderate to moderately severe pain: 50 to 100 mg q4-6h, not to exceed 400 mg/day (elderly: ≤300 mg/day; creatinine clearance <30 mL/min: dose q12h, ≤200 mg/day; hepatic impairment: 50 mg q12h); one 50-mg tablet is roughly equivalent to one Tylenol #3

Action: centrally acting, synthetic nonopioid analog of codeine that produces analgesia by weak μ-receptor agonism (has 10% of the affinity of codeine), serotonin/NE reuptake blockade, and enhancement of neuronal serotonin release; opioidlike CNS side effects and thus may be better tolerated in injured workers who wish to remain working

Contra: acute EtOH intoxication; use with opioids, psychotropics, or central analgesics

Warn/prec: seizure disorder, head trauma, increased ICP, concomitant MAOI or SSRI, pregnancy C, acute abdominal conditions, and opioid dependence

Adverse reactions: vertigo, nausea, constipation, headache, somnolence, vomiting, pruritus, asthenia, sweating, dry mouth, dyspepsia, diarrhea, syncope, orthostatic hypotension, and tachycardia

Trazodone (Desyrel, Apothecon; Oleptro, Labopharm) – [tabs 50, 100, 150, 300 mg]

Indic/dosage: depression: 150 to 400 mg in divided doses; off-label for aggressive behavior: 50 mg bid, titrate prn; take with food to enhance bioavailability

Action: triazolopyridine derivative antidepressant; mechanism not fully understood (serotonin reuptake inhibitor in animal models)

Contra: early post-MI period and pregnancy C

Warn/prec: CV disorders, nursing, and discharge before elective surgery

Adverse reactions: drowsiness, nausea/vomiting, dizziness, dry mouth, constipation, urinary retention, hypotension, bitter taste, fatigue, blurred vision, headache, arthralgia, incoordination, tremor, and priapism (≈1:6,000 to 10,000)

Sample Dosing of Selected Oral NSAIDs

Diclofenac (Voltaren) – [tabs 25, 50, 75 mg] 50 to 75 mg bid; Arthrotec (diclofenac/misoprostol) 50 to 75 mg/200 mg bid or 50 mg/200 μg tid
Etodolac (Lodine and Ultradol) – [tabs 200, 300, 400 mg] 200 to 400 mg po bid/tid
Ketoprofen (Orudis) – [tabs 25, 50, 75 mg] 25 to 75 mg tid/qid
Ketorolac (Toradol) – 15 to 30 mg IV/IM q6h or [tab 10 mg] 10 mg po q4-6h; total duration of ketorolac treatment not to exceed 5 days
Meloxicam (Mobic) – [tab 7.5 mg] 7.5 to 15 mg qd
Nabumetone (Relafen) – [tabs 500, 750 mg] 1,000 to 2,000 mg qd or 500 to 1,000 mg bid
Naproxen (Naprosyn and Aleve) – [tabs 250, 375, 500 mg] 250 to 500 mg bid
Oxaprozin (Daypro) – [caps 600 mg] 1,200 mg qd

Opioids

Morphinelike narcotic agonists have activity at the μ- and κ-opioid receptors and possibly the δ-receptors. The μ-receptors mediate supraspinal analgesia, euphoria, respiratory and physical depression, miosis, and reduced GI motility. The κ-receptors mediate spinal analgesia, sedation, and miosis. Unlike NSAIDs, which have a ceiling effect for anesthesia, opioids act in a dose-dependent manner and can control all intensities of pain with increasing doses up to the point of surgical anesthesia. The major drawback is side effects, which are also dose-dependent (Table 30-1).

TABLE 30-1 Equianalgesic Dosing Table.

	Equianalgesic				
Medication	**IM/IV**	**po**	**T1/2 (h)**	**Duration (h)**	**Sample initial dosing**
Codeine	120	300	3	4–6	15–60 mg po q4-6h
Fentanyl (Duragesic patch)	100 μg	—	—	—	25 μg/h patch, q3d
Hydrocodone (Lortab and Vicodin)	—	30	—	4–6	Various products/ dosing
Hydromorphone (Dilaudid)	1.5	7.5	2–3	4–6	2–4 mg po q4-6h
Meperidine (Demerol)	75	300	3–4	4–5	75–150 mg IV/ IM q3-4h

Methadone (Dolophine)	—	20	—	6–8	Various dosing
Morphine	10	30	2–4	4–6	10–30 mg po q4h
Morphine CR (MS Contin)	—	30	—	8–12	15 mg po q8-12h
Oxycodone	—	30 po 15 PR	—	3.5	5–10 mg po q4h
Oxycodone CR (Oxycontin)	—	30	—	8–12	10–40 mg po q12h
Pentazocine (Talwin)	60	180	2–3	4–6	30 mg IV/IM q3-4h

All dosing in milligrams except where noted. The dosing table should be used as follows: to convert from drug A to drug B, calculate the total number of milligrams of drug A given over a 24-hour period. Convert total to drug B using the columns under "equianalgesic." Administer that amount of drug B over 24 hours.

Loeser J, ed. *Bonica's Management of Pain.* 3rd ed. Hagerstown, MD: Lippincott Williams & Wilkins; 2000.

Injectable Corticosteroids

	Hydrocortisone	Prednisolone	Methylprednisolone
Relative potency	1	4	5
Onset	Fast	Fast	Slow
Duration of action	Short	Intermediate	Intermediate

	Triamcinolone	Betamethasone
Relative potency	5	25
Onset	Moderate	Fast
Duration of action	Intermediate	Long

Sample Steroid/Analgesic Injections

Shoulder Bursitis/Rotator Cuff Tendinitis (Lateral Approach) – Using a 1.5″ 21G needle, inject a 5-mL mix of 20 mg triamcinolone and local anesthetic to the lateral shoulder 2 cm anterior and inferior to the acromial angle at a depth of ≈2 cm below the skin.

Lateral Epicondylitis – Rest arm on a table palm down, elbow flexed 45°. Using a 1.5″ 23G needle, inject a 5-mL mix of 10 mg triamcinolone and local anesthetic into the most tender area about the extensor tendon attachment to the lateral epicondyle.

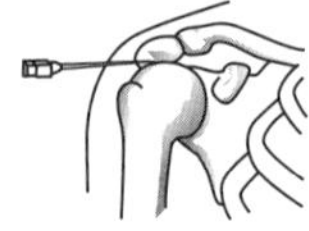

Figure 30-1

Courtesy of Steinbrocker O, ed. *Aspiration and Injection Therapy in Arthritis and Musculoskeletal Disorders.* Hagerstown, MD: Harper & Row; 1972.

Carpal Tunnel – Supinate the wrist and extend over a towel. Using a 1.5″ 25G needle, inject a 1-mL mix of 10 mg triamcinolone and local anesthetic directed distally at a 60° angle to the skin proximal to the distal wrist crease between the palmaris longus and flexor carpi radialis tendons. The needle is inserted 1 to 2 cm. Median n. anesthesia confirms proper injection; paresthesias may last 1 to 2 weeks. Volume is minimized to reduce postinjection discomfort.

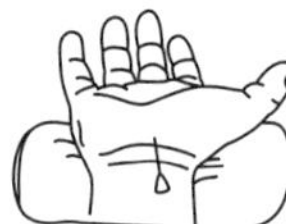

Figure 30-2

Courtesy of Steinbrocker O, ed. *Aspiration and Injection Therapy in Arthritis and Musculoskeletal Disorders.* Hagerstown, MD: Harper & Row; 1972.

De Quervain's Tenosynovitis – Place the forearm on a table on its ulnar side in ulnar deviation (support under the distal forearm with towels). Using a 1″ 25G needle, slowly inject a 5-mL mix of 40 mg triamcinolone and local anesthetic at a 45° angle along the APL and EPB sheaths to create a sausagelike wheal. If resistance is encountered, retract the needle to avoid tendinous injection.

Knee – Seat the patient with knees flexed 90° and the feet dangling. Using a 1.5″ 21G needle, inject a 5- to 6-mL mix of 20 to 40 mg triamcinolone and local anesthetic either medially or laterally to the patellar tendon toward the intercondylar notch. Discourage excessive postinjection ambulation × 24 hours.

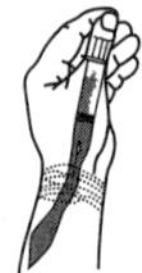

Figure 30-3

Courtesy of Snider RK, ed. *Essentials of Musculoskeletal Care.* Rosemont, IL: American Academy of Orthopaedic Surgeons; 1997.

Pes Anserine Bursa – With the patient supine and knee in extension, advance a 1.5″ 21G needle perpendicularly to periosteum at the point of maximal tenderness (medial leg) and then pull back slightly. Inject a 4-mL mix of 20 mg triamcinolone and local anesthetic.

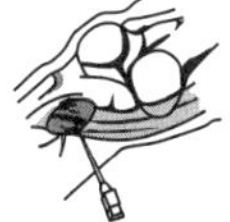

Figure 30-4

Courtesy of Steinbrocker O, ed. *Aspiration and Injection Therapy in Arthritis and Musculoskeletal Disorders.* Hagerstown, MD: Harper & Row; 1972.

Plantar Fascia – Place patient prone on a table with feet extending over the edge. Advance a 1.5″ 23G needle at the point of maximal tenderness near the medial attachment of the plantar fascia to calcaneus. Retract ≈2 mm from the periosteum and inject a 2-mL mix of 20 to 40 mg triamcinolone and local anesthetic.

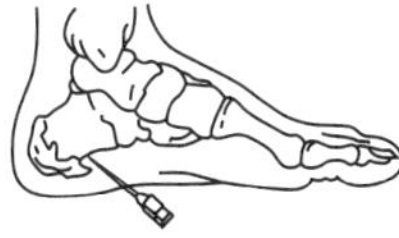

Figure 30-5

Courtesy of Steinbrocker O, ed. *Aspiration and Injection Therapy in Arthritis and Musculoskeletal Disorders.* Hagerstown, MD: Harper & Row; 1972.

REFERENCE

1. Silverstein FE. Celecoxib long-term arthritis safety study. *JAMA*. 2000;284:1247-1255.

Appendix

ABBREVIATIONS

AC acromioclavicular
ACC American College of Cardiology
ACh acetylcholine
ACJ acromioclavicular joint
ACL anterior cruciate ligament
ACPA anticitrullinated protein antibodies
ACR American College of Rheumatology
ACSM American College of Sports Medicine
AD assistive device
ADA Americans with Disabilities Act
ADLs activities of daily living
AFO ankle foot orthosis
AHA American Heart Association
AHRQ Agency for Healthcare Research and Quality
AIDP acute inflammatory demyelinating polyradiculoneuropathy
AKA above the knee amputees/amputation
ANA antinuclear antibodies
APL abductor pollicis longus
AROM active range of motion
AS ankylosing spondylitis
ASA acetyl salicylic acid
AT anaerobic threshold
ATFL anterior talofibular ligament
AVN avascular necrosis

BiPAP bilevel positive airway pressure
BKA below the knee amputees/amputation
BMI body mass index
BMD bone mineral density
BP blood pressure
bpm beats per minute
BTX botulinum toxin
BW body weight

CABG coronary artery bypass graft
CAD coronary artery disease
CC coracoclavicular
CFL calcaneofibular ligament
CHD coronary heart disease
CHF congestive heart failure
CIC clean intermittent catherization
CK creatine kinase
CNS central nervous system
COG center of gravity
COPD chronic obstructive pulmonary disease
CP cerebral palsy
CPAP continuous positive airway pressure
CPM continuous passive motion
CR cardiac rehabilitation
CRP C-reactive protein
CRPS complex regional pain syndrome
CSF cerebrospinal fluid
CT computed tomography
CTLA-4 cytotoxic T-lymphocyte antigen-4
CWS comfortable walking speed

DBP diastolic blood pressure
DER dynamic elastic response
DF dorsiflexion
DIP distal interphalangeal
DM diabetes mellitus
DMARD disease-modifying antirheumatic drug
DMOAD disease-modifying osteoarthritis drugs
DVT deep venous thrombosis
DXA dual-energy x-ray absorptiometry

ECG electrocardiogram
ECRB extensor carpi radialis brevis
EDX electrodiagnostic
EMG electromyography

EPB extensor pollicis brevis
ER external rotation
ESI epidural steroid injection
ESR erythrocyte sedimentation rate
EULAR European League Against Rheumatism

FARES fast, reliable, and safe method
FAST Fitness Arthritis and Seniors Trial
FDA Food and Drug Administration (US)
FES functional electrical stimulation
FEV_1 forced expiratory volume in 1 second
FM fibromyalgia
FRC functional residual capacity

GAIT Glucosamine/Chondroitin Arthritis Intervention Trial
GBS Guillain-Barré syndrome
GFR glomerular filtration rate
GRF ground reaction force

HDL high-density lipoprotein
HF hip flexion
HKAFO hip-knee-ankle-foot orthosis
HLA human leukocyte antigen
HO heme oxygenase
HO heterotopic ossification
HR heart rate
HRT hormone replacement therapy
HTN hypertension

IA intra-articular
IAPV intermittent abdominal-pressure ventilators
IASP International Association for the Study of Pain
IM intramuscularly
iNOS nitric oxide synthase
INR international normalized ratio
IP interphalangeal
IPPV intermittent positive pressure ventilators
ISCD International Society for Clinical Densitometry
ITB intrathecal baclofen
ITB iliotibial band
IVH intraventricular hemorrhage

JIA juvenile idiopathic arthritis

KF knee flexion

LEx lower extremity
LLQ left lower quadrant
LV left ventricle

MCA middle cerebral artery
MCP metacarpophalangeal
MI myocardial infarction
MRI magnetic resonance imaging
MS multiple sclerosis
MSK musculoskeletal
MTX methotrexate
MVA motor vehicle accident
MVV maximal voluntary ventilation
MWD microwave diathermy

NCV nerve conduction velocity
NIH National Institutes of Health
NMJ neuromuscular junction
NOF National Osteoporosis Foundation
NSAID nonsteroidal antiinflammatory drug
NTD neural tube defect
NYHA New York Heart Association

OA osteoarthritis
OP osteoporosis
ORIF open reduction and internal fixation
OT occupational therapy

PAS periodic acid–Schiff
PCI percutaneous coronary intervention
PCL posterior cruciate ligament
PF plantarflexion
PLSO posterior leaf spring orthosis
Po_2 oxygen partial pressure
PR pulmonary rehabilitation

PRICE protection, rest, ice, compression, and elevation
PRP platelet-rich plasma
PT physical therapy
PTB patellar tendon bearing
PTFL posterior talofibular ligament
PTT partial thromboplastin time
PVD peripheral vascular disease
PVL periventricular leukomalacia
PWB partial weight bearing

qid four times daily
QSART quantitative sudomotor axon reflex test

RF rheumatoid factor
RGO reciprocating gait orthosis
RICE relative rest, ice, compression, elevation
ROM range of motion
RPE rate of perceived exertion
RSD regional sympathetic dystrophy
RV residual volume

SACH solid ankle cushioned heel
Sao_2 oxygen saturation
SBP systolic blood pressure
SCI spinal cord injury
SCS spinal cord stimulator
SD standard deviation
SGA small for gestational age
SMA spinal muscular atrophy
SNAP sensory nerve action potential
SNRB selective nerve root block
SS symptom severity
SSRI selective serotonin reuptake inhibitor
SWD shortwave diathermy

TBI traumatic brain injury
TBSA total body surface area
TD terminal device
TENS transcutaneous electrical nerve stimulation
TF transfemoral
TFL tensor fascia lata
TG triglyceride
TH transhumeral
THA total hip arthroplasty
tid three times daily
TKA total knee arthroplasty
TLC total lung capacity
TMJ temperomandibular joint
TNF tumor necrosis factor
TR transradial
TSF tibial stress fracture
TV tidal volume

UEx upper extremity
UMN upper motor neuron
US ultrasound
UTI urinary tract infection

VC vital capacity
VC voluntary closing
VCUG voiding cystourethrogram
VMO vastus medialis obliquus
VO voluntary opening

WB weight bearing
WBAT weight bearing as tolerated
WC wheelchair
WHO World Health Organization

Note: Locators with *f* and *t* denotes figures and tables.